The Miracle of Stem Cells

How Adult Stem Cells are Transforming Medicine

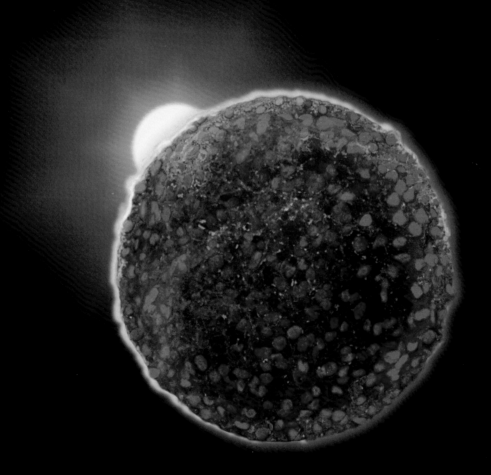

Roger J. Howe, PhD, Maynard A. Howe, PhD,

Nikolai I. Tankovich, MD, PhD, David A. Howe, MD,

with James R. Tager

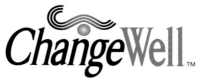

For more information:

Changewell, Inc.,

P.O. Box 7303, Rancho Sante Fe, CA 92067

www.changewell.com

info@changewell.com

T: 858-756-1491

F: 858-756-3467

ISBN 10: 0-615-29686-2

ISBN 13: 9780615196862

Front cover:

Image of cell is courtesy of Stemedica, Dr. Yuri Kudinov (MD, PhD). Design was done by Nancy Van Allen. Neural stem cell that was stained with membrane dye Dil and nuclear dye DAPI.

Back cover images from left to right:

Retinal Pigment Epithelial (RPE) cells image:

Embryonic stem cells differentiating into retinal pigment epithelium precursor cells . Nuclei are in blue, and pink indicates Pax6, a protein that is present in retinal tissues. The image was taken by David Buccholz. Copyright © 2008 The Regents of the University of California. All rights reserved. Used by permission.

Cardiomyocyte image:

Copyright (2003) National Academy of Sciences, U.S.A. Urbanek, K., Quaini, F., Giordano, T., Torella, D., Castaldo, C., Nadal-Ginard, B., ... Anversa, P. (2003). Intense myocyte formation from cardiac stem cells in human cardiac hypertrophy. *Proceedings of the National Academy of Sciences of the United States of America, 100*(18), 10440-10445.

All other images on the back cover are courtesy of Stemedica, Dr. Yuri Kudinov (MD, PhD).

TABLE OF CONTENTS

ACKNOWLEDGEMENTS

We are deeply indebted to the entire Stemedica team for their assistance in providing much of the clinical and laboratory science that forms the underpinnings of this book. Dr. Alex Kharazi (MD, PhD), Stemedica's Vice President and Chief Technology Officer, and his team helped us distill a complicated science into more readily understandable text for the reader. Dr. Eugene Baranov, (PhD), Vice President of Global Research, provided much of the background for and translation of the original Russian scientific work. His efforts in coordinating interviews with many of the pioneers of stem cell research and therapy from the former Soviet Union have proved invaluable in helping us uncover the historical body of stem cell science and technology. Our consultant, Dr. Maria Alexandrova (PhD), one of the pioneers of stem cell science, shared her insights with us. Dr. Alexandrova is the daughter of Anatoly Alexandrov one of the fathers of the "Russian Manhattan" project. We also appreciate the many professional scientists and physicians from the United States, Europe and Asia that provided content, guidance and review of the various sections of the book and to the patients that shared their personal stories of successful stem cell treatments.

We were also assisted by a top-level editor, Dr. Mark Tager (MD), and his team comprised of Sasja Tse, Nayana Jennings, William Rodarmor, Jordan Rothenberg and Irene Howe. Their editorial efforts, along with Nancy Van Allen and Marsha Slomowitz, who created the design, made the pages in this book come to life. Their considerable skills are represented in every chapter. Our thanks go out to Marcie Frank for her tireless support and effort to coordinate those involved in the production of the book.

We are forever grateful to Dr. Arlene Howe (DD), whose unfortunate accident provided the inspiration for us to form Stemedica Cell Technologies, Inc., and ultimately to write this book. Last, but certainly not least, we want to express our deep appreciation and respect for our brother, Dr. Ron Howe (DBA), who guided the care and recovery of his wife, Arlene. His personal struggle and the invaluable insights he learned as a caregiver demonstrated the dedication, courage and empathy required to live with and support an individual suffering from a debilitating medical condition. Stemedica has integrated Ron's important insights into the treatment protocols for patients participating in stem cell therapy. With our love and affection, we dedicate this book to Arlene and Ron.

Introduction
A Personal Story

At the end of 2004, starting another company was the furthest thing from our minds. We—Roger and Maynard—were easing into retirement. Over the last three decades, we had successfully launched five companies together. At this point in our lives, non-profit ventures occupied the majority of our time, punctuated by our active involvement in competitive hockey and an occasional round of golf at the courses near our San Diego homes.

We were not the only members of our family who had settled in Southern California. Our brother David, a physician, ran a thriving private practice in El Cajon. Our eldest brother Ron ran a quiet bed-and-breakfast with his wife Arlene in the small town of Julian. Our brother Bruce was president of a nutraceutical company. We remained close to our sisters Mary, Janet and Gloria who lived in other locations. We spent a significant amount of time together, and as the year drew to a close, we made plans to spend Christmas with each other, as a family. When we went to sleep on December 4th, 2004, we believed that our lives had settled into a familiar routine. The next day, this illusion was shattered.

The Accident

The people of Julian had not experienced a December snowstorm that strong in years. Snowflakes blanketed the roads, while furious winds made navigating the narrow winding roads almost impossible.

It was through this storm that our sister-in-law Arlene was driving her minivan. She had just picked up three workers to help clean the family's bed-and-breakfast. On the way back home, Arlene noticed that a sharp curve loomed in the road ahead. She applied the brakes, but the build-up of ice and snow was deeper than she thought.

The van suddenly went into an uncontrollable slide. In a second it had careened to the other side of the road. A brief moment later, the van was tumbling down an 80-foot ravine.

When the van stopped, Arlene lay motionless, suspended in the upside-down vehicle. The three other occupants were able to escape through the window, but Arlene remained pinned, her body trapped within the twisted wreckage of the automobile's front seat.

Another motorist had witnessed the crash and quickly called 911 for assistance. Several hours later, Arlene was in the emergency unit of the nearest hospital, while doctors anxiously determined her condition.

Meanwhile, Ron waited nervously for his wife to return home. After several hours had gone by, Ron called the husband of one of Arlene's passengers, who gave him the news that sent him rushing to the hospital.

Ron was soon to discover that Arlene's condition was critical. Her spinal cord had been severely damaged and her vertebrae cracked and separated from their normal alignment. He listened, shocked and numb, as her attending physician gave his prognosis: "If Arlene makes it, she will be a quadriplegic."

When we received the news, we rushed to be with our brother and sister-in-law at the hospital. After tearfully embracing us, Ron walked us over to Arlene's bed. We barely recognized her. Scores of tubes, bandages, and machines surrounded her bedside. Our conversation with her physician and nurses was very direct and extremely discouraging.

In the days and weeks following, our extended family and friends offered prayers, support and hope for Arlene's recovery. Her

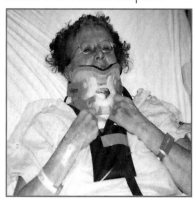

Arlene Howe in the hospital.

dedicated medical team worked around the clock to keep her with us. Arlene's courage and fortitude, persistence and faith gave her the strength to fight for life, and to begin the long and difficult road to recovery.

When Arlene finally stabilized, our family brought all our resources to bear to help her improve her condition. We drew upon our years of experience and networking in the medical field to arrange for the best physical therapy, hospital and home care available. In spite of these excellent resources, Arlene made very little progress. Her life seemed destined to confinement in a bed and a specialized wheelchair.

Watching our brother and sister-in-law struggle daily with her spinal cord injury, we were determined to do all we could to help. We asked all the medical experts we knew if there were treatment options besides physical therapy. A few of our physician friends admitted that there was some exciting work coming out of Russia that might offer hope for Arlene. They explained that physicians in Moscow had been successfully treating spinal cord injuries for a number of years using stem cell therapies.

Peering Behind the Iron Curtain

Moscow. For our generation, that word brought up memories of a childhood spent during the Cold War. We reminisced about the fears we had of the Soviet Union, remembering school day drills of ducking under the desks to protect ourselves from Soviet missiles. We reminded each other of the weeks we had spent digging a bomb shelter in our yard, fortifying it with concrete and steel walls and supplying it with enough food to last our family for days in the event of a nuclear attack.

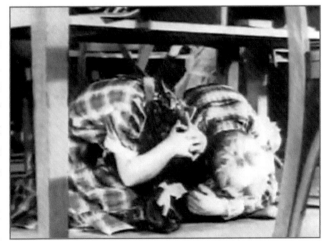

Children conducting a safety drill in the mid 1950s.

As a family growing up in the rural Midwest, we had been taught to view the Russians as the Soviet enemy. Our teachers, parents, and ministers had warned us that communism was spreading quickly and could one day take over the world. During our childhood, to think that Russian scientists and physicians could provide help to anyone in the United States would have been unimaginable. How ironic, we reflected, that the country we feared in our youth could offer hope and healing to our family later in life.

Nervous but resolute in our determination to improve Arlene's condition, we took the long journey to Moscow. There we met with Dr. Nikolai Mironov (MD, PhD), an internationally renowned neurologist who, through approved clinical studies, had performed hundreds of adult stem cell treatments. After examining Arlene, Dr. Mironov agreed to enroll her in a clinical study he was conducting, using adult stem cells to treat spinal cord injury. Later on in this book, we will reveal her results. But on that windy day in Moscow, we were not sure ourselves what to expect from Arlene's treatment.

Anxious and uncertain, we spoke to Dr. Mironov at length about the history of stem cell treatments in Russia. Our investigations did not stop there; we delved into an exhaustive examination of stem cells and their potential therapeutic uses. We spoke with respected scientists and physicians who had worked with stem cells. These were not second-rate doctors operating in fly-by-night clinics; instead, these were members of the Russian Academy of Science who maintained prestigious positions at top research institutes and hospitals across the country.

Although Russian researchers have been conditioned to be cautious after decades behind the Iron Curtain, slowly the Moscow scientists and physicians we spoke with began revealing the details of an amazing story.

The Russian Discovery

Physicians at one of the most prestigious hospitals in Moscow, these researchers explained, had saved the lives of Kremlin leaders and other top officials through stem cell therapies they had perfected over several years. Their early research and pre-clinical studies used fetal and bone marrow-derived stem cells. As their research progressed, they advanced their technology to include stem cells taken from healthy adult volunteers.

Realizing that any understanding of stem cell medicine was incomplete without the patient perspective, we asked if we could view some of the clinical results firsthand. We were encouraged by what we observed. Spinal cord injury patients presented a spectrum of improvement. Some seemed to have gained significant benefits, others moderate or fair benefits. Even more important, despite asking repeatedly, we did not uncover any problems with safety. After reviewing the spinal cord injury results, we were allowed to interview patients who had been treated for conditions such as

Alzheimer's, Parkinson's, stroke, serious diseases of the eye, and other debilitating conditions. Dozens of these patients described various degrees of clinical improvement, confirming what we had previously learned.

Medical doctors and researchers often use the term "anecdotal" when referring to these isolated case studies. Without large scale, well-designed clinical trials it is difficult to draw conclusions on how a treatment will impact a larger population. At this point, however, we could not ignore the body of positive clinical evidence presented to us—especially as it pertained to helping our sister-in-law.

Restoring Lives

After our return from Moscow, we began to report our findings to some of our business associates. In addition, we met with several physicians and scientists who expressed a great deal of interest but remained highly skeptical of our report.

The more conversations we had, the more we noticed a recurring theme. When sharing our story with a group of people, we would often mention other medical conditions for which stem cell treatments seemed especially promising. After we were done talking, a member of the group would invariably come up to us and acknowledge that they had a family member or a friend who suffered from one of these conditions. As this experience repeated itself, we began to realize the prevalence of some of these chronic diseases, for which adult stem cells may hold the answers. Together, we started brainstorming ways to make this revolutionary stem cell-based medicine available to wider segments of society.

While many physicians, scientists, businessmen, friends and associates tried to discourage us from moving forward with our efforts to build a stem cell company, our spirits were bolstered by many others who offered encouragement, financial support and professional guidance. Privately, many physicians confided in us that they were frustrated by the lack of medical options they could provide to patients suffering from incurable conditions. They expressed to us the hope that stem cell therapy would allow them to provide treatment to their patients. We were guided not only by their support, but also by the knowledge that a clinically validated stem cell product could potentially treat thousands, perhaps millions of people with debilitating, incurable conditions.

Privately, many physicians confided in us that they were frustrated by the lack of medical assistance they could provide to patients suffering from incurable conditions. They expressed to us the hope that stem cell therapy would allow them to provide treatment to their patients.

The tragedy and despair of Arlene's accident gave birth to a vision of hope and promise. This vision was to develop a medical technology dedicated to saving, restoring and improving the quality of life for patients who had no other significant options. Our vision led us to Dr. Nikolai Tankovich (MD, PhD), a surgical oncologist and physicist and former high-level Russian researcher, to form Stemedica Cell Technologies, Inc.

What You Will Learn

This book is a continuation of that vision, an attempt to better educate different audiences on the therapeutic potential of modern stem cell therapy. As you read through these pages you will discover that:

- Thousands of people have already received stem cell therapy in clinical studies around the world.

- Stem cells offer significant potential for renewal of injured or degenerated tissue.

- Stem cell research has a long and storied history, which encompasses decades of work on several continents.

- Stem cell-based treatments are likely to become widely available in the near future.

This information is useful for every member of society. But chances are, you picked up this book for more specific reasons. Different readers will be interested in different aspects of this book.

If you or a loved one are suffering from a condition for which current medicine offers little hope, this book will teach you:

- How stem cells may offer hope to "no-option" patients.

- How far stem cells have come along the path of "clinical translation."

- Which clinical trials have been, or are currently being, conducted for stem cell therapy.

- What to keep in mind when considering a stem cell treatment.

If you are a medical professional who wants to expand his or her knowledge of how stem cells are affecting the medical field, this book will assist you in understanding:

- The mechanism(s) of action by which stem cells can affect cellular repair.

- Which clinical conditions are most likely to respond to stem cell therapy.

- What research has already been completed on stem cells for clinical applications, and what conclusions can be drawn.

- Which stem cells are most suited for different clinical applications.

If you are a public policy professional, this book will help you assess:

- The magnitude and variety of societal health conditions that currently have no meaningful treatment options, for which stem cells may be clinically pertinent.

- How stem cell medicine could reduce health care costs and increase patient independence and quality of life, resulting in societal benefit.

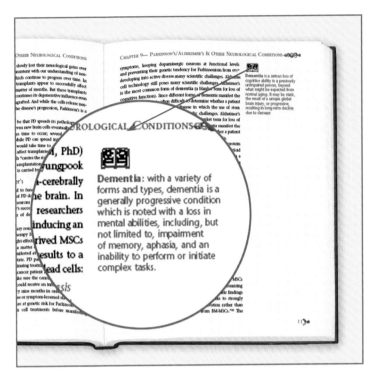

- How (and why) different research centers, educational institutions, and even national governments have embarked upon stem cell research programs.

If you are a financial analyst, this book will show you:

- The potential financial impact of even a single stem cell product.

- How stem cells may drastically affect the health care industry, biopharmaceutical industry, and insurance industry.

- How future innovation will almost certainly increase the effectiveness and availability of stem cell-based therapeutic options.

Given such a varied audience, many of the terms used in this book will be unfamiliar to some of our readers. You will find selected words **boldfaced** and defined in the margin.

Many of the terms used in this book will be unfamiliar to some of our readers. You will find selected words **boldfaced** and defined in the margin.

What is a Miracle?

In many ways, stem cells are the ultimate scientific mystery. Exploring how stem cells work provides a look at the healing process of our own bodies; of how we grow and age as human beings. When we look into the possibilities of stem cells, we are studying the highly versatile building blocks of life itself, as well as a set of the most powerful healing tools available to the human body. These tiny cells offer the secrets to the origins of life and the replenishment of our vitality.

When we look into the possibilities of stem cells, we are studying the highly versatile building blocks of life itself, as well as a set of the most powerful healing tools available to the human body.

Looking at these stem cells under a microscope, one can scarcely believe their incredible potential. Stem cells are how every one of us began our lives. That is one reason why this book is entitled, "The Miracle of Stem Cells." But a miracle is in the eye of the beholder. For a spinal cord injury patient who has not moved their arms or legs in months or even years, the ability to prepare their own meals is a miracle. For a stroke patient who was previously unable to speak, the chance to once again say even a few words is a miracle. For the diabetic retinopathy patient with degenerating vision, the ability to regain some measure of sight is a miracle.

If you were told that you could never walk again, how would you feel if you were able to graduate from a wheelchair to a walker? How would you react after learning that a family member who previously could not comprehend what they were reading, was now cognizant of everyday news events? Answer these questions honestly, and you will understand how the advance of stem cell research and the use of stem cell treatments may seem like a miracle to patients who have resigned themselves to a life with a serious and permanent condition.

So whether you are a patient or a doctor, a researcher or a health care consumer, if you wish to better understand the miraculous nature of these stem cells and the therapeutic options they provide, read on.

Chapter 1
Understanding the Promise of Stem Cells

On September 28, 1928, by complete accident, medical science made a tremendous leap forward. It was on that day that Scottish scientist Alexander Fleming discovered that he had made a mistake and forgotten to cover his petri dish from the night before. The dish was being used to grow Staphylococcus, a common bacteria, but Fleming's mistake had allowed a blue-green mold to grow on the dish. Before Fleming could throw out his contaminated results, he realized that the bacteria had stopped growing in the areas where the mold was present. This unexpected observation led to the realization that penicillin, the mold, could be used to treat bacterial infections, giving birth to the use of antibiotics as a medical treatment.

The accidental discovery of antibiotics saved millions of lives by enabling doctors to effectively treat bacterial infections for the first time. Before 1928, there was no effective treatment for

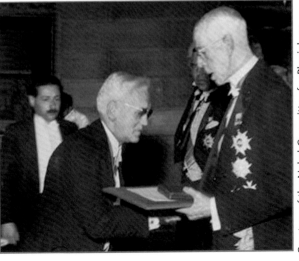

Alexander Fleming receiving the Nobel Prize in 1945 from King Gustavus Adolphus of Sweden.

Courtesy of the Nobel Committee for Physiology or Medicine.

Antibiotics and stem cells have much in common. Like penicillin, stem cells are poised to usher in a new medical revolution, one that will be used to treat some of the most prevalent and debilitating diseases of this century.

bacterial infection. It was not unusual for a minor wound to become life-threatening. In 1924, for example, President Calvin Coolidge's adolescent son died from an infected blister he had acquired while playing tennis. Antibiotics turned the impossible into the possible; medicine was suddenly able to offer solutions, instead of condolences. When penicillin became widely available in the 1940s, healthcare took a large and permanent step forward. Antibiotics were nothing short of a medical revolution.

Unlike antibiotics, stem cells were not discovered by chance; in fact, scientists have been researching stem cells for over a century. The word "stem cell" is almost 150 years old, and the first major stem cell discovery occurred over 100 years ago.[1] There was no fortuitous accident that made today's stem cell treatments possible. But antibiotics and stem cells have much in common. Like penicillin, stem cells are poised to usher in a new medical revolution, one that will be used to treat some of the most prevalent and debilitating diseases of this century.

Stem Cells: The New Medicine

Today, stem cells offer the possibility to effectively treat or stop the progression of dozens of diseases and conditions. Many of these conditions currently have no effective medical treatment. People who have experienced a spinal cord injury, for example, have limited ability to reverse their permanent neurological damage. Those who have lost sight from eye conditions such as retinitis pigmentosa or diabetic eye disease are rarely able to improve their vision. Human beings do not have the ability to regrow entire organs, or to heal significant wounds without disfiguring scars.

Millions of people suffer from conditions that lack effective treatment options. Almost one million Americans with diabetic retinopathy have vision that is considered threatened.[2] Over 50,000 Americans die each year from traumatic brain injury.[3] Stroke affects another 795,000 annually.[4] In the U.S. and around the world, people are crying out for another medical revolution.

Stem cells will be the penicillin of the 21st century. Adult stem cells have already been used to successfully treat a range of conditions, from spinal cord injury to stroke to cardiac disease. The possible applications of stem cell treatment may well be limitless. In fact, stem cells are being tested for many conditions. In this book, we will confine our discussion to research and treatment being done in four areas:

1. *Neurological conditions*, such as stroke, traumatic brain injury, Alzheimer's, Parkinson's and spinal cord injury.

2. *Cardiovascular conditions*, such as heart disease and peripheral artery disease.

3. *Ophthalmic (vision-related) conditions*, such as diabetic retinopathy, macular degeneration, and retinitis pigmentosa.

4. *Wound care*, such as burns, and chronic skin ulcers related to diabetes, vascular disease or pressure sores.

In these areas especially, medical science has made significant strides with adult stem cells, and there is a growing consensus that stem cell therapy may offer solutions to previously unsolvable medical dilemmas.

A search of the National Institutes of Health's (NIH's) database of clinical trials reveals over 3,000 clinical trials using stem cells to treat various conditions in the United States alone.

"Ten Years Away?"

Stem cell research has advanced to the point where many major universities and research centers have set up their own stem cell laboratories. Thousands of scientists are involved in bench-top research that advances the scientific community's understanding of how these cells work. Seen through the viewpoint of the bench-top researcher alone, stem cell treatments may seem a decade away. But theirs is not the only viewpoint to take into account. There is also an entire community of clinicians and medical specialists, including the FDA, who are currently exploring innovative new ways to treat disease with stem cell-based therapies. In order to understand how close we are to a legitimate set of stem cell treatments, it is necessary to look beyond the laboratory benchtop.

Stem cells have been used, and are currently being used, in hundreds of clinical trials and studies around the world. In fact, a search of the National Institutes of Health's (NIH) database of clinical trials reveals over 3,000 clinical trials, in the United States alone, using stem cells to treat various conditions.[5] This list includes clinical trials that will occur in the future, are ongoing, or have already been completed. And the NIH's list only shows clinical trials that occur within the United States; trials have been, and continue to be, conducted in other countries as well.

While there is still progress to be made before stem cells transition to mainstream treatment, it is already a fact that thousands of patients around the world have been treated, or are currently being treated, with stem cells. Behind each patient is a face, a name, a

Cell Based Therapy
Stem cells fall into the larger category of cell-based regenerative medicine products. Since 1988, approximately a third of a million patients have received treatment with regulatory agency approved cellular products. These treatments involved over 675,000 units of Good Manufacturing Practice produced therapies.[6]

Disclaimer

Patient names and personal information have been changed in order to protect and maintain confidentiality. Relevant medical history has not been altered and was used and provided with permission.

This text is provided solely for the purpose of disseminating information on stem cells and stem cell medicine. Accordingly, nothing contained within this text is to be interpreted as claim of effectiveness of stem cells for the treatment of any medical condition.

story. Within the pages of this book, the reader will uncover the stories of:

- A former professional athlete who suffered a serious and debilitating stroke. Stem cell treatments helped him regain his freedom of movement, ability to speak, and active lifestyle.

- A real estate developer from Montana who was diagnosed with Parkinson's several years ago. Stem cell transplantations drastically reduced his symptoms and have allowed him to maintain an active lifestyle almost a decade after his diagnosis.

- An award-winning engineer from Russia who faught diabetes all his life, eventually losing much of his sight to the disease. Stem cells improved his vision, cut his insulin dosage in half, and allowed him to return to work.

- A housewife from southern California who acquired cerebral palsy during her birth, and who suffered from severe spasms, muscular pain, lack of mobility and other neurological complications for over 49 years. After receiving stem cell treatment she regained balance, significantly reduced her muscle spasms, decreased her pain and regained some range of motion.

Their results give testimony to the fact that stem cell treatments are not "ten years away." The case studies mentioned above demonstrate that stem cells offer tangible promise for these "no-option" patients.

For the lay reader, these results will probably arouse a sense of basic curiosity: Where do stem cells come from? How do scientists isolate and cultivate them? What stem cell types are most likely to make the transition into mainstream medicine?

None of these questions can be answered without first providing a response to the most basic question of all: What are stem cells?

A Stem Cell Overview

Every living organism is made up of cells; they are the fundamental building blocks of life. A simple bacteria may be composed of five to ten cells, while the human body is formed by perhaps 100 trillion cells (although scientific opinions vary on how many cells make a human body), but these two organisms are like a small house and a skyscraper; they are both built with the same materials.[7]

In order to grow and regenerate, cells reproduce by a process of division; one cell becomes two, and so on. This allows an organism to grow, and for organs to replenish themselves. Cells within a taste

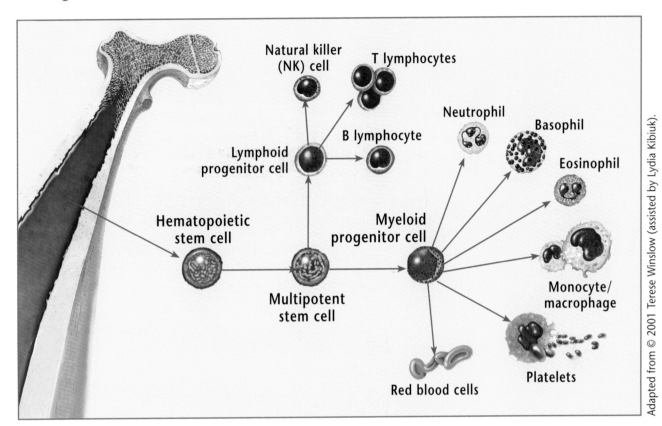

Adapted from © 2001 Terese Winslow (assisted by Lydia Kibiuk).

bud, for example regenerate every 10-14 days. Skin cells turn over every 14-28 days.

Hematopoietic stem cells can differentiate into red blood cells, white blood cells or platelets.

There are many different types of cells within the human body. Blood cells are different from neuronal cells, which are different from the cells that compose muscle or fat. The distinctions go even further, as these general cell categories are broken down into even more specialized cell types.

In fact, it takes many different types of cells to make a human body function correctly. But these different cell types have a common originator. Just as separate branches will grow from the same tree trunk, so will different cell types arise from a common cell progenitor. These progenitor cells, the tree trunk from which different branches of cells arise, are what we refer to when we use the term "stem cells."

The Definition of a Stem Cell

In order to be considered a stem cell, two criteria must be met: differentiation and self-renewal. Differentiation refers to a stem cell's ability to transform into a different type of cell. For example, a hematopoietic stem cell (often referred to as an HSC) is a stem cell that grows in the bone marrow and is the common originator for all blood cells. Discovered by Russian scientist, Dr. Alexander Maximov (MD), (whose story will be explored in the next chapter), an HSC can differentiate into red blood cells, white blood cells, or platelets. Once created, these more specialized blood cells can only reproduce into copies of themselves; a platelet can only form platelets, and so on. But with differentiation, stem cells are capable of amazing transformations that make their presence invaluable to the health of the human body.

In addition to differentiation, a stem cell must also have the capacity for self-renewal. If differentiation is a stem cell's ability to give birth to another type of cell, then self-renewal is its ability to give birth to more stem cells. After all, if stem cells could only turn into other cell types, then one day we would all run out of stem cells. However, all stem cells have the ability to go through cell division without differentiating into other cell types. A stem cell that has not transformed into another cell type is referred to as an "undifferentiated stem cell," or a stem cell in an "undifferentiated state." It is in this state that stem cells are capable of self-renewal. Once a stem cell gives rise to another cell type, those new cells cannot naturally transform back into stem cells.

While all stem cells have the same capacity for self-renewal, not all stem cells have the same level of differentiating ability. Put simply, some stem cells have the ability to differentiate into more cell types than others. The term "potency" describes the range of differentiation options available to a stem cell, and different stem cells have different levels of potency.[8]

Stem Cell Sources: Embryonic Stem Cells

One source of stem cells comes from human embryos. These embryonic stem cells (ESCs) are cultivated from the innermost cell of a blastocyst, a four-day-old fertilized egg. These stem cells are known to possess high potency levels, and when it was discovered that human ESCs could be isolated and grown in cell cultures, many scientists believed they had found the perfect cell source for clinical use.

However, embryonic stem cell research is a controversial issue within a wider society. The source for most of these stem cells are embryos stored in fertilization clinics; when couples decide not to use their embryos, they may donate these embryos to scientific research. Scientists who support embryonic stem cell research point out that blastocyst-derived cells are a valuable source of stem cells,

Colored scanning electron micrograph (SEM) of an embryonic stem cell. Embryonic stem cells are pluripotent; they are able to differentiate into almost any cell type.

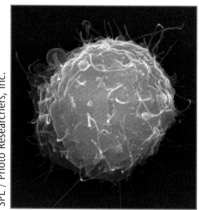

SPL / Photo Researchers, Inc.

and allow for the possibility of advanced scientific breakthroughs that would later translate into life-saving treatments.

Opponents of embryonic stem cell research argue that it is unethical to use embryos, potential human lives, as a mere means to perform research. Pro-life advocates often equate embryonic research with abortion. Some religious traditions perceive embryonic research as a slippery slope that devalues unborn human life in favor of scientific advancement.

While society debates the ethical and religious considerations of embryonic stem cell use, clinicians have all but abandoned the idea of putting embryonic stem cells in human beings. Currently, there are few clinical trials underway that use embryonic stem cells to treat human beings for any disorder or condition. The reason has less to do with societal opprobrium, and more to do with the therapeutic unsuitability of the cells themselves.

Teratomas

The essential problem in using ESCs is this: these powerful stem cells appear to be too potent—and hence, uncontrollable. Embryonic stem cells can form any cell within the adult human body, which is incredibly exciting from a research standpoint. When placed within a patient, however, there is a likelihood that they will run amok, and cause a type of tumor known as a teratoma.

The word teratoma comes from the Greek word for "monstrous tumor," and that is exactly what they are; monstrous tumors that arise when stem cells disobey the cues from their environment and begin forming random tissue. Usually manifesting as a congenital defect, these teratomas may be present at birth, and often contain tissue or organ components. Teratomas have been found containing hair or teeth; in some rare cases, even entire organs have been found encapsulated in these tumors.

While it has been established that teratomas may arise as a potential consequence of embryonic stem cell use, media and scientific attention has not focused on this possibility. A partial explanation for this lack of focus may be because teratomas are not often well known beyond medical circles. Teratomas usually result in spontaneous abortions, meaning that they are rarely seen in living humans.

Since teratomas are caused by misbehaving stem cells, it stands to reason that embryonic stem cell therapy might introduce the danger of inducing teratomas in a patient. Unfortunately, that fear is not unfounded. In a British study on laboratory rats, researchers attempted to use embryonic stem cells to treat Parkinson's disease. While the results were very encouraging, there was a disheartening side effect: 20% of the treated rats developed teratomas. Doctors who reviewed the results were forced to admit that, with such a high instance of dangerous side effects, human trials were out of the question.[9]

Embryonic stem cells lend themselves well to basic scientific research, and in fact appear to be an exciting new tool for drug discovery. Different scientific teams have begun working on the hypothesis that newly created drugs could be tested on these cells, which would be designed to simulate different cell populations within the human body. Thus, medicinal researchers could note the efficacy of the drug, and its side effects, all without running a clinical trial. The societal benefit of using these cells for drug discovery may be enormous, as it will drastically reduce the amount of money and time needed to bring a new drug to market.

All of these considerations ensure that embryonic stem cells will play a vibrant role in the burgeoning stem cell research movement, but with such a high incidence of potential side-effects such as teratomas, they simply cannot be trusted as a potential therapeutic option for humans. An ideal stem cell would be easier to control, with well-established lines of differentiation. It is this rationale that has led scientists and clinicians to adult stem cells as the most promising source for treating patients.

Adult Stem Cells

A recent *Fortune* magazine article accurately highlights some of the major conclusions that the scientific community has arrived at regarding the clinical suitability of adult versus embryonic stem cells:

When it comes to stem cells, the public—and the media—tend to focus on embryos. But researchers and analysts say marketable therapies already are emerging from less controversial work with stem cells.

Adult cells make up the lion's share of the stem cell space, mainly because they are easier to come by than embryonic cells, and less expensive to run in clinical trials. They are also derived from mature tissue, like bone marrow or umbilical cord blood, so they avoid the ethical debate that surrounds embryonic cells.

To be sure, many researchers consider embryonic stem cells to be more versatile, and they may someday be more useful than adult stem cells in treating diseases. But researchers also hope adult stem cells can help them combat a variety of maladies from diabetes to heart disease.

In fact, adult stem cells are currently the only type of stem cells used in transplants to treat diseases, such as cancers like leukemia.

Furthermore, researchers are far closer to commercializing drugs based on adult stem cells than any product based on embryonic stem cells.[10]

All these points underscore the fact that, while embryonic stem cell research offers advantages of its own, the significant thrust of medical advancement currently lies with adult stem cells, which are more useful for clinical application and are removed from the ethical controversy and medical complications that surround their embryonic counterparts. After years of tests with adult stem cells, with multiple clinical trials on thousands of patients, there have been only a handful of reports of tumor formation. Furthermore, a review of these reports reveals that all but one of these tumors were caused by hematopoietic stem cell transplantation, in a phenomenon known as donor cell leukemia.[11] This procedure is very similar to a blood or bone marrow transplant; in fact, bone marrow transplants can also cause donor cell leukemia.[12] Just as with a bone marrow transplant, proper screening of blood samples for pre-leukemic indicators can negate the risk of donor cell leukemia during a hematopoietic stem cell transplantation.[12] The remaining situation of donor-derived tumorigenic tissue (see page 26) resulted from a case where the patient should not have been eligible to receive stem cells, and where the cells were apparently improperly cultivated.

Given an understanding of context, the current risk of donor-derived tumor formation from adult stem cells appears to be negligible. These figures stand in stark contrast to embryonic stem cell pre-clinical trials, which have shown ESCs to be unsuitable for use in humans, due to their unsuitably high likelihood of side effects.

Adult Autologous Cells

Adult stem cells used for therapeutic purposes can come from two sources: the patient's own body, or a donor. These stem cells

Bone Marrow Transplantation

One of the primary ways that a bone marrow transplantation works is by replenishing the patient's supply of stem cells. In fact, a bone marrow transplantation can be seen as one of the earliest forms of stem cell treatment.

The first American bone marrow transplantation was performed almost 50 years ago. In a touching though bittersweet story, a five-month old boy was saved from a terrible immunodeficiency syndrome through a successful transplant of bone marrow stem cells. The boy, who had lost eleven members of his family to the same disease, grew up to become a healthy adult.

Dr. Robert Good (MD), who performed the surgery back in 1962, is considered one of the trailblazers of modern immunology. Since his groundbreaking procedure, bone marrow transplants have been an option for patients suffering from leukemia, Hodgkin's lymphoma, aplastic anemia, and even radiation poisoning.[13]

Senescence: the state or process of growing and becoming old. Specifically, a cell's loss in the ability to divide and grow.

are referred to as autologous and allogeneic stem cells, respectively. Autologous stem cells are taken from the patient's body, and then reinserted back into the patient.

When dealing with any autologous stem cell source, the major advantage involves immunocompatibility. There is no danger that the patient will reject an autologous stem cell transplant, since they are the patient's own cells. However, there are some disadvantages that complicate autologous use. For many autologous stem cells that are cultivated from older or ill patients, there is the problem of **senescence**, which reduces the quality and potency of the cells.

People often wonder why, the older someone is, the longer it takes them to heal from a wound. As we age, the number of stem cells in our body diminishes. In addition, the stem cells that remain in our body become weaker. Simply put, the older the stem cells are, the less effective they will be. Thus, while there may be value in using an autologous source of cells from an older patient, an optimal source would contain a population of younger cells with less senescence.

Senescence is not the only disadvantage to autologous stem cell treatment. If a patient is being treated for a degenerative condition, then the effectiveness of an autologous procedure may be limited. Parkinson's disease, for example, may contain a genetic component, and the patient's own stem cells would contain the same Parkinson's-prone malformation as the cells they are attempting to replace. For these and other reasons, therapies using allogeneic stem cells may provide a better alternative for a positive clinical response.

Adult Allogeneic Stem Cells: Stem Cell Medicine

With allogeneic stem cell therapy, cells are taken from a donor and administered to a patient. There are several advantages that allogeneic sources have over autologous sources. Allogeneic sources, if properly cultivated and developed, are less senescent than autologous stem cells, as the allogeneic cells are often from significantly younger donors. They also show more promise for treating degenerative disease. This is because allogeneic cells, if properly screened, will not be prone to the same condition as cells from a patient with a degenerative disorder.

Similarly, many diseases negatively affect the potency of a person's endogenous stem cells, making the difference between autologous and allogeneic stem cell therapy even more pronounced.

As well, autologous stem cells can only be used to treat one patient. That means that there is little incentive to perform rigorous testing of the cell population, or go through cell culturing and priming techniques that could enhance the efficacy of the cells.

In contrast, one population of allogeneic stem cells—known as a master cell bank—could be used to treat hundreds of thousands, if not millions, of patients. For that reason, proprietary and cutting-edge cultivating techniques are used to make sure these cells are as therapeutically effective as possible. In the same way that pharmaceutical companies will utilize a variety of proprietary techniques to make sure that their products are better than the generic brand, so can allogeneic stem cells be of superior clinical benefit when compared to autologous cells from an aged donor.

The process of ensuring that allogeneic stem cells are both effective and safe is a long one; scientists must isolate a population of stem cells from donated tissue, develop a master cell bank, and cultivate the cells for pre-clinical or clinical use. Throughout, the cells need to undergo several rounds of comprehensive safety testing. It all starts with the stem cell sources themselves.

Where do Allogeneic Stem Cells Come From?

A stem cell donation program is very similar to any other donation program; in fact, stem cell donations must follow the same guidelines as an organ transplant. This is because allogeneic stem cells are all cultivated from donated organs. From donated brain tissue, for example, scientists can isolate neural stem cells. From the bone marrow, they can derive mesenchymal stem cells as well as hematopoietic stem cells and endothelial progenitor cells, three distinct and potent cell lines.

Although it was previously an axiom of medical science that most organs could not regenerate themselves, we know today that

Below are some of the sources of allogeneic stem cells.

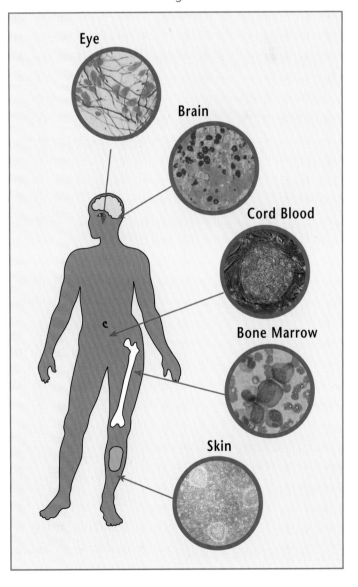

Eye

Brain

Cord Blood

Bone Marrow

Skin

Fetal Stem Cells

It may seem confusing that fetal stem cells are placed in the category of adult stem cells. Fetal cells are considered adult cells because, unlike embryonic cells, they are advanced to the point where they can only differentiate into cells of one primary tissue type. The blastocyst is divided into three primary tissue layers, and any adult cell will fall into one of these three categories.

This distinction helps us understand why embryonic stem cells are prone to teratoma formation, while fetal stem cells are not. Teratomas usually contain tissue from all three primary tissue layers, something that could only result from a misbehaving embryonic cell.

Given the confusion over the term adult stem cell, some scientists prefer to use the term somatic stem cell in its place. This book will utilize the former term.

With proper cultivating techniques, one fetal tissue donation can yield enough stem cells to treat hundreds of thousands of potential patients.

many organs contain their own source of stem cells. Scientists have a variety of tissue sources to choose from if they want to cultivate a stem cell population. However, different populations appear to be more effective for different medical conditions. The stem cells of the heart, for example, are more effective for treating cardiac conditions. Other stem cell types, such as mesenchymal stem cells, have a wider range of utility from a therapeutic standpoint. This issue will be covered in depth in later chapters, but for now it suffices to know that if a scientist is aiming to develop stem cells for use in a variety of conditions, he or she will need a variety of tissue sources.

Fetal Stem Cells

In addition to utilizing tissue from adult donors, allogeneic stem cell researchers sometimes use fetal cells as a tissue source. These fetal stem cells come from miscarriages or therapeutic abortions. In the same way that parents may donate their children's organs if the child passes away, organs from fetuses can also be donated. Organ donation is tightly regulated by the Federal Government. With proper cultivating techniques, one fetal tissue donation can yield enough stem cells to treat hundreds of thousands of potential patients.

Fetal cells are a particularly powerful stem cell source. These cells have not even begun the process of senescence, and thus are more powerful than cells that come from other adult tissue sources. Furthermore, it takes time for the fetus to develop the HLA proteins that determine immunogenicity, the signals by which the immune system recognizes resident versus foreign tissue. If the stem cells are removed before the fetal tissue has developed its HLA, then these cells will not encounter the same histoincompatibility issues as other adult cells. These characteristics make them very useful from a therapeutic standpoint.

A paper published in the journal *Stem Cells* illustrates all these points. A team of researchers, led by Dr. Zhi-Yong Zhang (PhD) of the National University of Singapore, compared stem cells taken from fetal bone marrow to stem cells derived from fully formed adult bone marrow. The stem cell type for both sources was mesenchymal stem cells, a type this book will discuss in greater detail. Zhang et al. found that the fetal stem cells reproduced more than three times as quickly as the more adult stem cells (32.3 hours versus 116.6 hours, on average). The fetal cells were also more likely to form cell colonies, proliferated more readily, and were apparently more potent than their adult counterparts. Furthermore, the research team confirmed that the fetal cells were more immunocompatible than adult cells.[14]

All of these characteristics represent significant advantages for using fetal stem cells during allogeneic transplants. The cells' greater potency and proliferative capacity means that they can effect a greater clinical result, while their immunocompatibility makes it more likely that the body will not reject the transplantation.

> **In Vitro vs. In Vivo**
> Scientists use twin terms to discriminate between cells that are inside or outside of the human body. Cells within the body are *in vivo*, or "in the living." Cells outside of the body are known as *in vitro*, or "in the glass."

Eliminating Tissue Dependency

Stem cell researchers often struggle from tissue dependency; they must have a source of tissue with which to isolate their stem cells. For autologous stem cell scientists, this is an especially serious problem. For autologous stem cells, one tissue source equals one treatment: doctors draw out the patient's bone marrow, isolate the stem cells, and then treat the patient. Because most facilities are not allowed to manipulate cells, if the doctor wants to provide a second treatment, they would need to draw more bone marrow. And if they wanted to treat a different patient with that bone marrow, then they would no longer be operating within the realm of autologous treatment. Autologous stem cells from some sources, such as fat or cord blood, can be harvested in larger quantities and banked for later use.

Allogeneic stem cell researchers are able to cultivate many different treatments from one tissue source. The number of treatments that can be derived from one source varies, depending on the cultivating techniques used. Using proprietary technology, the most skilled allogeneic stem cell researchers can develop a population of stem cells which can be used to treat hundreds of thousands of individuals, all from one tissue source.

Since one tissue source can yield so many treatments, it is important that the original tissue source be a healthy one. For this reason, scientists arrange their first round of tests at this stage of the stem cell production process. The patient and the donated tissue are screened for a battery of viral and infectious diseases, all before the stem cells are isolated. Only if the donated tissue passes through this gauntlet of safety tests does the process move on to the isolation phase. (See the figure on page 25.)

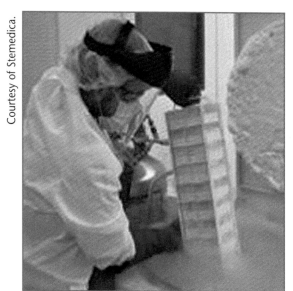

Courtesy of Stemedica.

Photo of a cryogenically preserved master cell bank.

Building a Master Cell Bank

Using centrifugal techniques and magnetic beads, researchers isolate the desired stem cell population from other cell types. Isolation of the stem cell population is fairly straightforward, but a lot of thought goes into developing proper centrifugal techniques. A previous generation of stem cell isolation techniques used mechanical segregation, while today the stem cells are isolated using a series of enzymes. With enzymatic separation, dead cells are also removed from the cell population, resulting in a healthier group of stem cells.

After isolation, another round of testing is initiated. The stem cell population is examined in detail, in order to determine all of the cells' characteristics. Researchers measure which bio-markers are expressed, whether the cells appear to contain immune-privileged capacities, whether there are any chromosomal abnormalities that might lead to adverse events, and so on. In the same way that a doctor might give a new patient a comprehensive physical exam, researchers study all the qualities of these newly isolated cells. The entire population is also examined as a whole, to make sure that no other cell types are present. This ensures that, during clinical studies, clinicians only inject the appropriate cell type.

After their basic properties are determined, the stem cells are tested for potency. Their ability to differentiate into various cell types is measured and analyzed. The cells are also tested for their migratory ability: if injected *in vivo*, will they successfully reach the area of injury?

If the answer to this question is yes, and if the stem cell population performs superlatively in all other areas, then the researchers can begin building a master cell bank. The master cell bank, the population of allogeneic stem cells from which all treatments will later derive, should be marked by high potency, immuno-privileged status, and appropriate bio-markers. Above all else, however, it should contain no abnormalities that would suggest the possibility of adverse events or side effects. This includes key safety tests for tumorigenicity, as well as acute and chronic toxicity. These tests will be repeated several times over to ensure that the cells are not prone to tumor formation or the creation of a toxic environment when used *in vivo*. Once a master cell bank of safe and effective stem cells has been created, the stem cells can be further expanded, and prepared for use in pre-clinical or clinical trials.

Expansion

Expansion involves putting these cells through a number of cell passages, with each pass representing a multiplying of the number of cells.

At this point researchers must be especially careful to avoid senescence. Just as senescence occurs in stem cells within the human body, it can also occur *in vitro*. After a certain number of passes, the stem cells will have hit their peak; each subsequent pass will make the stem cells more senescent, and thus less effective. Thus, many research institutions and private companies have struggled with the trade-off: should they make fewer doses of stem cells at therapeutic strength, or create larger numbers of weaker stem cells?

Thankfully, given the right techniques, a cell population can be cultivated in large numbers without losing potency. Advances in proprietary technology have brought us to the point where stem cells can be expanded to therapeutic amounts without sacrificing their strength. Again, this requires rigorous testing, with researchers measuring the characteristics of their cell population after it has been expanded. This testing of the cells at the expansion phase also further ensures that no abnormalities have developed.

After expansion, the cells are ready to be cryogenically preserved and stored for later clinical or pre-clinical use. But there is one more optional process that these cells can undergo if researchers wish to exert further control over their behavior, a process known as cell priming.

Cell Priming

Through the process of priming, scientists can affect a stem cell's behavior, making its effects more predictable. Stem cells can be primed to preferentially differentiate into a certain type of cell. For example, if a scientist wanted to create a stem cell treatment for Bernard-Soulier syndrome, which affects platelet formation and function, he may wish to induce hematopoietic stem cells to differentiate into platelets only. Through cell priming, this is possible. Other examples

Photo of primed neuroprogenitor cells.

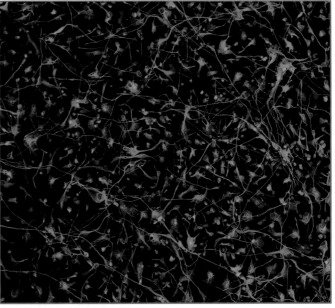

Courtesy of Stemedica, Dr. Yuri Kudinov.

Minimal Manipulation

Many autologous cell proce-dures fall into the category of the practice of medicine. An example is removing fat from a patient and, during the same procedure, trans-planting the fat (and stem cells) to another area of the body. The FDA exerts its authority when the cellular product has gone beyond what they term "minimal manipulation." Citing the Federal Food, Drug, and Cosmetic Act (FDCA) and/or the Public Health Service Act (PHSA), the FDA asserts that cellular expansion and adul-teration must take place in the carefully controlled and regulated cGMP environ-ment. The FDA is currently prosecuting a case against Regenerative Sciences for non-cGMP manufacturing.[16]

of cell priming might include inducing stem cells to release large amounts of certain growth factors, known as up-regulation, or to not release those factors at all.

How is this accomplished? One way involves changing the attributes of the cells themselves. Another way involves creating a specialized medium for the cell culture. Scientists can place differ-ent nutrients or biochemical signals, such as specific growth factors, in the cell medium. The stem cells will differentiate distinctively, based on what is available to them and on what signals they receive. In the same way that feeding a human being a certain diet will change that person's body shape, feeding stem cells a certain mix of nutrients will change their behavior.

In manipulating the cultured medium, scientists can also insert communication molecules into the culture, exerting a further level of control over what commands the stem cells receive. In order to coordinate their actions, cells will communicate using specific molecules. Dr. Larry Goldstein (PhD), director of the University of California, San Diego's Stem Cell Program, refers to these coor-dination-molecules as a "molecular call signal," allowing cells to recognize other cells of the same type.[15] With the right call signal, scientists can better prime their stem cells. It is through these tech-niques and others that scientists can effect a greater measure of control over the stem cells' actions when placed within the body.

After expansion and priming (if priming is necessary), the cells are cryopreserved; different research institutions and companies have developed proprietary technologies to ensure that the cells are appropriately stored and viable upon thawing. When scientists and clinicians around the world need a source of stem cells, they now only need to thaw out the cells, and administer them to the patient.

Why is This Important?

Through appropriate cultivating, expansion, and priming tech-niques, scientists can develop a stem cell line that is uniquely suited to treat a range of diseases. By consistently testing for safety and efficacy, these researchers can work to develop a high-quality line of stem cells with enhanced efficacy and proliferative capacity. Only after the master cell bank has yielded enough stem cells to form a working stem cell line, and after these cells have been repeatedly tested and approved by the appropriate government regulatory agencies and organizations, only then are they ready for *in vivo* use.

This process may seem lengthy and complicated, and it is, but it is also a vitally important step in bringing us much closer to mainstream stem cell treatment.

It is impossible to correctly ascertain how effective stem cells are as a treatment without ensuring that they were manufactured correctly. While different companies and research institutions have unique manufacturing processes, regulations and accreditations allow for a measure of uniformity that is necessary for examining a stem cell treatment's clinical results. One important regulatory step involves ensuring compliance with current good manufacturing practices (cGMP). Good manufacturing practice guidelines aim to establish, among other things, that:

- Manufacturing processes are clearly defined and controlled, with explanations for any later changes to the process.

- Manufacturing staff has the necessary training and qualifications to competently perform their jobs.

- Records are kept to make sure that the manufacturing process does not deviate from standard procedure.

- The product is consistently evaluated to ensure safety and efficacy.

ASSURING STEM CELL SAFETY

1. DONOR SCREENING: Donor is tested prior to tissue collection for viral & infectious diseases in accordance with FDA Safety Panel: HIV (Types I&II), HBV, HCV, HTLV (Types I&II), WNV, CMV, Syphilis, Mycoplasma.

2. TISSUE SPECIMEN PROCESSING & CELL EXPANSION: Karyotyping of cells for any chromosome abnormalities and Mycoplasma testing are conducted.

3. MASTER CELL BANK: Full safety, purity, potency testing per applicable US Federal guidelines including HIV (Types I&II), HBV, HTLV (Types I&II), CMV, EBV, B19, Contaminant & Adventitious Viruses, Syphilis, Sterility, Mycoplasma, Endotoxin.

4. PRE-TRANSPLANTATION PREPARATION: Prior to release, cells undergo a final set of safety testing for sterility, Mycoplasma and Endotoxin. For MSCs VEGF production is also tested.

5. TUMORIGENICITY & ACUTE/CHRONIC TOXICITY TESTING: Cell lines are tested in independent GLP certified labs and audited by a third party certified auditing lab.

The Importance of Patient Selection and Safe Cells

In 2009, a study conducted by an international group of researchers, led by Dr. Ninette Amariglio (PhD), was published in the *Public Library of Science* (PLoS) journal, the results of which struck stem cell scientists like a bombshell.[17] A thirteen-year-old Israeli boy with ataxia telangiectasia had developed benign tumors after receiving fetal neural stem cells. Amariglio et al.'s brain study revealed that the tumors were undoubtedly a result of the stem cell transplantation.

Ataxia telangiectasia (A-T) is a neurodegenerative disorder that results from a genetic disability. This disability also predisposes patients to genetic mutations that could cause tumors, a clear contraindication for cell-based treatment. Given A-T's propensity towards genetic mutation, many clinicians believe this patient should never have been considered a viable candidate for stem cell therapy.

Even more shocking, the protocols that were used to make the stem cells were poorly established and seriously flawed. The stem cell manufacturers skipped mandatory safety testing procedures, and used potentially toxic antibiotics during the manufacturing process. Furthermore, the stem cells were crudely cultured.

Given the patient's particular condition, it is possible that even properly cultured cells could have caused an adverse effect. Currently, this is the only known case of a donor-derived brain tumor, and more investigation is needed. Either way, the "PLoS case," as it is often referred to in research circles, is a clear indication that proper manufacturing techniques are vital to ensuring the health of future patients.

In California, the state Food and Drug Branch has the right to grant cGMP certification to stem cell manufacturers. The cGMP license demonstrates that the manufacturing facility is compliant with all applicable state and federal laws and that the cells are ready for human use once governmental permission is obtained.

Not just in the United States, but in countries around the world, governments have increasingly realized the significance of regulation for the stem cell industry, and have insisted that companies become cGMP compliant in order to be considered legitimate. This license is one important step towards establishing uniformity in the stem cell manufacturing field.

Currently, not enough stem cell manufacturers have gone through the process of becoming cGMP licensed. This is a serious issue for clinicians and patients around the world who study the results of other clinical trials in order to enhance their own understanding of how stem cells can work therapeutically.

Without knowing how the cells were made, clinicians cannot reach firm conclusions about the safety and efficacy of these trials, regardless of whether the findings were exemplary or lackluster. In a field where clearly understood clinical results are essential, improperly regulated manufacturing slows the rate of progress.

With stem cells, however, the necessity for proper manufacturing procedures is even more pronounced. Poor manufacturing processes can result in a stem cell product of dubious safety and efficacy. In the same way that the ingredients of a drug must be correctly mixed together, a stem cell *must* be appropriately manufactured. There is no excuse for manufacturing stem cells without going through the appropriate safety and regulatory processes.

Translational Medicine

A properly regulated manufacturing process allows for examination of the cell's behavior *in vitro*, and provides researchers with a preliminary understanding of how the cells might behave in the human body. It is only after the cells are manufactured that they are ready for *in vivo* use, and that is when the clinical work begins. Scientists and clinicians the world over have been using autologous and allogeneic stem cells to perform hundreds of clinical trials, testing their ability to treat various medical conditions. The cell sources and protocols may be different, and there are debates over which diseases are most likely to respond to treatment, but stem cell clinicians share the same goal: to use these cells to create a new, more effective medicine for the millions of people suffering from serious diseases.

There is a term for translating scientific research into medical treatment, and appropriately enough it is called "translational medicine." Translational medicine refers to the journey between an original scientific discovery and an available drug or treatment option that is ready for widespread use. It is often a long road from bench to bedside, but for this particular voyage, the destination is far closer than many people think. Stem cell treatments are not ten years away; in fact, for thousands of people across the globe who have participated in clinical studies, these treatments are already here. And soon, they will be available to society at large.

Without knowing how the cells were made, clinicians cannot reach firm conclusions about the safety and efficacy of these trials, regardless of whether the findings were exemplary or lackluster.

In subsequent chapters we will detail the results of pre-clinical and clinical studies which demonstrate how stem cells can provide a therapeutic effect for different diseases. We will show how dedicated scientists and doctors around the world have painstakingly laid the groundwork for a future where stem cells can be used to treat catastrophic conditions and change lives for the better. But before that, we would like to share with you the remarkable and true story of how stem cell research began.

Chapter 2
A Russian Story

It was 1917, and Alexander Maximov needed to get out of Russia.

The Bolsheviks were seizing control of the country in a series of bloody revolutions. The turmoil had begun in Maximov's home city of St. Petersburg, when the members of the Russian Parliament, known as the Duma, declared that they would no longer answer to the emperor.[A] The Imperial military, already embroiled in the midst of World War I and facing waves of mutinous soldiers, was power-less to stop the coup. Czar Nicholas II abdicated and Russia was left in a precarious balance of power, with the Provisional Government directing policy while the Soviets mobilized the people.

This balance of power shifted in November, when the Bolsheviks overthrew the Provisional Government and declared communist rule. Again, the epicenter of the revolution was St. Petersburg, where Maximov was born and where he had been teaching for over a decade. As a professor at the Military Medical Academy,

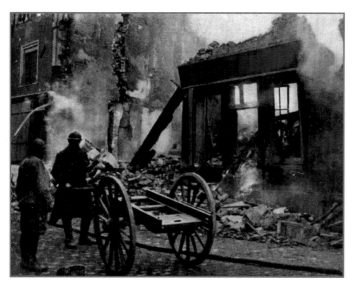

Bolsheviks overthrew the Provisional Government and declared communist rule. As a professor at the Military Medical Academy, Maximov was put in a precarious position.

Maximov would have been in the middle of the swirling political violence that made scientific pursuit impossible. On December 19th, 1917, he wrote to a friend in America:

The recent events going on in Russia have not only interrupted my scientific work, but they have rendered life altogether impossible for a University professor or any cultured man. I have one hope left—to emigrate at the first possibility after the end of the war and to apply elsewhere my scientific knowledge and experience.[1]

This decision signified the beginning of a new chapter in Maximov's already storied life. As a brilliant artist, an avid mountain climber, and a Russian nobleman, Maximov was a true Renaissance man. But his grand passion and greatest legacy was his lifelong pursuit of science.

Maximov certainly had the opportunity to pursue whatever vocation he wanted. Born to a noble family in St. Petersburg in 1874, young Alexander began life with the Russian equivalent of a silver spoon. Being a member of the Russian nobility ensured that he would be one of the privileged few allowed to study at prestigious educational institutions. Growing up in St. Petersburg meant that he was at the very capital of the powerful Russian Empire.

Little is known about Maximov's parents; it is known that Alexander shared an affectionate relationship with his older sister Claudia, who took seriously the role of the supportive older sibling. This relationship would later invert itself, with Claudia following her younger brother into self-imposed exile from Russia.

While no one could have predicted the upcoming communist rule, Russia in the late 19th century was already a hotbed of political dissent and social change. In 1861, a mere thirteen years before Alexander's birth, the czar had ended the institution of serfdom, effectively abolishing slavery in the Empire. Along with the Industrial Revolution, an influx of newly freed serfs swelled the boundaries of St. Petersburg. A growing anarchist movement preached violent resistance to Imperial power. In March 1881, when Maximov was just seven years old, an anarchist wielding home-made hand grenades assassinated the Russian czar. The assassination, conducted in full view of the public in the streets of the city, was a hint of future violence to come.

However, the same social upheaval that was destabilizing Russia as a nation also ushered in a flowering of Russian culture. The growth of a new group of young, educated Russians brought in a "Silver Age" of artistic expression.[2] It was during this time that Tchaikovsky, Stravinsky, and Rakhmaninov began to create their music, Dostoevsky and Tolstoy penned their great works of literature, and Chekhov embarked on his career as a playwright.

The world of science also grew by leaps and bounds. Dr. Ivan Pavlov (PhD), the Nobel Prize-winning scientist, conducted his seminal experiments on conditioned behavior, training dogs to salivate at his command. Dr. Dmitri Mendeleev (PhD), the inventor of the periodic table, refined his theories on chemistry from his post at St. Petersburg University. Russian scientist, Dr. Ilya Mechnikov (PhD), undertook his experiments in immunology in Odessa, for which he would later win his own Nobel Prize. Mechnikov served as scientific director of the Pasteur Institute in France. During a difficult financial time, he was able to keep the Institute afloat with funds from his Nobel Prize.

It was into this world of distinguished scientific pursuit that Alexander Maximov entered when he began studying at the Imperial Military Medical Academy in 1891. The Military Academy, situated at the heart of St. Petersburg on the banks of the Neva River, was the premiere institution for medical study in Russia. Impossibly out of reach for all but the select few, the Academy offered a top-notch scientific education and the opportunity for rapid advancement through the ranks of the Russian military. These two factors ensured a successful and distinguished career in Imperial Russia; if you could pass muster at the Academy, you could make your mark on the world of science.

However, Maximov did not just succeed at the Military Medical Academy; he excelled. He was awarded a gold medal for his student work on **amyloid** degeneration of the liver, and graduated in 1896 at the head of his class.[3] As a reward his name was engraved on a marble plaque in the main building of the Academy. At the age of 22, Alexander had already distinguished himself as one of the most promising young scientists that Russia had to offer.

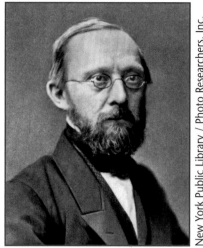

Rudolph Virchow is referred to as "the father of pathology." His often cited phrase, "Omnis cellula e cellula" means "Every cell originates from another cell."

Amyloid: a waxy protein substance generally formed in straight, nonbranching fibrils. These may be arranged in either bundles or meshwork, and are comprised of identical polypeptides. Amyloids may deposit in organs or tissues due to abnormal conditions, such as Alzheimer's.

Maximov continued his studies by gaining his medical degree, working as an assistant professor in the Academy's Department of Pathology, and writing and defending his doctoral dissertation. Having successfully passed all the academic hurdles that the Academy had to offer, the young scientist moved to Germany in 1900 in order to study embryology and experimental pathology.[4] At this point in his career, Maximov began to distinguish himself in histology, the study of tissues and cells.

On the Frontlines of Science

While our scientific understanding of human cells has been greatly developed in modern times, in Maximov's day histology was a relatively new field. The theory that all plants and animals are formed by tiny building blocks called cells (a theory that is commonly accepted today) was proposed in 1839 by the German scientists, Drs. Theodor Schwann (MD) and Matthias Jakob Schleiden (PhD). Dr. Rudolf Virchow (MD), another German scientist, expanded upon the theory decades later.

Virchow, a controversial figure among his contemporaries due to his radical politics, made several important advances in various scientific fields. In 1858 he published the essay, "Omnis cellula e cellula." This Latin phrase, meaning, "Every cell originates from another cell," reflected his theory that cell division is responsible for the creation of new cells. Before Virchow there were disparate theories about the origin and growth of certain organisms; one popular belief was that maggots could suddenly appear, fully formed, in rotten food. Virchow's pronouncement of cell division as the origin of new cell formation discredited this myth, and also filled in the missing piece of classical cell theory.

When Alexander Maximov began studying histology in Germany, cell theory had only existed as a unified concept for less than half a century. The field of histology may have been established, but it still needed new pioneers to blaze a trail of discovery. In Germany, Maximov created the term "polyblasts," which he used to refer to the wandering white blood cells within the body.[3] Much of his work focused on inflammation, the body's natural reaction to injury.

It is almost certainly during his time in Germany that Maximov learned of the research of Dr. Valentin Häcker (PhD), the German zoologist whose work with crustaceans had created an interesting new concept for biologists. Häcker, who had been studying the reproductive biology of the Cyclops crustaceans, examined the early embryonic cell of these millimeter-length creatures. Drawing from the vision of mid-nineteenth century German biologist, Dr. Ernst Haeckel (MD, PhD), who saw the fertilized egg as a stem which branched off into different reproductive cell lineages, Häcker dubbed this humble crustacean embryo a "stammzelle."[5] Häcker's proclamation occurred in 1892; shortly afterwards, Häcker's fellow zoologist, Dr. Edmund Beecher Wilson (PhD), of Columbia University, published a book which translated the German neologism into "stem cell."[4, 5] While many scientists of the time first came across this new word in Wilson's book, it is more likely that Maximov learned of the concept of a "stammzelle" through Häcker's original discovery.

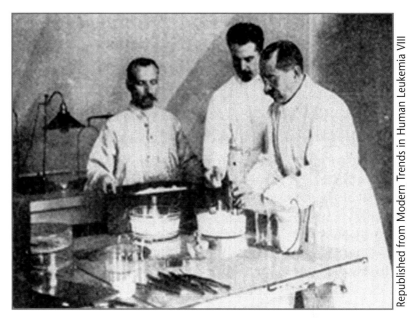

Republished from Modern Trends in Human Leukemia VIII (1989), R. Neth, R. C. Gallo, M. F. Greaves, et al. Springer Science & Business Media.

Maximov (right) in his tissue culture laboratory at the Military Medical Academy in St. Petersburg (1915).

It is also almost certain that Maximov's work in Germany brought him into contact with the work of hematologist, Dr. Artur Pappenheim (PhD), the German physician who would go on to found the great scientific journal *Folia Haematologica*. Pappenheim was one of the first scientists to ask whether blood cells came from a single common source. This single source, Pappenheim believed, could be considered a "stammzelle" in its own right.[5] Pappenheim pursued all his studies in Germany, and was conducting some of his most important research during the time that Maximov was in the country. There is no proof that the two like-minded scientists ever met personally, but Maximov was surely aware of the German doctor's work. It was Pappenheim's hypotheses that would provide much of the underpinnings for Maximov's subsequent scientific theories.

In 1903, Maximov returned to the Military Medical Academy in St. Petersburg as a Professor in Histology and Embryology. In just seven years, he had gone from being a graduate of the prestigious Academy to a respected professor at the same institution. Here his interests broadened; he continued to study the process of inflammation and its effects on the body, but also began studying blood and connective tissue.

Courtesy of Prof. Andrey Novik and Prof. Tatyana Ionova, founders of the A. A. Maximov Memorial Foundaiton.

This bust of Maximov shows him as a general in the Russian Imperial Army. The bust is placed at Pirogov National Medical Surgical Center's Department of Hematology and Cellular Therapy in Moscow.

Hematopoiesis: the formation and development of blood cells. In the embryo and fetus this occurs in a multitude of areas throughout the body including the liver, spleen, lymph nodes, thymus and bone marrow. Throughout the remainder of life, it occurs mainly in the bone marrow, with a portion occurring in the lymph nodes.

During this time Maximov rose to the position of a general, or state councilor in the Russian Imperial Army.[3] He was, after all, a respected and influential teacher at one of Russia's most prestigious military institutions. Maximov's bust at the Pirogov National Medical Surgical Center in Moscow, shows a serious and meticulous young man wearing his military uniform. With his high forehead, well-groomed mustache and elegant attire, Maximov cut a dashing figure that would have fit well within Russian high society. But it was his scientific work on blood and tissue that proved to be Maximov's enduring legacy, as well as the birthing ground of one of his most exciting and respected discoveries: the unitarian theory of **hematopoiesis**.

The Unitarian Theory of Hematopoiesis

The term hematopoiesis refers to the formation of blood cells in the body, and until Maximov, it was undetermined how different types of blood cells were formed. While red blood cells, which carry oxygen throughout the body, are the most common type of blood cells, there are also white blood cells, which are a major part of the body's immune system, and platelets, which are an integral part of wound healing. Since the blood cells were so different, it was assumed that the cells originated from different sources. Through his research Maximov uncovered the fact that, while blood cells may develop differently and thus become completely distinct from each other, they actually have the same origin as other kinds of blood cells.

During his experiments, Maximov came upon one type of cell that acted like no other blood cell type. These "primitive blood cells," as he first called them, were completely separate and unique from other parts of the blood. As Maximov explained in a lecture:

These primitive bloods cells, which is what I call them, contrary to what would commonly be expected are not erythroblasts [a type of red blood cell] but completely undifferentiated elements with a round bright nucleus and narrow basophilic cytoplasm. These are neither red nor white blood corpuscles.[6]

He went on to observe their behavior, realizing:

These primitive blood cells differentiate into two kinds of cells. One type—which makes up the majority—produces hemoglobin in their cytoplasm, and thus become the so-called primitive erythroblasts....Another fraction of the primitive blood cells remains hemoglobin-free. These cells now possess a large, bright nucleus with nucleoli, and a thin, ameboid, strongly basophilic rim of cytoplasm. In histological terms, they resemble large lymphocytes. These are the first embryonic leukocytes that first appear as lymphocytes.[6]

Maximov was fully aware of the wide-ranging implications of what he had witnessed. A previously unexplored cell transformed into both red blood cells and white blood cells; thus, it was the origin for different lineages of blood cells.

Subsequent research revealed that these "primitive cells" were actually responsible for all the various cell types within the blood. For Maximov, this cemented his realization that he had discovered something monumentally different from other blood cells. In 1909, while speaking of his research with chicken blood, he warned his listeners not to think of these "primitive cells" as just another type of red blood cell:

Despite the fact that these lymphocytes produce erythroblasts, they should not be considered erythroblasts themselves; as, in addition to the production of hemoglobin-containing cells, they also give rise to megakaryocytes [platelets] and diverse other elements in the yolk sack, which have nothing to do with the red blood corpuscles.[6]

Drawing by Maximov of cells as viewed through his microscope.

Maximov's research convincingly demonstrated that all blood cells had a common origin. This original cell was able to exist as a unique cell type, but also proved to be the stem from which the different branches of blood cells would all grow. With this concept in mind, Maximov knew exactly what to call his new discovery.

In the early 20th century, German was the scientific language of the day. So Maximov, whose native language was Russian and who also spoke German, French, and English fluently, decided to publish his results in the language that would allow scientists from all over the world to

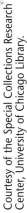

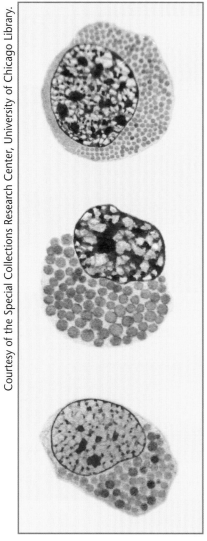

Courtesy of the Special Collections Research Center, University of Chicago Library.

Drawings by Maximov of cells as viewed through his microscope.

study them. Thus, in 1909, Maximov submitted a summary of his research to Pappenheim's,[7] *Folia Haematologica*, under the wordy German title "Der Lymphozyt als gemeinsame Stammzelle der verschieden Blutelemente in der embryonalen Entwicklung und im post fetalen Leben der Säugetiere." The title translates to "The Lymphocyte as a Stem Cell, Common to Different Blood Elements in Embryonic Development and During the Post-Fetal Life of Mammals."[6]

In all the dry scientific language, it is easy to miss the presence of one word, "stammzelle," or stem cell. It was a word that, only fourteen years before, had been used mainly to refer to the embryonic cell of a crustacean that was barely visible with the naked eye. Maximov had taken this exotic and little-known concept of a stem cell and placed it squarely within the human body. He had breathed life into a concept that offers, even today, exciting new prospects for science, medicine, and technology.

In his lecture on June 1st of that year, Maximov proudly concluded: "In mammalian organisms a single type of cell exists... which both looks different and may produce a variety of differentiation progeny depending on their current location and survival factors."[6] The lecture, given at a special meeting of the Berlin Hematological Society, announced Maximov's unitarian theory of hematopoiesis and established his position as a founding father of stem cell research.

That is not to say that Maximov's new theory wasn't controversial. Dr. Alexander J. Friedenstein (PhD), the discoverer of mesenchymal stem cells and ideological defender of Maximov, explained that "Maximov's theory was far ahead of its time and, although Maximov was highly respected by the scientific community, his concept of local stromal conditions was met with skepticism."[7] In fact, Maximov had declared himself squarely on one side of a scientific controversy which had been brewing for decades.

Stem cell scientists Drs. Miguel Ramalho-Santos (PhD) and Holger Willenbring (MD, PhD), both of the University of California, San Francisco, believe that the debate began in 1879. At that point, the two co-authors explain in a 2007 paper, newly developed cell-staining techniques "enabled the identification of different white blood cell lineages, splitting investigators of hematopoiesis into two camps. Dualists did not believe in the existence of a stem cell common to all hematopoietic lineages."[4]

"By contrast," the authors continue, "according to the unitarian model of hematopoiesis, a cell existed that represented the common origin of erythrocytes [red blood cells], granulocytes, and lymphocytes [both white blood cell types]. Thus, Unitarians were naturally poised to introduce a term that captured the developmental potential of such a cell."[4]

With his presentation, Maximov proudly declared that "stammzelle" was the term that Unitarians were looking for. In fact, Maximov explicitly rejected the dualist point of view, declaring in his presentation: "There is no reason to assume the existence of two clearly distinct cell types, i.e., the myeloblasts and the lymphoblasts."[5] Though Maximov's theory made him a hero to those who suspected that various blood cell types came from a single source, other scientists refused to accept his results. However, contemporary accounts make it clear that even die-hard dualists who did not accept Maximov's conclusions held only the highest esteem for his reputation.

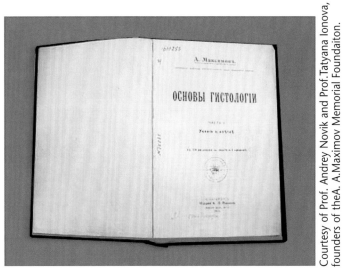

Courtesy of Prof. Andrey Novik and Prof. Tatyana Ionova, founders of the A. Maximov Memorial Foundaiton.

Maximov's book *The Essence of Histology* published in 1914.

A Homeland in Turmoil

While the 1909 meeting in Berlin demonstrated that Maximov's professional life was on the rise, other events signaled success in his personal life. Cementing his position on the high rung of Russia's social ladder, Maximov married a ballerina of the Russian Imperial Ballet and adopted her son from a previous relationship.[2] Maximov was now a family man, whose scientific successes offered not just prestige but a measure of financial security for his loved ones.

Maximov began writing down some of his observations and theories regarding histology, turning to the content of his academic lectures for inspiration. He was hoping to write a textbook, which would both demonstrate his academic prowess and provide a lasting gift to future generations of doctors. He accomplished his goal in 1914, when *The Essence of Histology* was published. It quickly became the standard text for Russian histology students. Basking in his literary success, Maximov took a summer trip to South America.

In his absence, his homeland and the continent of Europe exploded into violence. On July 28, 1914, Austria-Hungary declared war

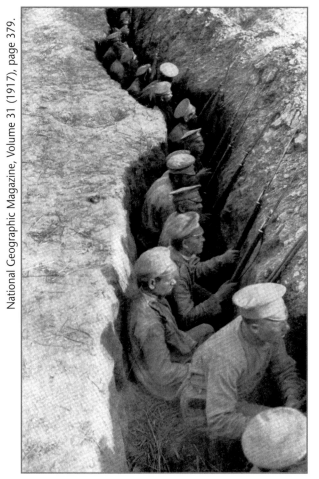

National Geographic Magazine, Volume 31 (1917), page 379.

Russian troops awaiting German attack.

on the tiny nation of Serbia, exactly a month after a Serbian patriot had assassinated the Archduke of Austria and his wife. Serbia, which had long resented being cast under the shadow of the powerful Austro-Hungarian Empire, stood little chance of winning any conflict alone.

Days before the conflict, Prince Regent Alexander of Serbia sent off a desperate telegram to the czar of Russia, explaining that Austro-Hungarian demands were "unnecessarily humiliating for Serbia and incompatible with her dignity as an independent State."[8] Expecting war, the Serbian leader begged the Russian czar for aid:

It is impossible for us to defend ourselves, and we supplicate your Majesty to give us your aid as soon as possible. The highly prized good will of your Majesty, which has so often shown itself toward us, makes us hope firmly that this time again our appeal will be heard by his generous Slav heart.

In these difficult moments I voice the sentiments of the Serbian people, who supplicate your Majesty to interest himself in the lot of the Kingdom of Serbia.[8]

The impending war forced Russia's hand. A powerful and aggressive Austro-Hungarian Empire, poised on Russia's border, was a threat impossible to ignore. In contrast, Serbia had always been a loyal ally to the Russian Empire. But beyond that, the Serbian people were ethnically Slavic, just like the Russians. It was more than a question of realpolitik; it was a question of blood.

On the same day that war began between Serbia and Austria-Hungary, Russia prepared to fight. Recruiters fanned across the country, ordering young men to heed the call of their motherland. Russia's large territory made mobilization a costly and time-consuming enterprise, but its large population would result in overwhelming military force.

Germany, fully cognizant of Russia's potential power and loyal to its Austrian allies, declared war on the czar just days later. On

August 3, 1914, German troops invaded Russia. Maximov's homeland was suddenly and irrevocably plunged into the midst of a great war.

Maximov learned about the outbreak of World War I while he was in Rio de Janeiro.[3] A loyal patriot and lover of his country, he immediately returned to Russia, knowing that his skills as a doctor and as an army officer would be needed in the motherland.

World War I was almost certainly a stressful time in Maximov's life, a catastrophic event that presaged worse times to come. Upon arriving in Russia, Maximov would have learned of the harrowing ordeal of Dr. Nikolai Anichkov (MD), one of his brightest pupils and dearest friends. Studying in Germany at the outbreak of the war, Anichkov was promptly arrested by German authorities and thrown into a prisoner-of-war camp. After his German colleagues arranged for his release, Anichkov escaped to Sweden in order to return to the Russian army.[9] Maximov would have no doubt been amazed by Anichkov's escape, never suspecting that his old pupil would later help him make a similar bid for freedom.

Anichkov went quickly to the front line, serving as head physician for a medical evacuation train.[9] Similarly, Maximov's pupils, who were all trained in a military academy, were expected to serve the motherland in the war that had mobilized the entire country. Maximov had this constant fear over his head; any day, he might receive the news that one of his students had been killed by an enemy bullet.

Unfortunately, the Great War was the first in a chain of events that would irrevocably change the future of Russia, bringing an end to Imperial power and divorcing Maximov from the land of his birth. During Maximov's life, Russia had already been embroiled in several wars: The Russo-Crimean war of 1877-1878, which occurred just years after Maximov's birth; The Boxer Rebellion of 1900, in which Russian troops fought against a widespread Chinese rebellion; and the Russo-Japanese War of 1904-1905, in which Russia was soundly defeated and put to shame by an Oriental power. But all of these wars were limited in their effect; the military was involved, but the people were scarcely touched.

Not so in World War I, a war in which Russia was invaded by a powerful German army intent on bending Russia to its will. The Soviet demographer Boris Urlanis put the number of Russian military deaths at over 1,800,000.[10] Perhaps more staggering is the estimated 1,500,000 civilians who died during the war, due to famine, disease, warfare

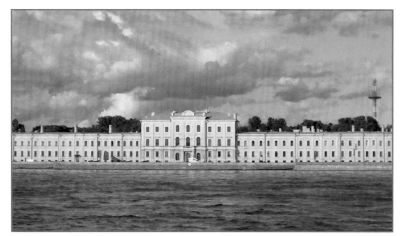

Miliary Medical Academy in St. Petersburg where Maximov was a professor.

and the first use of toxic gas by the Germans.

Even in a country as large as Russia, the loss of so many people was shocking. But the Russian Empire was hit with another blow that shook the foundations of the country. Domestic unrest had been fomenting for over a decade. Anarchists assassinated prominent supporters of the Imperial regime; at their height, these radicals were killing thousands of people each year.[11] Labor forces went on strike, with occasionally violent results. Knowledge spread that the Communists, who had already spearheaded an abortive revolt in 1905, were again gathering power.

It is in the context of this impending doom that Maximov struggled to continue his life as a peaceful man of science. Even during the war, Maximov was able to continue his work and maintain his coveted position as Professor of the Department of Histology and Embryology at the Military Medical Academy in St. Petersburg.[12]

This hope was dashed during the 1917 Revolution. That year the violence spilled into the streets. The city of St. Petersburg became a war zone, and when the dust cleared, the Bolsheviks were in power.

Maximov held no illusions that he would be treated well by the Bolshevik regime. He had been a high-ranking army officer in the Imperial Army. Even worse, he was of noble birth. If there was any question as to how the nobles were to be treated during the start of the Communist regime, "the answer would be obvious—the Bolsheviks exterminated them brutally… just like other 'enemies of the revolution'," explains Vladislav Kalyuzhny, member of the Russian Nobility Association in America.[B] With the Russian regime change, Maximov suddenly became a target.

At the same time, Maximov's reputation as one of Russia's foremost scientists afforded him a powerful measure of protection. His professional status, already greatly admired, continued to rise. In 1920, he was chosen as a member of the Russian Academy of Sciences. His nomination for membership was supported by none other than the Nobel Prize-winning Professor Ivan Pavlov.[12]

Maximov had become a fixture of Russia's scientific establishment, an event that normally would ensure one's status as completely untouchable by the government. But in a society where everything was judged by the State, no one could assume that they were beyond the reach of the Communist Party. Maximov, whose powers of observation had been honed by years in the laboratory, could not have missed the signs that his position of Imperial privilege had suddenly shifted.

But even without the Soviet threat of punishment hanging over his head, Maximov's life under Soviet rule was miserable. Although the Communists quickly signed a peace treaty ending their involvement in World War I, the Bolshevik takeover did not end the fighting in Russia. Anti-Bolshevik forces fought to regain the country, plunging Russia into a civil war that took six years to resolve.

Conditions inside St. Petersburg were abysmal. Dr. Igor Konstantinov (MD, PhD), a cardiac surgeon at Australia's Royal Children Hospital and chronicler of Russian medical history, writes that between 1914 and 1920, "Russia suffered more from starvation, civil disorder, physical and mental suffering than all the nations combined, exhibiting a higher mortality from disease than it had sustained from the World War and subsequent bloodshed. During the famine period 10 million died from starvation alone."[13]

Maximov's position as a scientist allowed him to survive the famine, but still substantially lowered his standard of living: "In the larger cities, learned professors shoveled snow and stood in the bread line while the less-favored tried to be put in jail to be rationed."[13]

For Maximov, who grew up in urban nobility, who had rubbed shoulders with some of the most powerful men in the world and married a privileged ballerina, the sudden descent into poverty would have been a painful psychological blow. Maximov began to send letters to his friends outside the country, begging to get out. In a telling display of the man's personality, he complained not about his own poverty-stricken state, but only about how the country's conditions had made it impossible for him to continue his research. Such was his dedication to his work.

Escape

In desperation Maximov turned to his friend Dr. George Huntington (MD), a professor at Columbia University and a fellow man of science. Huntington and Maximov, who shared an

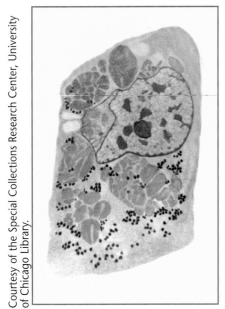

Cellular drawing by Maximov.

academic and professional interest in anatomy, appear to have met at a conference in Boston in 1908.[2] Years later Maximov wrote his American colleague to ask "as to whether it be possible to receive a suitable position as University professor of Histology and Embryology or some similar post in the United States or elsewhere in the wide world."[1]

Maximov first wrote his friend for help in 1917. Huntington appears to have diligently taken up the scientist's cause by contacting Professor Robert Bensley, Professor Emeritus of Anatomy at the University of Chicago, and exhorting him to act on his friend's behalf. Professor Bensley, realizing the significant contribution Maximov could make to the University, offered Maximov a position.

It took Maximov until 1919 to learn that he had been offered a position in America. In a letter in March of that year, Maximov wrote to Bensley:

Dear Professor Bensley:

From a letter from Professor I have learned that you have been so kind as to offer me a position in the University of Chicago. But your letter never reached me. We have no postal communication at all as the other countries do so I use a very rare opportunity to post this letter somewhere in Finland or Sweden. But, for reasons that you will certainly understand I am unable to write more than I do. I wish to express you my sincerest thanks for your kind offer. Unfortunately there is no physical possibility of leaving Petrograd now. I hope to remain alive until there will be such a possibility, and then perhaps there will still be found somewhere a suitable position for me. In any case my resolution to leave this country remains more fixed than ever.

Yours very truly,

A. Maximov [C, 14]

Maximov's situation was far from unique; for scientists and intellectuals trapped in Soviet Russia, escaping the country was nearly impossible. Sergei Fedorov, another Russian scientist, wrote to his American friends during that time, "I have no hope at all of ever having a chance to visit America. Firstly, because we are not allowed to leave Russia and, secondly one needs money for traveling. You are probably aware that all valuable property and money have been confiscated and, naturally, the same fate has overtaken all I had."[13]

While other scientists resigned themselves to their fate, Maximov was not content to remain in a country where he could no longer carry out his life's work. In the winter of 1922, he hatched a plot to escape the country.

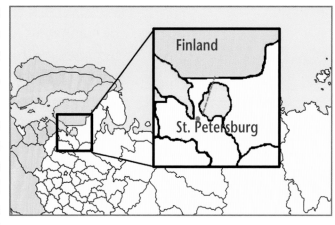

Crossing the frozen Lake of Ladoga.

Leaving his remaining belongings with his pupil Nikolai Anichkov, the professor took his wife, his sister and his adopted son up to the Lake of Ladoga.[13] The frozen lake stretched from the north of St. Petersburg almost all the way to the Finnish border. If Maximov could cross the lake, he would be able to escape Russia. Of course that was contingent on his ability to cross the frozen lake, in the middle of the merciless Russian winter, with his family in tow.

Having been parted from almost all that he owned, Maximov had very little with which to bribe the border guards who patrolled the edges of the lake. Thankfully, the guards were more than happy to accept what he did have: alcohol, perhaps originally used for lab purposes.[13] Maximov and his family then sledged across the frozen lake, braving the cold in order to escape to non-Soviet Finland. Even taking the short-est route, Maximov would have had to travel almost two hundred kilometers with his family in order to cross the lake itself. From there, the Maximovs continued on foot past the Finnish border to freedom.[13]

The Brief, Second Life of Alexander Maximov

From Finland, Maximov crossed into Sweden and arranged trans-port to Chicago.[13] Once there he was surely relieved to discover that his American colleagues had remained true to their word, offering him a job as Professor of Anatomy at the University of Chicago. Grateful for the opportunity to renew his life's work, Maximov threw himself into his duties as a professor and as a scientist. He began work on a definitive textbook of histology. The *Bloom and Fawcett: A Textbook of Histology*, as it is now called, has been used by biomedical investigators for more than three-fourths of a century. Maximov, who based the textbook on his earlier Russian writings, used his own handmade drawings for many of the scientific depic-tions of cells.

Maximov was a gifted artist and his drawings demonstrate the depth of both his poetic spirit and his highly disciplined, scientific mind.

In a time when cameras were still uncommon, Maximov drew precise illustrations of tissue that could only be seen with a microscope. His drawings, which can be seen as works of art as well as medical materials, are still studied today by aspiring doctors.

But Maximov's work at the University was not confined to pieces of paper. In the laboratory he was recognized as a dedicated professional, while his American students soon came to think of him as a brilliant but demanding tutor. Contemporary descriptions of the professor insist that he was a captivating teacher, "always surrounded by his young disciples," who at the same time held his pupils to an exacting standard.[3] One such pupil was William Bloom, a star student who completed the histology textbook after Maximov's death.

No one could have predicted that Bloom and Maximov would work so closely together. For one thing, before Maximov's arrival, Bloom had believed that Maximov was dead. In Bloom's introduction to a histology course, his professor, Dr. Florence Sabin (PhD), had described the discoveries of the great Alexander Maximov, before going on to explain that Maximov had died in the Russian Revolution. One can imagine Bloom's shock when he later learned that Maximov was not only alive, but teaching at the University. Recognizing an opportunity to study under a master scientist, Bloom convinced a reluctant Maximov to become his mentor. It was the beginning of a relationship that would affect both men for the rest of their lives.

With Bloom by his side, Maximov soon threw his hat back into the ring of scientific controversy. With both a detached scientific demeanor and a calm determination, he battled those who disagreed with his theories, including many learned men who rejected his unitarian theory of hematopoiesis. Contemporary documents show that even scientists who were familiar with Maximov's work disagreed with his findings. In a 1929 letter to one of Maximov's pupils, the German professor, Dr. Karl Aschoff (MD), writes, "As much as I respect Maximov, I cannot agree with him on the origin of polyblasts from lymphocytes."[D, 13]

Maximov's role was that of a warrior with few allies, tirelessly studying the origins of different blood cells in order to defend his theories against his academic detractors. While he never managed to achieve scientific consensus on his theories during his lifetime, through his own struggles Maximov was able to bring other scientists to his point of view.

Especially illuminating is a letter to Maximov from Professor Nathan Chandler Foot (MD), who taught at the University of Cincinnati, College of Medicine. Dr. Foot, who had publicly disagreed with Maximov, had written to apologize:

Your work with lymphocytes, reinforced by that of your pupil Bloom, has astonished me and has forced upon me the fact that I owe you a public acknowledgment; you will remember that I stated, in 1925, that if you would relinquish your claims as to the lymphocytic origin of the 'polyblast', no better name for this cell could be devised. How completely have you confounded me! Now that you have not only failed to relinquish your claims, but have actually proved them, there is nothing left for me to do but crawl into a hole and hide my shamed head! However, you know that I was perfectly sincere and unbiased in my criticism and that I shall be most glad to acknowledge my mistake, both to you and in public.[15]

Dr. Foot, who also compliments Maximov on the stunning quality of his scientific drawings, continues to offer his humblest apologies:

This necessity for recasting all my conceptions has come to me like an epoch-making event, to you it will be merely one more scalp to your belt... Thanking you again for your kindness in sending me these interesting papers and hoping that you won't laugh too immoderately when you read this letter (I say this ruefully) I remain, with admiration and best regards,

Very sincerely yours,

Chandler Foot[15]

In keeping with the humility of his character, Maximov did not gloat over his victory, simply writing back:

My dear Dr. Foot,

Please accept my thanks for the kind letter you wrote me. I am very glad that you have acknowledged the developmental abilities of the lymphocyte. I am glad not because I have advanced this theory years ago, but because your change of attitude will certainly tend to clarify one of the most important and confused questions of morphological hematology and pathology.[16]

Maximov's response was written on June 22, 1927. A little over a year later, he passed away from coronary sclerosis and myocarditis.[13]

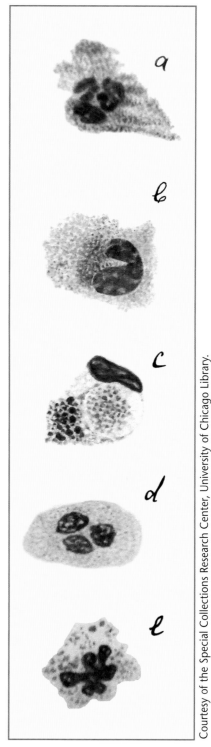

Drawings by Maximov of cells as viewed through his microscope.

During the later part of his life, the Professor suffered from severe coronary arteriosclerosis, an ironic fact considering that Maximov's prize pupil Nikolai Anichkov was one of the pioneers in exploring the causes of this disease.[13]

Maximov's condition did not keep him from his passion of mountain climbing; the summer before he died, he traveled to Madonna di Campiglio, a mountain resort in the Italian Alps. Dr. Bloom, who accompanied him on the trip, wrote of his mentor, "By 1928, hiking at this altitude was too strenuous for him, but he was able to enjoy the magnificent scenery as he rode on a mule along the steep trail to the foot of one of the glaciers."[2] For Maximov to even travel to such a high altitude, with his serious cardiovascular conditions, demonstrates his firm resolve to enjoy life regardless of his ill health.

Correspondences by his friends make it equally clear that Maximov knowingly sacrificed his health to further the pursuit of his scientific studies. Dr. Hal Downey (PhD) of the University of Minnesota wrote to Bloom after Maximov's death, saying, "Your report on Maximov's condition makes him more of a hero than ever. It is difficult to understand how a man could work at such high pressure with the pathology he had."[17] Maximov was a scientist until the end; at the time of his death, he was performing a series of experiments on *in vitro* collagen formation. He was also close to finishing his textbook of histology.

Unfortunately, he would not live to see the completion of either project. Alexander Maximov died in his sleep on December 3, 1928. He was 55 years old. While the scientific world was dismayed by the loss of a legendary researcher, Maximov's closest friends and family suffered another stunning blow just days later. On December 18th Maximov's sister, Claudia, took her own life. Contemporary accounts describe Claudia as devoted to her successful younger brother; she often worked as a lab assistant in his experiments. Claudia also reportedly felt alienated from Maximov's demanding and pampered wife.[2] She was buried next to her brother in Chicago's Oak Wood Cemetery.[2]

While many medical and academic professionals were present at Maximov's funeral, it took decades for the scientific establishment to uniformly accept Maximov's theory of hematopoiesis. It would take until the 1960s for Maximov's theory to be vindicated. Two Canadian scientists, Drs. Ernest McCulloch (MD) and James

Till (PhD), published a paper proving the existence of stem cells. Their results demonstrated the veracity of Maximov's findings from over half a century before. McCulloch and Till, who began their research by studying the effects of radiation on mice, eventually discovered "multipotent" cells from which colonies of cells originated. Similarly, it was not until 1988 that Maximov's more specific hypotheses concerning the hematopoietic stem cell were confirmed by pathologist Dr. Irving Weissman (MD), a Stanford University professor who isolated the hematopoietic stem cell in both mice and humans. While appreciation for their own work is duly earned and well recognized, we feel obliged to mention that these eminent researchers were exploring a trail that had been blazed by Maximov decades before.

Alexander Alexandrowitsch Maximov was a general, a mountain climber, an artist, a socialite, a professor, and a Russian nobleman. But above all, he was a superlative man of science, who dedicated himself to answering some of the most perplexing medical problems of the day. His work, performed with exacting discipline and immersive academic curiosity, advanced the frontiers of medical science and provided the origin of our understanding of how stem cells work. For this, we consider Maximov to be the father of stem cell research.

Letter from Maximov
On the next page is an image of the previously discussed letter that Maximov sent to Professor Huntington at the University of Chicago. The image is courtesy of the Special Collections Research Center, University of Chicago Library.

Dear Professor Huntington,

The recent events going on in Russia have not only interrupted my scientific work, but they have rendered life altogether impossible for a University professor or any cultured man. I have one hope left — to emigrate at the first possibility after the end of the war and to apply elsewhere my scientific knowledge and experience. I hope you won't mind my asking your advice as to whether it be possible to receive a suitable position as University professor of Histology

CHAPTER 3
From Disaster to Recovery

After Maximov's death, the stem cell story becomes inextricably tangled with the intrigue and danger of the Cold War. Separated by the immovable barrier of the Iron Curtain, Maximov's students in the West were cut off from his scientific inheritors in the Soviet Union. American disciple, Dr. William Bloom (MD) dedicated himself to finishing his teacher's textbook, which would eventually run to seven editions. *Bloom and Fawcett: A Textbook of Histology*, as it is now known, is still in use today, albeit in a substantially altered form. The textbook has been Maximov's enduring legacy to the field he loved.

In the USSR, however, Maximov's name was almost forgotten, the result of Soviet policy. As Communist ideology permeated the Russian scientific establishment, biologists were judged not by their merits but by their political affiliations. Dr. Boris Afanasyev (MD, PhD), Director of St. Petersburg's Institute of Child Hematology and Transplantology, explains, "In the history of histology and hematology in the USSR, Maximov's name had been given a negative

The Purge

In 1928, the year Maximov died, a Soviet scientist named Trofim Lysenko proposed a new agricultural technique that catapulted him to Soviet stardom.

Eventually, those who disagreed with Lysenko's view of science were sent to the gulag, no matter their research. Lysenko held a special contempt for biologists, accusing them of deliberately undermining Sovietism.[2] This policy greatly contributed to Maximov's post-mortem fall from grace in his homeland.

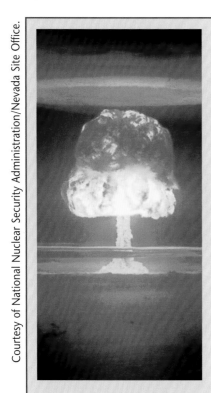

Courtesy of National Nuclear Security Administration/Nevada Site Office.

In 1942, Soviet scientist Georgii Flerov informed Stalin of his suspicions that the Americans were building a powerful weapon. Flerov had noticed that scientists in Allied countries had stopped publishing any papers on nuclear fission; it was as if all nuclear research in America and Britain had simply stopped. Flerov correctly concluded that the American government had begun a project to harness nuclear technology for military use, and he urged the Soviet Premier to do the same. Thus began the Soviet effort that would eventually lead to their successful production of a nuclear weapons arsenal.

connotation when he was mentioned together with a group of other 'reactionary' scientists."[1] With Maximov viewed as a traitor to the Communist cause, his good name, and more importantly his work, was on the verge of falling into obscurity.

The irony was that while Maximov was all but forgotten in Russia, his insights into the human body had become more important than ever. In both the Soviet Union and America, politics would soon push stem cell research to the forefront of the government's consciousness. Our understanding of stem cells would not be nearly as advanced as it is today, were it not for the outbreak of the Cold War.

The Rising Threat of Radiation

In the aftermath of World War II, the entire world realized the devastating consequences of the atomic bomb and the enormous monopoly of power that it conferred upon the United States. That monopoly was short-lived. Russia tested its first atomic bomb in 1949, and suddenly the world had two nuclear superpowers. Both sides realized that atomic warfare had become a real and terrifying possibility.

Soviet leaders were already academically aware of the damage that a nuclear explosion could cause. Besides being able to vaporize entire cities, atomic bombs release life-altering radiation energy. Radiation has a devastating effect on the human body: organs fail and the body's systems shut down. Large doses of radiation can kill a human being almost immediately, but even smaller doses can have disruptive effects. Many people who survive the initial exposure later develop immune problems, cancer, and other serious medical conditions. As well, the effect that radiation has on DNA means that terrible mutations may occur in children of those who were previously exposed.

To better understand the consequences of radiation, Russia sent hundreds of their key scientists to Japan to study the victims of the atomic bomb. But, the Soviets gained firsthand experience of radiation's lethal effects in 1957. In an incident that was kept secret by the Soviet government for decades, the USSR suffered its first radiation contamination disaster. Even today, few people know about the harrowing events that occurred in the closed town of Ozyorsk, near the Ural Mountains. What happened there affected thousands of people, and provided an impetus for Soviet research into radiation.

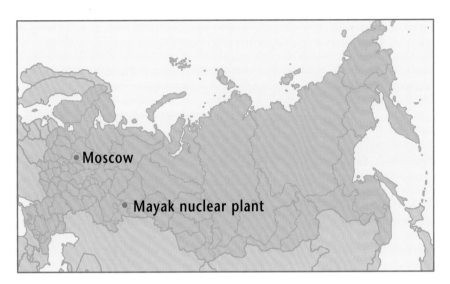

Kyshtym: The Unknown Radiation Disaster

In September of 1957, the cooling system at the Mayak nuclear fuel reprocessing plant failed, and the temperature in one of the storage tanks began to rise uncontrollably. The resulting non-nuclear explosion released a massive radioactive cloud into the air, which eventually spread hundreds of kilometers from the reprocessing plant.

The Mayak nuclear plant was located deep within Russia, near the Ural Mountains. The plant itself was not placed on any maps; nor was the town of Ozyorsk, which officially did not exist. The nearest open town was Kyshtym, a small town which nevertheless held thousands of inhabitants.

The spread of radioactivity threatened the lives of everyone in the vicinity, and the Russian authorities responded inadequately. It took the government a week to evacuate the 10,000 people near Kyshtym. Even today, details on how many people died in this accident are hazy. In 1977, Dr. Leo Tumerman (PhD), the former head of the Biophysics Laboratory at the Institute of Molecular Biology in Moscow, who at that point was living in Israel, reported that the nuclear disaster had killed and injured hundreds.[3] Dr. Zhores Medvedev (PhD), another high-level Russian researcher and Soviet dissident, would go on to expose the Kyshtym explosion to the world in 1979, years after being exiled from the Soviet Union; his book, *A Nuclear Disaster in the Urals*, paints a harrowing picture of the massive fallout.[4]

The Kyshtym disaster can be seen as the Soviet Union's wake-up call. Reports of the radiation brought home to Soviet officials the

But what if radiation could be combated? What if the human body contained its own defense mechanisms against radiation? Could medical science find a way to fight the effects of radiation exposure, thereby limiting one of the major effects of nuclear fallout?

fact that a single nuclear accident had the potential to essentially destroy part of the country. The prospect of nuclear war, furthermore, meant a likelihood of radiation that could devastate entire regions, poisoning millions of people. Without an effective medical response to radiation, the Soviets were looking at the possibility that a single technical or political misstep could destabilize the regime and cause massive damage.

But what if radiation could be combated? What if the human body contained its own defense mechanisms against radiation? Could medical science find a way to fight the effects of radiation exposure, thereby limiting one of the major effects of nuclear fallout? The Soviet government was eager to answer this question, and to have a medical treatment that would give them the edge in any potential nuclear war.

One American scientific researcher, Dr. Bruce Carlson (MD, PhD) of the University of Michigan, concluded after visiting the USSR during 1965-66, "The restoration of function in irradiated tissues has been a priority subject in many areas of Soviet biomedical research for a number of years."[5] Carlson went on to describe the "considerable effort" that had been put into the field.[5] While prevention was best, Soviet researchers also hoped to treat radiation exposure, if and when it occurred. To this end, Soviet scientists looked for biological protectors against radiation.

In searching for these cellular protectors, researchers followed three lines of inquiry, searching for cells that could:

- *Reduce DNA mutation.* Nuclear radiation can break apart DNA strands, or alter the nucleotide building blocks of DNA, the result is genetic mutation. Soviet researchers looked for ways to arrest radiation's effect on the DNA.

- *Scavenge free radicals.* Ionizing radiation creates unstable molecules, which look to stabilize themselves by stealing electrons from other molecules. The resulting chain reaction disrupts cells and weakens the body. We know today that a diet rich in antioxidants helps clean up free radicals; scientists were looking for other ways to do so.

- *Replace damaged cells.* Radiation blasts the cells of the body into oblivion. Entire organs, like the thyroid, can be destroyed. Important somatic systems shut down. The body is suddenly robbed of the mechanisms it needs to function.

The Soviet government aimed to accomplish the third goal by replenishing the blood system. A treatment that could accomplish this, they reasoned, could theoretically be developed into a therapeutic regimen that could fight against the effects of radiation. To accomplish this monumental task, the Soviet government turned to their most distinguished researchers, biologists and histologists who had risen to the top of the Soviet scientific establishment. A good part of this scientific dream team consisted of researchers who had made significant stem cell breakthroughs.

Chief among this number were two Jewish microbiologists from the Military Medical Academy in St. Petersburg. Dr. Joseph Chertkov (PhD) would make important contributions to our understanding of the stem cell microenvironment. Alexander Friedenstein would almost single-handedly resurrect Maximov's work, and also make one of the most important cellular discoveries of the century: that of the bone marrow stromal cell, better known as the mesenchymal stem cell, or MSC.

Alexander Friedenstein: Another Russian Giant

Alexander Friedenstein began his medical career in the venerable halls of Maximov's old university, the Military Medical Academy in St. Petersburg, and began studying epidemiology and microbiology in the 1950s. Friedenstein's work, which focused on the interaction between the bone marrow and the blood, led him unwaveringly to Maximov's extensive body of research.

While Friedenstein, seen as "the other giant in Russian hematology," did not always agree with Maximov's conclusions, it is clear that he had a great respect for his Russian predecessor.[6] Friedenstein "can be credited today for having contributed to the restoration of Maximov's good name by highlighting the great significance of Maximov's fundamental studies in hematology," explains Dr. Boris Afanasyev, a Russian stem cell clinician.[1] Later in life, Friedenstein published a paper focusing on Maximov's ideas, describing the scientist's theory as "far ahead of its time" and defending Maximov against his detractors.[7]

Friedenstein's respect may have been motivated by more than just professional courtesy; like Maximov, Friedenstein was mistrusted in the USSR by virtue of his birth. Maximov was a nobleman in a profoundly anti-elitist system; Friedenstein was a Jew in a country that held deep-rooted anti-Semitic prejudices. Dr. Robert Gale (MD,

Multipotent Cells

As for the original cells that gave birth to entire MSC colonies, Friedenstein awarded them another name: colony-forming-unit fibroblast, or CFU-F.[8] The concept of a colony-forming unit is an especially important one for the current generation of stem cell researchers, who need to grow entire colonies of cells in order to run scientific studies and clinical trials. Because all stem cells are able to self-replicate, any mesenchymal stem cell is theoretically capable of becoming a colony-forming unit. One CFU, if removed from its natural location and put into an *in vitro* environment (or another organism) can grow an entire colony of cells.

When measuring a patient's overall health, doctors will sometimes measure the person's colony-forming efficiency, or CFE. A below-average CFE within the bone marrow would imply a sub-standard number of mesenchymal stem cells. Dramatic CFE changes can indicate blood disorders such as leukemia or anemia, or that the body has been exposed to radiation. As a human being ages, the CFE number drops as the person's stem cell population becomes more senescent.

PhD), a distinguished American transplant surgeon and friend of Friedenstein, explains, "Anybody who was Jewish and wanted to leave the USSR to emigrate to Israel was known as a 'refusnik'. If they received permission to immigrate," Gale continues, "they would immediately be fired from their jobs."[A] Essentially, expressing a desire to move to Israel was considered a lower form of treason in the eyes of the Politburu. Although Friedenstein did not appear to be a refusenik himself, the Soviet government kept him on a tight leash, unwilling to lose such an important researcher.

Despite the pressure he may have felt, Friedenstein continued his work without any signs of discontent. He served in a high capacity, heading an immunomorphological laboratory at the N. F. Gamaleya Institute of Epidemiology and Microbiology in Moscow for over a quarter of a century. At the same time, he enjoyed performing the routine work of the lab; personal and academic accounts describe him as "a true bench-worker, personally doing tissue culture and transplantation experiments, preparing tissue sections, performing immunochemical stainings, etc."[8]

Dr. Alex Kharazi (MD, PhD), Chief Technology Officer at Stemedica Cell Technologies, Inc. and a former Soviet researcher who worked with Friedenstein's laboratory group on several collaborative projects over the years, concedes that Friedenstein "could come off as a bit of an intense personality, at times."[B] Nevertheless, Kharazi declares, the biologist "was tremendously respected in Russian scientific circles. His work was well known even in the medical community, although he wasn't a medical doctor. The man was universally acknowledged to be a genius." With his thin frame, slender hands, high forehead and intelligent eyes, Friedenstein was every inch the figure of the brilliant scientist.

Discovering Mesenchymal Stem Cells

Friedenstein's brilliance manifested itself in his research. During the course of his examinations into the working of the bone marrow, he discovered a type of cell he had never seen before. It appeared to be some type of stem cell, but Friedenstein quickly realized that it was not a hematopoietic stem cell, which was the only known stem cell type at the time.

The scientist prepared several of these mysterious cells for *in vitro* experiments, hoping that each cell would grow into a fully functional colony of cells that would lend itself to further study.

And grow these cells did; within 10-12 days, there were thousands of cells in each colony.[8]

Examining his results, Friedenstein realized that these newly grown cells were multipotent, able to differentiate into several distinct types of cells. In contrast to hematopoietic cells, these new cells were responsible for forming connective tissue rather than blood cells. Later studies, by Friedenstein and others, would reveal an additional ability; these cells could greatly aid in healing already-damaged tissue.

Friedenstein named his new cells BMSC, or "Bone Marrow **Stromal** Cells." He was reluctant to use the term "stem cell" for his new discovery, possibly so that it would not be seen as merely an expansion of Maximov's work. In fairness to Friedenstein, however, the term "Bone Marrow Stromal Cell" is an accurate encapsulation of the cells' origin and basic function. Later, the cells would just be called MSC, or marrow stromal cells. As time progressed, the acronym MSC shifted, and now many scientists use the term **MSC** to mean **mesenchymal stem cells**.

As previously discussed, mesenchymal stem cells, or MSCs, are potent stem cells that are responsible for forming the connective tissue of the body. They are multipotent, and thus able to differentiate into a variety of cell types. For example, MSCs can become chondrocytes and instigate collagen repair. They can become osteoblasts, the type of cell responsible for bone formation. Or they can form adipocytes, those much-maligned cells that are responsible for storing fat.

Friedenstein measured mesenchymal stem cell activity in mice, rats, guinea pigs, and other species, including human beings. His experiments led not only to the discovery of MSCs, but also to an understanding of their ability to self-propagate both within and outside of the body.

Chertkov and the Microenvironment

Across town from the Gamaleya Institute, Friedenstein's colleague Dr. Joseph Chertkov (MD, PhD) studied different aspects of both hematopoietic stem cells and MSCs. Even after the discovery of MSCs, very little was known about them. Chertkov was the first to describe the physiological characteristics of MSCs—the aspects of their composition that allowed them to carry out their basic functions. His research deepened our understanding of the differences

Stroma: the framework or surrounding substance (which is usually made of connective tissue) of which an organ is made. It is also the protoplasmic framework from which some cells may be made, e.g. red blood cells.

Mesenchymal stem cell (MSC): a pluripotent stem cell. More specifically, cells that are undifferentiated and have the capacity to become a variety of other cells, including, but not limited to: osteoblasts (bone), chondrocytes (cartilage), and lymphocytes (lymphatic).

The stem cell is informed by its niche as to "whether or not it will start to regenerate, generate new offspring, try to repair tissue, or build new tissue."

between HSCs and MSCs, cementing the fact that there are different types of stem cells. But Chertkov, who was Senior Scientist at Moscow's Hematological Scientific Center, was particularly interested in studying the stem cell's microenvironment.[9]

The stem cell microenvironment, sometimes referred to more loosely by researchers as the stem cell niche, is a location that gives the cells their marching orders. As Dr. David Scadden (MD), Professor at Harvard Medical School, explains, the stem cell is informed by its niche as to "whether or not it will start to regenerate, generate new offspring, try to repair tissue, or build new tissue. In that case," he continues in an online interview, "a niche is a combination of a functional and an anatomic definition."[12] The stem cell niche provides an important role in managing the stem cell's behavior within the body.

We owe a good deal of our understanding of stem cell niches to Chertkov, who studied the stromal microenvironment and its effect on HSCs. His 1984 paper entitled "Hematopoietic Stem Cell and its Microenvironment" was a seminal work in developing an understanding of how stem cells interact with their microenvironment.[9, 13] Chertkov's work helped demonstrate that the niche was another variable in the ever-evolving stem cell equation.

Pushchino

Friedenstein, Chertkov, and others were not working in a vacuum; they were leaders of highly disciplined teams of scientists who had been assembled by the Soviet government. They were given whatever equipment they needed; money and resources were no object. The study of stem cells was given top priority by the Soviet government.

Friedenstein and others had already realized that it was possible to grow new organs with stem cells; although Friedenstein's greatest inventions occurred in the 1960s, according to some Russian scientists, he was already growing new bone from gall bladder stem cells back in the 1950s.[c] He believed that stem cells had amazing healing powers that, combined with medical application, offered an ingenious method for treating radiation exposure.

Friedenstein headed the stem cell research effort at the N. F. Gamaleya Institute for Microbiology and Epidemiology, but this was just one of the institutions that had been tasked by the Soviet government with the monumental directive of discovering anti-radiation protection mechanisms, including stem cell treatment.

There was the Research Center for Blood Transfusion and Bone Marrow Transplants in Moscow, where Chertkov did much of his work. Researchers there studied how to effectively perform transplants from donor to patient. The Institute of Biophysics studied the effects of radiation, in order to learn how to combat it. In Oblinsk, which contains the world's first nuclear power plant, scientists performed *in vivo* animal radiation studies. Together, these four centers had hundreds of scientists working on research related to stem cell treatments.

But if one wants to understand the magnitude of this scientific undertaking, one should remember only one word: Pushchino. This city, one hundred twenty miles south of Moscow, was simply a sleepy town for hundreds of years. But in 1962, the government changed all that.

That year, members of the National Academy of Sciences met to discuss their various projects. Undoubtedly, the Kyshtym incident, which had occurred a mere five years earlier, was on the minds of many of the scientists. As well, some of the researchers would have heard about a cutting-edge study coming out of Canada, with two scientists claiming to have proven the existence of stem cells within the bone marrow. At their meeting, these prestigious associates of the Academy decided that they needed to found a new research center, one that would:

Allow for the creation of a new powerful center of biological research, having the necessary physical plant and supplied with state-of-the-art equipment. The creation of such a center will provide great possibilities for the use of biophysics and biochemistry in various branches of biology and for the conduct of deep, integrated theoretical research, the results of which will serve as the basis for the development of practical recommendations for the application of the achievements of the biological sciences in agriculture and medicine.[14]

The Academy decided on Pushchino, which was close enough to Moscow to provide for constant communication, but far enough from any major urban center to escape the notice of prying eyes. Overnight, the small town became a city of scientists, existing almost solely for the purpose of advancing research into the effects of radiation and how to combat them. Pushchino enjoyed another advantage being located twenty kilometers from, at that time, the largest cyclotron in the world.

The Stem Cell Niche

Chertkov was not the discoverer of the stem cell niche. That honor goes to Dr. Raymond Schofield, a British scientist who conducted much of his research at the renowned Paterson Laboratories (now the Paterson Institute for Cancer Research). In 1978, Schofield was studying the actions of hematopoietic stem cells in the spleen. He realized that the HSCs acted differently in the spleen than they did in other parts of the body. In order to explain this discrepancy, he hypothesized that the stem cell's behavior was partly determined by the cells around it. It was in his 1978 paper on the subject that he applied the term "stem cell niche" to his hypothesis.[11] Although previous experiments had suggested the existence of a stem cell niche in animal models, Schofield was the first to apply it to mammalian hematology.[12]

A review of both Chertkov and Schofield's work demonstrates how great scientific minds may often focus on the same problems. It also brings up the question: how much more quickly would stem cell research have advanced, if researchers had not been divided by the Iron Curtain?

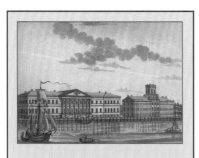

In 1925, the Russian Academy of Sciences, which had existed since 1724, was renamed the Academy of Sciences of the USSR. The Soviet government afforded the Academy a great deal of respect, recognizing it as the premiere scientific organization in the Union. That did not stop it from forming a government commission in 1929 to purge the Academy of counter-revolutionary elements. After that point, Soviet control over the agenda of the Academy was solidified.[15] Recently declassified CIA documents demonstrate that, during the Cold War, the goals of the Academy were very much in keeping with the goals of the Soviet government.[16]

Even with governmental interference, the Academy of Sciences remained the elite scientific organization of the USSR. Today, the organization is once again known as the Russian Academy of Sciences.

Almost a third of the scientists living in Pushchino were biologists. While not all of these scientists were assigned to stem cell projects, a significant portion of them were focused on research that directly or indirectly advanced Soviet knowledge of stem cells. These teams of researchers worked in isolation from the outside world, though they communicated frequently with their counterparts in Moscow.

The USSR's willingness to establish an entire city dedicated to scientific research dealing with the problem of nuclear fallout shows how seriously they were considering the concept of stem cell treatment. Stem cell researchers were given every consideration; no expense was considered too lavish. The entire state was focused on making sure the scientists had everything they needed.

The Canadian Discovery

The Soviets were not the only ones who recognized the potential of forming cellular "protectors" to combat the effects of radiation. America and its Cold War allies were also hard at work encouraging their own scientists to make breakthroughs in regenerative science. In fact, one of the most important pieces of the stem cell puzzle fell into place neither in the USSR nor in America, but rather in Canada.

In 1961, two Canadian scientists, Drs. James Till (PhD) and Ernest McCulloch (MD) were conducting studies with the goal of measuring the effects of radiation on mice; like their Soviet counterparts, they were motivated by the possibility of discovering ways to survive nuclear war. Till declared in an interview, "This was the late-1950s, early 1960s. The memories of Hiroshima and Nagasaki were still fresh. There was much concern about the threat of nuclear weapons, that we might have to fight an atomic war. So, being able to ameliorate the effects of total-body irradiation by having a bank of marrow was a big deal." Till acknowledged that their research was supported by the government, declaring "Some of our very early funds came from the Defence Research Board of Canada."[17]

Till and McCulloch knew that their work was timely, but they could not have predicted the result of their study. What started as an attempt to reduce the effects of radiation turned into a eureka moment not unlike Fleming's discovery of antibiotics. Examining the spleens of irradiated mice, McCulloch noticed clumps of cells that corresponded with the bone marrow injections the mice had been given. The two researchers, after further study, decided they had stumbled upon some of "the active cells" in the bone marrow.[17] They realized that these miraculous cells were responsible for the formation of entire cell colonies. Their announcement to the world, entitled "Cytological Demonstration of the Clonal Nature of Spleen Colonies Derived from Transplanted Mouse Marrow Cells," vindicated Maximov's work and provided the impetus for stem cell research. Two years later, the duo fleshed out their theory and presented it to the world at large.

There is no doubt that Till and McCulloch's discovery was a fundamental event in the course of stem cell research. Friedenstein discovered bone marrow stem cells after Till and McCulloch's findings, for example. Perhaps if he had not been inspired by Till and McCulloch's work, he may never have delved into such an exhaustive investigation of this previously undiscovered cell type. These two Canadian researchers were the architects of a new scientific field; they took the barely blazed trail of stem cell science and paved the way for future breakthroughs.

But to see Till and McCulloch as the scientists who began stem cell science is to forget that Friedenstein, Chertkov and others had been following similar lines of research before the Canadians had their breakthrough. It is to ignore previous pioneers, like Maximov and Virchow, who laid the first stones of this great scientific edifice. It is to forget the long train of scientific inquiry that began over a century ago, and is still ongoing in centers around the world.

As much as the USA and USSR may have wanted it to appear that their respective sides in the Cold War were solely responsible for the scientific breakthroughs that characterize the beginning of stem cell science, a complete picture must include both Westerners and Soviets.

Governments at War, Scientists at Peace

Much of the work on stem cells during the Cold War era was classified. Scientists who pursued involvement with stem cells saw portions of their research withheld from the public and from fellow scientists. Official reports on clinical studies would sometimes be altered, limiting the number of people who knew the true results. Important Soviet researchers, rarely traveled abroad; the government did not want to let these state assets out of their sight.

But there were some startling moments of peace and mutual cooperation between stem cell researchers during the Cold War.

One would like to think that Russian and Western scientists were able to work together because of some inherent altruism in the heart of the political bureaucrats. The motivations were probably more pragmatic; government leaders on both sides realized that if they wanted scientific breakthroughs, they had to encourage scientific innovation.

The scientific journals remained open, and American researchers were able to learn about Soviet advances through the pages of such publications as Washington, D.C. based *Science News.*[8] Similarly, Russian scientists read about the advances in research that occurred in North America, including Till and McCulloch's seminal work.

Not all scientific cooperation occurred indirectly, through the pages of scientific journals. Some scientists did brave their governments' disapproval and travel abroad. Friedenstein, despite his valued status as a top-notch Russian scientist, was able to attend a few European scientific conferences.[19] Americans traveled to Russia to work side by side with Soviet scientists, although they each felt the troubling sensation that they were under constant surveillance. One American doctor even flew to Russia to assist the country during one of its darkest hours.

This American doctor, Dr. Robert Gale, recalls, "We were all very anxious to have scientific collaboration," but he admits that some scientists were more accessible than others. "People who were part of the [Soviet] system, scientist apparatchniks, you could collaborate with openly. In fact, that was even encouraged. I had many collaborations with Soviet hematologists, and those collaborations were encouraged and funded by the United States, and encouraged by the Soviet government. But non-apparatchniks were not encouraged; you could not openly work with them."

Friedenstein was one such non-apparatchnik, Gale remembers. "We could have social discussions in his apartment, but if we wanted to have any serious discussion, we would have to conduct that conversation in the street."

Still, the amount of cooperation between these two opposed powers was remarkable, given the political climate. One would like to think that Russian and Western scientists were able to work together because of some inherent altruism in the heart of the political bureaucrats. The motivations were probably more pragmatic; government leaders on both sides realized that if they wanted scientific breakthroughs, they had to encourage scientific innovation. Stifling academic cooperation, by keeping their researchers from participating in wider scientific forums, would only ensure intellectual stagnation. In essence, a breakthrough treatment for radiation poisoning was too valuable a goal for either side to risk failure by playing politics as usual.

The Mystery of Soviet Clinical Studies

Both Soviet and American researchers performed hundreds of tests on irradiated subjects. Of course, the vast majority of these subjects were animals; scientists could not ethically expose humans to life-altering radiation in order to conduct their experiments.

At a certain point, however, human subjects were required to advance scientific understanding of the ways in which ionic radiation interacted with the human body. In the Soviet Union, there were a plethora of citizens who were exposed to radiation. Those affected by the Kyshtym disaster numbered in the thousands. Recent research has revealed that even before the disaster, people who worked in or lived near Kyshtym were exposed to radiation. The nuclear fuel reprocessing plant had very few security measures in place to protect its workers, and much of the nuclear waste was dumped into the nearby river, which affected communities downstream.[20]

Furthermore, the Communist authorities responded to the Kyshtym disaster by sending over 1,000 ethnic Tatar families to perform clean-up operations. Some of these liquidators have since taken the Russian government to court, and they describe a harrowing story of farmers with bleeding hands and discolored bodily fluids, victims of radiation.[21]

From this instance alone, we know that Soviet stem cell researchers would have been able to find a patient population for clinical trials. Did they do so? Because so many documents remain classified, any assumption that they did perform stem cell treatments of any kind on Soviet subjects suffers from lack of evidence. There are, however, indications that clinical studies did occur. Dr. Valentin Grischenko (MD, PhD), a former member of the National Academy of Sciences of the Soviet Union (now a member in the Academy of the Ukraine) has reported that late in his life, the Russian Premier Leonid Brezhnev received stem cell therapy in order to augment his failing health.[22] Speaking to the well-regarded Russian newspaper *Komsomolskaya Pravda* about Brezhnev's treatment, Grischenko explained, "That medication was called 'Elixir of Immortality' and was produced from bone marrow. Theoretically, that cell therapy should stimulate all defense forces of organism [sic] and rejuvenate it."[22]

Similarly, Andrey Bredikhin—the Press Secretary of the Laboratory of Immunology of the Scientific Center for Obstetrics, Gynecology,

Pluripotent: able to change into a variety of capacities—particularly, differentiating into one of several different cell types. Also, a cell's ability to possibly differentiate into a multitude of tissues or organs.

and Perinatology at the Russian Academy of Medical Science—confirmed to the newspaper *Pravda* that Soviet Premier Boris Yeltsin had also received cell therapy, and named another prominent member of the Academy as the doctor who administered the treatment.[23] For Soviet scientists to perform this procedure on two separate heads of state implies that they had knowledge of how stem cells would act within the human body.

Acute Radiation Syndrome (ARS): The Problem

For their leaders, the Soviet clinicians were simply attempting to turn back the clock. For Russian villagers and workers who were exposed to radiation, the targeted condition was acute radiation syndrome.

Of all the organs damaged by acute radiation syndrome, the blood system is the hardest hit. Even a small dose of radiation (25 rems in a short period of time) will lead to changes in the blood. White blood cells die, leaving the body more susceptible to infection. Red blood cells die, and the body is no longer receiving the nutrients it needs to function. The bone marrow is decimated; the body is no longer able to renew its blood supply. Without functioning bone marrow, production of mesenchymal and hematopoietic stem cells plummets. The body is unable to repair the damage it has suffered.

When the bone marrow is functioning correctly, however, it has the ability to help regenerate the body. German radiobiologist, Dr. Albright M. Kellerer (PhD) points out:

*A large number of studies have made it clear that bone marrow stem cells are remarkably **pluripotent**, that a substantial fraction—of the order of 1%—circulates in the peripheral blood, and that they can migrate to various tissues to proliferate and differentiate there.[20]*

Stem cells from the bone marrow, with their high potential for differentiation, make an excellent "emergency response team" for the body.

Cold War-era scientists hoped this cellular emergency response would include a way to treat some levels of acute radiation syndrome (ARS), the clinical name for the changes which occur to the body in the wake of radiation exposure. For an ARS-affected patient, the hypothesis was that both hematopoietic and mesenchymal stem cells could not only cleanse the blood stream but could eventually help other areas of the body struggling with radiation poisoning by differentiating into needed cell types. Stem cells could be the protector cells for regenerating damaged tissue that everyone had been looking for.

When someone is exposed to radiation, however, the stem cells suffer just like any other cell. With the bone marrow thoroughly irradiated, there are not enough stem cells to replenish the body's damaged tissues. The bone marrow needs to go through a process of myelopoiesis, reforming itself and producing new blood cells. But in the meantime, the bloodstream is left without a source of new blood cells. No new HSCs or MSCs are being produced. The body is unable to use its stem cells, one of its most powerful regenerative tools, to fight radiation sickness.

The more the Soviet researchers learned about stem cells, the more they realized how vital a role they played within the body. Increasingly, they began to wonder if a transplant of stem cells to the bone marrow of the afflicted patient could battle acute radiation syndrome. Fortunately, a new procedure had recently been developed to do just that.

Bone Marrow Transplantation

In a bone marrow transplant (BMT), the patient's compromised bone marrow is injected with stem cells. If the body does not reject the transplant, then the stem cells can proliferate and differentiate, seeding themselves in the depleted bone marrow and providing a jump-start to the body's blood system. It is a reset button for the body, which cannot be healthy without a functioning blood system.

In the United States, the first bone marrow transplants began in 1939. They were highly experimental, and mainly utilized animal studies, although there were a few small-scale clinical studies.[24] Meanwhile, Friedenstein, Chertkov, and others were conducting similar studies in the Soviet Union. Early on, authorities from both sides of the Cold War recognized the importance of this research. Dr. Edward Donnall Thomas (MD), the Nobel laureate who conducted much of the seminal research on BMT, acknowledged in his Nobel lecture that "because of concern about irradiation exposure our early funding came through the Atomic Energy Commission."[24] In many ways, this funding from the Atomic Energy Commission paralleled the Soviet efforts to support regenerative research in the Soviet Union.

The Soviets and the Americans were paying especially close attention when five Yugoslavian researchers from the Vinca research reactor were flown to France to undergo experimental bone marrow transplantation. The five researchers had been exposed to deadly doses of radiation when the reactor unintentionally went critical. The French transplant team, led by Dr. Georges Mathé (MD), managed to save four of the five patients, but critics believed that the benefits of the operation were marginal, at best.[24, 25]

Another major breakthrough occurred when the first successful bone marrow transplant for treating immune deficiency syndrome was performed on a young boy at the University of Minnesota in 1968. Soon after, BMT was used to treat lymphoma. Studying the recent advances that had been made in the bone marrow transplant protocols, doctors around the world began to wonder if BMT could be used to replenish irradiated bone marrow cells and fight the effects of radiation.

While both American and Soviet doctors were attempting to better understand the possibilities of BMT, it took a terrible tragedy before medical science was offered an opportunity to clearly study the results. In May 1986, thirteen patients received bone marrow transplants at the simply named Moscow Hospital 6. The attending doctors included some of the best hematologists and transplant surgeons from both the United States and the USSR.

In contrast to the multinational character of the attending medical team, the thirteen patients all came from a small Ukrainian town named Pripyat. Pripyat, with a population of only 50,000, had been founded in 1970 to house the workers who operated the nearby nuclear power plant. The power plant, which supplied much of Ukraine's electricity, went by the official name of The V. I. Lenin Nuclear Power Station. But it is better known by its other name: Chernobyl.

CHAPTER 4
Crests and Falls

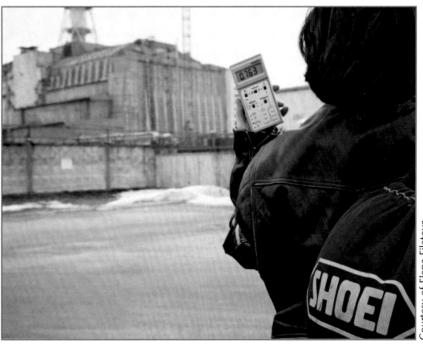

A view of the Chernobyl Nuclear Power Plant. The Geiger counter shows even after 15 years had passed (date of the image) there were still detectable levels of radiation.

Courtesy of Elena Filatova.

Chernobyl

In an event that has highlighted for the world the dangers of nuclear power, on the morning of April 26, 1986, the Chernobyl Nuclear Power Plant experienced a catastrophic accident. An explosion at reactor Number 4 released a significant amount of radioactive material into the air. Plant workers were immediately exposed to high doses of radiation, resulting in textbook cases of acute radiation syndrome (ARS). More than 30 separate fires broke out; some of these fires threatened to consume the other three nuclear reactors, an event that could have caused subsequent explosions.

Firemen, knowing full well the possible deadly consequences of radiation poisoning, rushed to the scene.[1] Russian analyst, Robert Ebel, explains that these heroes put themselves in harm's way to limit the effect of the blast:

The danger that the fire would travel along the roof of the turbine hall meant that the initial fire-fighting efforts were concentrated on the roof. It was during this action that many of the firefighters received what were eventually fatal doses of radiation... The firemen lacked proper protective gear, the roof was built of highly flammable materials, and the fire-fighting trucks were not equipped to attack fires on buildings of this height, in some places reaching 235 feet. The chance of survival for those firemen who made it to the rooftop was minimal; it was for many a sentence of death.[1]

Firefighters, plant workers, doctors and even passersby—those who were near the power plant that day received fatal doses of radiation. While the Pripyat citizenry were evacuated, the ARS victims needed immediate medical attention. Eighty-four patients were treated at hospitals in nearby Kiev, Ukraine. Another 115 patients were sent to Moscow. In fact, almost all of the most seriously ill patients went to Moscow. The very worst cases were sent to one hospital in particular, Moscow Hospital 6.

Moscow Hospital 6 was primarily known as a hematology-oncology ward. But it had an unusual specialty: treating radiation-afflicted patients. The evening of April 26, deputy director, Dr. Angelina Guskova (MD, PhD), was connected to Chernobyl medical officials via a direct hotline. Dr. Guskova was assisted by American transplant surgeon, Dr. Robert Gale, who had offered his services to the Soviets upon learning of the nuclear disaster. Gale and Guskova were looking at individuals who had taken on an incredible amount of radiation. Twenty of the patients had suffered from Level IV exposure—between 6 and 16 Grays (Gy) of radiation. The chance of survival from ARS becomes negligible when exposure exceeds 6 Gy. For others who had experienced 4-6 Gy, the chances of survival were less than 50%.

Facing such dire medical circumstances, the doctors decided to perform bone marrow transplants on several of the patients, hoping that new stem cells would reverse bone marrow failure and give these patients a chance at life. They chose only the patients who were suffering from "an extremely severe and irreversible degree of myelodepression."[2] (Myelodepression is the clinical term for compromised bone marrow activity.) Thirteen patients, all suffering from Levels III and IV doses of radiation, received stem cell injections.

Unfortunately, for most of the patients, it was too little, too late. The patients had all suffered severe radiation burns. Seven of the thirteen patients died from injuries to the skin, gastrointestinal tract, and lungs, while four others died from viral-bacterial infections. While the bone marrow transplants may have been able to help restore the patients' bone marrow function, they proved unable to save the patients' lives.

Of the thirteen patients who received bone marrow transplants in the aftermath of Chernobyl, two survived. These two were distinctly fortunate; they both had sisters whose bone marrow could be used for donation. Even then, the bone marrow transplants were only a temporary measure; both patients rejected the donated cells after several weeks, but by then, they had begun producing their own stem cells.[2]

Another six patients received fetal liver cell transplants, with the hope that this source, rich in stem cells, would be less likely to trigger graft-versus-host disease and that they would be accepted by the body. Unfortunately, all but one patient who received these transplants died from skin and intestinal injuries. The last patient, who had received between 8-10 Gy of radiation, clung to life for several days after her transplant, before finally passing away. Her autopsy revealed that her own cells had begun the process of myelopoiesis (production of bone marrow, bone marrow cells, or blood cells in bone marrow); her body had begun forming new bone marrow. Given the complexity of the situation, doctors were unable to determine whether the results were from the transplant.

For the two patients who survived, it is impossible to know whether the transplants were the reason for their recovery, or whether they would have survived without the stem cell injection. Dr. Guskova decided that "in an emergency situation like the one described, the group of persons for whom bone marrow transplants would be indicated with a reasonable prospect of success is extremely limited."[2]

Comparison of the BMT-patients with the non-treated control group leads to few conclusions. In both groups, receiving over 9 Gy

Beyond Chernobyl

After Chernobyl, Western doctors as well as analysts and policymakers asked themselves: how did the staff of Moscow Hospital 6 know so much about radiation exposure?[1] Dr. Gale admits that he was exposed to information that had not previously traveled outside the confines of the Soviet Union, saying, "The value of having me accurately report the accident results, in the eyes of [Soviet Premier] Gorbachev and the Politburu, was far greater than the value of withholding prior information from me."[A]

It was partly through scrutiny of the actions of Moscow Hospital 6 that the world became more aware of the fact that the Soviet Union had amassed a significant body of knowledge pertaining to radiation exposure, a fact that further indicated that the Soviets had been less than open about previous nuclear incidents within their borders.

was an automatic death sentence. For those who received between 6.5-9 Gy, one patient from each group survived. But for those receiving less than 6.5 Gy, survival rates were better for those who did not receive a bone marrow transplant. All five patients in this category, without the transplant, survived. In contrast, out of four patients who received BMT, only one lived.[2]

It seems that in several cases, the stem cell transplants were rejected, resulting in graft-versus-host disease (GVHD), which further weakened the body. This disease, combined with infection, was established as the cause of death for several patients. Dr. Gale explained in a report published soon after the accident that these patients might have developed graft-versus-host disease precisely because they had not received higher doses of radiation. As Gale describes, the higher probability that the lower dose of radiation did not completely ablate the patients' bone marrow made it more likely that there would be enough cells remaining to provoke an immune reaction from the donated bone marrow.

The more irradiated the bone marrow is, the less likely it is to reject bone marrow transplants from non-matching donors. It is imperative to use stem cells that are less likely to be rejected by the body. Dr. Gale had hoped that transplantation with fetal liver cells could be effective in the Chernobyl patients, explaining that, "Since the immune system is not fully developed at this time, histo-incompatible fetal liver cells are less likely to cause graft-versus-host disease than comparable mismatched adult bone marrow cells." Whether they would have worked on the Chernobyl patients is impossible to know; the patients all died from unrelated causes. Dr. Gale was reluctantly forced to conclude that this may always be the case:

Regardless of the interpretation of these cases, it is certain that bone marrow transplantation can only save a small proportion of victims of radiation accidents; irreversible damage to other organs is likely to limit the success of this approach.[3]

Further, the transplant surgeon was compelled to acknowledge, "Although transplantation of hematopoietic stem cells can facilitate bone marrow recovery, this procedure is associated with such complications as graft-versus-host disease, interstitial pneumonitis, and iatrogenic immune suppression."[3] In other words, it was still a dangerous treatment option that exposed the patient to GVHD and potential infection.

It would be disingenuous to call Chernobyl a success in the advancement of stem cell treatment, but it was still an important event for stem cell research. It was one of the first times that stem cell treatments were performed on more than a few individuals, and it provided both Soviet and Western doctors an opportunity to refine their procedures. It also demonstrated how much researchers had yet to understand before stem cell-based therapy offered a legitimate treatment option.

Chernobyl was just one event within the wider backdrop of the Cold War, which spurred stem cell research on both sides of the Atlantic. Tragically, the atmosphere of mutual mistrust meant that many scientists who could have worked together as colleagues instead kept the full extent of their discoveries classified. Still, there were significant moments of cooperation, breakthroughs in stem cell research, and an early exploration of the concept of the stem cell as a treatment option for serious disease. As the Iron Curtain fell, however, there were still major hurdles to overcome. It would take another generation of medical scientists to develop stem cell treatments that would forever relegate these early results to the annals of history.

The Fall of the Iron Curtain

With the fall of Soviet Russia, there began a new era of stem cell research. Reminiscent of Russia in 1917, the collapse of the Soviet Union and subsequent political upheaval meant that funding for scientific research disappeared, practically overnight.[4] Dr. Vadim Repin (PhD), a former Soviet researcher and current correspondent member of the Russian Academy of Medical Sciences, acknowledges that with the transition, "It was very difficult to live in Russia without a decent base of funding and support."[B] Repin is the author of two excellent stem cell books published in 2003 and 2010. Repin transitioned into a private company in Russia, but for many of his colleagues, there was no pressing reason to continue research at home when the facilities of the entire world were available. Soviet researchers suddenly had the freedom to travel, and with the technological expertise they had, the world was at their fingertips. The Soviet diaspora provided an impetus for burgeoning stem cell research programs around the world.

Removed from the context of the Cold War, there was no longer any urgent reason to continue stem cell research. But scientists had already had a glimpse at the tantalizing prospects of stem cells, and they knew that there was more to accomplish.

The next decade was marked by a dazzling series of scientific breakthroughs that awakened widespread interest and brought stem cells to the forefront of public discourse. From a research standpoint, these breakthroughs have been tremendous, and they represent some of the most fascinating discoveries in all of science.

From a therapeutic standpoint, however, their effect has been less pronounced. Several of the most exciting breakthroughs involve the isolation of a new source of stem cells, an event that inevitably presaged a wave of optimism and excitement. Later, as researchers turned a more skeptical eye to the new cell source, they would realize that it was unsuitable for clinical applications, or useful for treating only a small collection of rare diseases, at best.

This roller-coaster of expectations has characterized the world's understanding of stem cell research since the late 1990s. The event which was perhaps most responsible for expanding public knowledge of stem cells was the isolation of embryonic stem cells (ESCs).

Embryonic Stem Cells

Stem cell research has a long and storied history that stretches over a hundred years. However, it was only in 1998 that stem cells exploded onto the front page of the newspapers and the forefront of public consciousness. It was then that University of Wisconsin professor, Dr. James Thomson (PhD, VMD) isolated cells from the inner cell mass of human blastocysts, or early-stage embryos. Using these cells, sometimes referred to as the embryoblast, Thomson created a line of embryonic stem cells. These cells had the advantages of differentiating into almost any other cell type; they were pluripotent.

That same year, Dr. John Gearhart (MD), professor and director of Pediatric Urology at Johns Hopkins University, discovered another source of pluripotent stem cells, derived from cells in fetal human tissue.[5] More specifically, these cells came from the germ cells of fetal reproductive tissue.[6] Using different cells, both Thomson and Gearheart's teams had created a new source of pluripotent stem cells that offered a tantalizing possibility of future scientific breakthroughs. It was the end of the twentieth century, Dolly the sheep had been cloned only two years earlier, and suddenly the future seemed more like a utopian science fiction novel, thanks to stem cells. A 1999 issue of *Science* magazine declared pluripotent stem cell research to be the scientific breakthrough of the year.[6] Embryonic stem cell research captured the public's imagination, and, as we know, also set off a firestorm of controversy that rages to this day.

Thomson, when interviewed by MSNBC in June of 2005 regarding his legacy, admitted that "embryonic cells would play a more important role in fundamental research than in transplantation therapies."[7] He also acknowledged that different stem cell lines were needed for breakthroughs in translational medicine, stating that the stem cell lines at the time were not adequately suited for such applications.[7] Thomson believed that ESCs (which at that time he called ESs) would be a useful platform for testing experimental drugs. In fact, he went on to found a biotechnology company in order to follow this line of inquiry. Thomson explained that:

> [Embryonic stem cells] will be a pervasive research tool that anybody interested in understanding the human body will use. And that will lead to knowledge, for the development of new drugs or whatever, that has absolutely nothing to do with transplantation. This will change human medicine in ways that don't make the front pages. And people will not even realize it's happened. My prediction is that that will be the long-term legacy of these cells.[7]

It is Thomson himself, who is considered the founder of the embryonic stem cell concept, who argues, along with many others in the scientific community, that the role of ESCs is in research, not translational medicine. There are a few clinical trials in the United States that are using ESCs or ESC derived products. So from what avenue can we find breakthroughs in stem cells' ability to offer medicinal benefits? The answer to that question appears to lie with adult stem cells.

Dr. Darwin J. Prockop (MD, PhD), Director of Texas A&M's Institute for Regenerative Medicine, explained in 2006 that:

> ...adult stem cells may be more useful for repairing damage to tissues by trauma, disease, or perhaps uncomplicated aging. Recent observations are providing increasing evidence for the concept that adult stem cells are part of a natural system for tissue repair.[8]

Despite the fact that embryonic stem cells are more poised for breakthroughs in the field of scientific inquiry than medical advancement, the furor regarding ESCs was responsible for a renewed surge of academic interest in the field. The events of 1998 caused scientists to take another look at the possibilities that stem cells offered. A 2002 special report on stem cells in the *Journal of Pathology* summates:

It is Thomson himself, who is considered the founder of the embryonic stem cell concept, who argues, along with many others in the scientific community, that the role of ESCs is in research, not translational medicine.

Induced pluripotent stem cell (iPS): adult stem cells that are genetically altered into becoming embryonic stem cells, and expressing the traits that are inherent to embryonic stem cells.

Ever since the first reports 4 years ago that pluripotential embryonic stem cells can be extracted and successfully propagated from early human blastocysts and aborted fetuses, both the general public and the scientific community have been gripped by the potential promise of stem cell-based therapies for the treatment of a wide variety of diseases that affect our vital organs.[9]

It is ironic to think that the discovery of human embryonic stem cells has helped fuel further research into the clinical uses of human adult stem cells, but it also demonstrates the extent to which the academic community has been focused on this field in the last couple decades.

Induced Pluripotent Stem Cells

In 2006, Dr. Shinya Yamanaka (MD, PhD), Professor at the Institute for Frontier Medical Sciences at Kyoto University, declared that he had discovered a way to regress fully formed adult mice cells into a stem cell-like state. The next year, he announced that he had performed a similar procedure with human cells, transforming adult fibroblasts into stem cells. His announcement was followed soon after by Professor Thomson's, who again made headlines by announcing that he had created a similar stem cell population. The resulting stem cells, termed **induced pluripotent stem cells** (iPS cells), had the potency of embryonic cells, without being derived from human embryos.

The media quickly announced that a "truce" had arrived in the "stem cell war" between those who favored ESC research and those who opposed it. With iPS cells, there was no need to destroy human embryos in order to access pluripotent stem cells.

Scientific enthusiasm, however, faded somewhat after a research study by biologist, Dr. Robert Lanza (MD), suggested that iPS cells were more senescent than embryonic stem cells. Lanza's research also indicated that iPS cells had less proliferative capacity, and were more likely to commit apoptosis (cellular death), than their embryonic counterparts.[10] Lanza declared soon after his study was completed that, "There was a 1,000 to 5,000-fold difference" between the proliferative ability of these two cell types.[11]

While iPSs allowed scientists to sidestep the ethical debate surrounding stem cells, their reduced proliferative ability hinted that they were not an effective therapeutic option.

Furthermore, iPS cells are even more prone to safety concerns than their embryonic counterparts. A Japanese research team, which included Dr. Yamanaka, acknowledged in the *Proceedings of the National Academy of Sciences* that "iPS cells are likely to carry a higher risk of tumorigenicity than ES [embryonic stem] cells, due to the inappropriate reprogramming of these somatic cells, the activation of exogenous transcription factors, or other reasons."[12]

The process of reverting an adult cell into a pluripotent stem cell is a complicated one; the cell is essentially being coaxed to do something against its nature. This is not the case for cancer cells that revert backwards from a differentiated state to a nondifferentiated one. The cell is artificially aged as it goes through different cell culturing procedures which forces it to drastically alter its behavior. Some or all of these factors may contribute to the iPS cell's greater likelihood of malformation.

Researchers continue to test different iPS cell lines on animal models, and so far there are certain lines that have not shown any tendency to turn tumorigenic.[12] It seems possible that, if the iPS cells are cultivated differently, they may become more suitable for potential therapeutic uses.

Umbilical cord blood (CB–cord blood): blood that is contained in the umbilical cord, which connects mother to fetus throughout pregnancy. This blood is rich in stem cells, and is either stored for later use or discarded after birth.

Umbilical Cord Blood and Placenta Banking

Concomitant with embryonic stem cell research, scientists began wondering if the stem cells within **umbilical cord blood** (CB) could be used to treat serious disorders. Umbilical cord blood, it was revealed in 1978, contained its own source of hematopoietic stem cells. Using this knowledge, a medical team led by Dr. Elaine Gluckman (MD, PhD), of the Hematology Hospital Saint Louise in Paris, used umbilical cord blood-derived stem cells to treat a young boy with Fanconi's anemia.[13] The stem cells came from the boy's HLA-identical sister, making the first umbilical cord stem cell treatment an allogeneic one.

After a baby is delivered, the mother's body releases the placenta, the temporary organ that transfers oxygen and nutrients to the baby while in utero. Until recently, in most cases the umbilical cord and placenta were discarded after birth without a second thought. But during the 1970s, researchers discovered that umbilical cord blood could supply the same kinds of blood-forming hematopoietic and mesenchymal stem cells as a bone marrow donor. With umbilical cord stem cells, it is possible to perform either autologous or allogeneic treatments: families can bank their child's cord blood and use it

The debate still rages as to whether umbilical cord blood contains enough stem cells to affect a therapeutic result.

if the child becomes ill, or turn to a registry of HLA-matched donors otherwise. And so, umbilical cord blood began to be collected and stored.

A group of Cleveland researchers, led by Dr. Mary J. Laughlin (MD), helped bring this cell source closer to a clinical translation in 2001, when they used CB from an allogeneic source to treat leukemia and aplastic anemia in adults. Before then, medical science had already established umbilical cord blood as a treatment option for children with blood disorders. But as Dr. Laughlin explained, "Researchers have wondered whether the small amount of stem cells in cord blood can create a whole new immune system in fully grown adults, who are also more likely than children to reject a less-than-perfect transplant."[14]

As Laughlin describes, the concerns of the scientific community were manifold. But one of the major concerns had to do with incompatibility. If the stem cells were allogeneic, would the host's body just reject the transplant? This concern was definitively addressed by Laughlin's study, which demonstrated that "just two ounces of blood harvested from an umbilical cord can create a new blood-producing system, and we do not even need a perfect match for a successful transplant because of the immature nature of cord blood stem cells."[14] Laughlin's study showed 90% of the treated patients growing new, healthy blood cells after the transplant.[c] The incidence of GVHD, a significant concern in stem cell transplants, was also lower than expected.

Cord Blood Stem Cells: The Limitations

Today, there have been over 20,000 cord-blood transplants performed to treat a variety of disorders.[15] However, it is worth noting that cord-blood transplantations are most often performed in lieu of bone-marrow transplantations; that is to say, their use may be restricted to certain types of blood disorders. In fact, umbilical cord blood and placental stem cells are considered most valuable for treating chronic blood-related disorders, and scientists note that their ability to differentiate into non-blood-related cells is "far from proven in a clinical sense."[15, 16]

The debate still rages as to whether umbilical cord blood contains enough stem cells to effect a therapeutic result. While Laughlin et al.'s study showed clinical benefit for adult patients, scientists, like Indiana University, School of Medicine's professor, Dr. Hal Broxmeyer (PhD), still worry that CB contains a "low, and sometimes limiting, number of cells collected in single donor units which can be less than optimal for engraftment of many adults and higher–weight children."[15]

Despite these difficulties, successful cultivating techniques may be able to produce enough cord blood-derived stem cells to create a therapeutic benefit. But for now, it seems that umbilical cord blood and placenta-derived stem cells are useful mainly for treating blood disorders.

Pushing the Field Forward

In a 2010 forum on stem cell research and its potential affect on the healthcare industry, Dr. George Daley (MD, PhD), the Samuel E. Lux IV Chair in Hematology at Harvard Medical School, was asked to determine whether embryonic or adult stem cell research was more important to the stem cell field. His answer: "Scientists don't engage in those debates. Scientists see all this research as very fertile space, which all needs to be pushed forward."[D]

Politicians and media figures are quick to describe researchers of different stem cell types as opposed to each other's work. Metaphors like the "stem cell war" and the "stem cell race" depict the main dynamic among researchers and clinicians as antagonistic. The truth is that a breakthrough in one area of stem cell research advances the knowledge base of the entire field.

Embryonic stem cells and induced pluripotent stem cells may not be the right choice for therapeutic applications, while umbilical cord-derived stem cells may be limited to blood-borne disorders. But the discovery of these cell types has led to an explosion of interest in stem cell research, which has ultimately brought us closer to stem cell-derived treatment applications. The research that has been done with these cells, and the research that is continuing to be performed, offers the scientific community a collection of unique insights that help all researchers perform their jobs more effectively. Each stem cell discovery provides inspiration to other researchers, and creates kinetic energy which pushes the field inexorably forward.

Adult stem cell researchers have also created their own kinetic energy, advancing their knowledge base at a dizzying rate. Since the days of Chernobyl, the field of adult stem cells has made a quantum leap. A new generation of hematologists, neuroscientists, pathologists and others have discovered new adult stem cell types and made clinical breakthroughs that make allogeneic stem cell therapy possible today.

The truth is that a breakthrough in one area of stem cell research advances the knowledge base of the entire field.

CHAPTER 5
A Quantum Leap

Advancing to Allogeneic Treatment

Drawing from the lessons of bone marrow transplants, stem cell researchers who hoped to use adult stem cell treatments in a clinical setting realized two things. First, a source of healthy allogeneic stem cells could be useful in a medical emergency. Second, these allogeneic cells would only be useful if they were accepted by the body and, in the case of bone marrow-derived stem cells, if they refrained from initiating graft-versus-host disease.

With bone marrow transplantations, the risk of rejection is reduced through the use of immunosuppressant drugs and serotype matching. Unfortunately, immunosuppressants can leave transplant patients vulnerable to infections. Similarly, patients must wait until an organ that matches their serotype becomes available, an event that often occurs too late.

For allogeneic stem cell treatment, the ultimate goal has been to develop a master cell bank that can be used to treat anyone, without

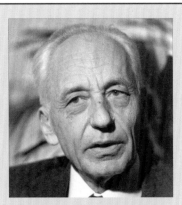

Although research into the function and behavior of HLAs advanced notably with the advent of genomic mapping, scientists have been aware of leukocyte antigens for over 50 years. It was in 1958 that Dr. Jean Dausset (MD), who was the head of the Immuno-haematology Laboratory at the National Blood Transfusion Centre of France, discovered the first leukocyte antigen, HLA-A2. Seven years later, he would discover that these antigens were part of larger genomic groups, which he dubbed the Major Histocompatibility Complexes (MHC). These and other discoveries earned Dr. Dausset the Nobel Prize in 1980.

danger of rejection and without the need for serotype matching or immunosuppressants.

A better understanding of how to accomplish this goal requires a better understanding of the problem. How does the body know which cells are its own, and which cells are foreign? The answer can be summed up in three letters: HLA.

Human Leukocyte Antigens (HLAs): The Body's Secret Passwords

In the 1990s, private and public groups began work on mapping the human genome. The decoding of the genome, completed at the turn of the millennium, was a massive project, the ramifications of which affected scientists of various disciplines. One result of these genome sequencing projects was an advanced understanding of nucleotide sequencing. More specifically for stem cell researchers, these scientific advancements helped them better identify the different HLA proteins which act as identification signals to the body. HLAs, or human leukocyte antigens, are still not completely understood today, but research has allowed us to reach certain conclusions.[1]

HLA are like the body's secret passwords: the human leukocytes encode proteins that appear on the outer portion of the body's cells. Killer T-cells, the white blood cells tasked with ridding the body of foreign pathogens, interpret these proteins as signals. The right signal leads to acceptance; the wrong signal causes the T cell to attack. In a transplant, the HLA that are of the same type as the patient will be accepted by the body. HLA that encode a different protein will send off the wrong signal. Conversely, in GVHD, if the body does not have the right type of HLA proteins as the bone marrow transplant, the donated T-cells will attack.

But if T-cells only react if the wrong signal is given, what happens if there is a poor or no signal at all? T-cells are engineered to react only when they recognize an HLA-encoded protein. But stem cells, if cultivated early enough and with the proper methodology, will not develop much HLA. During Chernobyl, the Russian clinical team used fetal liver cells on several patients, partly because, "During the second trimester of gestation, [the] fetal liver is a rich source of hematopoietic stem cells. Since the immune system is not fully developed at this time, histoincompatible fetal liver cells are less likely to cause graft-vs-host disease than comparably mismatched adult bone marrow cells."[2] But, these fetal tissue transplants represented a cross-section of cells that may have already been in more advanced stages of tissue development.

With a better understanding of how HLA proteins work, scientists were able to better understand why previous transplant procedures failed. Drawing from this, stem cell researchers have since worked to determine the optimal parameters for cultivating immune-privileged fetal-derived stem cells, ones that would remain multipotent and controllable without inducing an immune response from the patient's body. By doing so, some researchers have found a solution to transplant rejection, simply by circumventing the HLA proteins that make other transplant procedures risky.

A good understanding of how fetal stem cells work has also required a better understanding of fetal cell biology. Dr. Vadim Repin, the former Soviet researcher who has published several reviews on fetal cell therapy, points out that "fetal cell biology is a very specific area that combines areas of knowledge from genetics, embryology, biochemistry, modern cell biology, and medicine."[A]

With such an interdisciplinary focus required, it was not an easy task to determine the suitability of fetal stem cell transplant procedures. Today, however, we know that fetal stem cells—when harvested at the proper time and under the appropriate procedures—are not only immune privileged, but also have more proliferative capacity and less senescent tendencies than their counterparts, qualities that make them ideal for stem cell treatment. Dr. Repin stated, "If you have the possibility of receiving a treatment from an available bank of fetal [stem cell] tissue, that would be the primary echelon of treatment." But not all stem cells come from fetal origins. Bone marrow-derived stem cells, for example, usually come from adults. In the United States, treatments with fetal-derived stem cells are not currently available; so, could clinicians develop a therapeutic adult stem cell regimen that would not rely on fetal tissue?

It turns out that they can. There is one stem cell type that can be used in the treatment of a broad variety of diseases, and does not need to be cultivated from fetal sources in order to bypass the body's immune response. In the 1980s and 1990s, several teams of researchers would reveal the surprising attributes of mesenchymal stem cells, one of the most valuable stem cell type for clinical use.

How does the body know which cells are its own, and which cells are foreign? The answer can be summed up in three letters: HLA.

Mesenchymal Stem Cells and Continued Research

After Friedenstein's groundbreaking discoveries in the 1960s and 1970s, a biophysicist from the United Kingdom took up the baton and considerably advanced our knowledge of mesenchymal stem cells. Dr. Maureen Owen (PhD), of the Department of Orthopaedic Surgery at the Nuffield Orthopaedic Centre in Oxford, England, was already a well-recognized expert in the field of bone tissue research when she started investigating MSCs. Poring over Friedenstein's research, she quickly realized the full potential of these cells.

Alone and in collaboration with Friedenstein, Owen started looking more closely at the possibility of modifying mesenchymal stem cell behavior by modifying their *in vitro* conditions.[3] For example, Owen would use epidermal growth factor to increase the colony size of cell populations, or use hydrocortisone to prime the cells to differentiate into osteocytes, the cells which comprise bone.[4] Her research created a solid understanding of how to work with MSCs and prepare them for eventual *in vivo* use.

Another researcher, Dr. Arnold Caplan (PhD) of Case Western Reserve University, ushered in a new era for mesenchymal stem cells by using them to perform clinical trials in the United States. During the early '90s, Caplan's focus on mesenchymal stem cells was so exhaustive that other scientists began referring to MSCs as "Caplan cells."[5] Recognition of Caplan's efforts provided these cells with a nickname, but it was Caplan himself who gave them the name "mesenchymal stem cells" in a 1994 paper published in the *Clinics in Plastic Surgery* journal.[6] Friedenstein had used the term bone marrow-derived multipotent marrow cells, while Owen preferred the name "stromal stem cells."[3] But it was Caplan's name that eventually stuck, giving us the nomenclature we use today, and explaining the use of the acronym MSC.

In 1995, Caplan led the Phase I clinical trial which demonstrated to the world that mesenchymal progenitor cells (MPCs) could be isolated, expanded and placed *in vivo*, thus establishing a potential protocol for stem cell-based treatments. Twenty-three patients received autologous MPCs which were cultivated and then re-injected into their bone marrow. Caplan's team proudly concluded in a *Bone Marrow Transplantation* paper that "no adverse reactions were observed with the infusion of the MPCs. MPCs obtained from cancer patients can be collected, expanded *in vitro* and infused intravenously without toxicity."[7] Caplan's results demonstrated that MSCs were ready to begin the process of transitioning into the clinic.

The MSC as a Peacemaker

Caplan's work put Case Western Reserve University on the cutting edge of mesenchymal stem cell research, and more clinical trials began. In 2000, a Case Western Reserve University team began a clinical trial to study the effects of MSCs in breast cancer patients who had received high doses of chemotherapy.[8] The researchers, led by Drs. Omer Koç (MD) and Hillard Lazarus (MD), again used autologous MSC transplantation on a group of patients. The doctors were hoping that the MSCs might assist in "hematopoietic stem cell rescue," bringing HSC levels up. And it worked; hematopoietic stem cells recovered rapidly, and platelet and neutrophil (a type of white blood cell) levels rose.[9] The researchers could not safely attribute their results to the mesenchymal cells, however, as the patients had received the MSCs as part of an ongoing treatment regimen.[9] With the patients receiving other blood cells as well, there were too many variables for scientists to reach any firm conclusions.

But this and other studies helped open the floodgates. A 2001 article pointed out "the pivotal role of MSCs in the bone marrow microenvironment and their ability to support hematopoiesis first sparked *Bone Marrow Transplantation* physicians' interest in these cells."[9] Physicians wondered: How can the insertion of MSCs into the bloodstream activate hematopoietic stem cells, an entirely different type of stem cell?

Part of the answer has to do with an unexpected property of MSCs. These cells are immunomodulators; they have the potential to lessen the immune system's response to a perceived threat.[10] With this ability, MSCs can play the role of the peacemaker in a transplant operation, preventing host tissue and donated tissue from going to war with each other.

In contrast to a full bone marrow transplant, which contains a collection of different cells with varying levels of HLA, a mesenchymal stem cell transplant will not trigger immune rejection or GVHD. The implications of this discovery were significant; if MSCs were able to accomplish some of the benefits of a bone marrow transplant without any of the drawbacks, then they could lend

Dr. Koç and others explained that these miraculous cells offered "potential therapy to enhance allogeneic hematopoietic engraftment and prevent graft-versus-host disease."

themselves to therapeutic regimens for dozens of diseases. Koç and Lazarus pointed out back in 2001 that "the number of MSCs is estimated to be too few in an average bone marrow graft," suggesting that additional injections of just MSCs could be useful for BMT patients.[9] In a subsequent paper, Koç and others explained that these miraculous cells offered "potential therapy to enhance allogeneic hematopoietic engraftment and prevent graft-versus-host disease."[11]

A Treatment for Acute Radiation Syndrome (ARS)

This new generation of studies had revealed a useful treatment for acute radiation syndrome: using MSCs in conjunction with, or instead of, bone marrow transplants. Repin, who has written several books on stem cells, explained that:

During the Chernobyl tragedy, we didn't have the necessary knowledge regarding the real potency of stromal cells during irradiation damage. Without this knowledge, there was not much the doctors in Moscow could do to help, especially because the radiation was so high; the patients received megadoses of radiation; it was Armageddon.

It was only later, maybe 15 years later, that we learned the role of mesenchymal stem cells. Now we have the knowledge to apply mesenchymal stem cells in the case of acute radiation syndrome.[B]

Studies from Case Western Reserve University and other institutions have demonstrated that MSCs have four mechanisms of action which can be used to combat acute radiation syndrome:

1. *Anti-inflammatory effects:* Following ARS, the immune system is damaged and fails to provide regular immunomonitoring functions. This in turn leads to the increased incidence of infection and an inflammatory response. MSCs are proven to produce anti-inflammatory factors such as IL-10 (interleukin 10), which may alleviate pathological consequences and symptoms.

2. *Support for hematopoiesis:* As a result of acute radiation, the blood cells are damaged and need to be restored. Bone marrow-derived MSCs can accelerate new blood cell production by either direct interaction with hematopoietic stem cells in the bone marrow or by production of chemical factors such as G-CSF/GM-CSF (colony stimulating factors.)

3. *Mobilization of the patient's own stem cells:* Injected MSCs have a capability to migrate inside damaged organs and attract the patient's own stem cells to the site of injury by producing factors such as SDF-1 (stromal cell-derived factor 1). This may significantly enhance post-radiation regeneration.

4. *Anti-apoptotic effect:* Radiation can induce cell death via apoptosis. MSCs can rescue the damaged cells from apoptotic death by forming a gap junction with these cells and delivering anti-apoptotic factors such as SDF-1 and G-CSF.

These four mechanisms of action are beneficial in many conditions, not just the treatment of ARS. For example, brain trauma often causes a hypoxic (oxygen deprived) environment and results in cell apoptosis. Anemia of chronic disease can lead to a depletion of blood cells. Congenital conditions are often marked by a malfunction of the body's own, endogenous, stem cells.

Originally, research into MSCs was motivated by a desire for cellular protectors against ARS. Today, a collection of leading clinicians believe that allogeneic MSCs can be viewed not just as protectors, but as cellular repairmen, working to undo the damage caused by trauma or degeneration.

Allogeneic MSCs can be viewed not just as protectors, but as "cellular repairmen."

Regulating the Microenvironment

Yet another advantage of MSCs is that they appear to have a beneficial role in forming and regulating the stem cell microenvironment, or niche. Ever since Schofield and Chertkov's exploration of the idea of the niche, scientists have continued to investigate how a stem cell's interaction with an environment can help shape the eventual role the cell will have in the body.

The microenvironment is one of the main mechanisms through which stem cells receive their marching orders, responding appropriately to the needs of a certain area of the body. As a *Transfusion Medicine and Hemotherapy* paper explains:

Various intrinsic programs and pathways facilitate the unique characteristics of stem cells, and these programs, in charge of everything from maintenance, to proliferation, to eventual differentiation of the stem cells, have to be tightly controlled by the microenvironment.[12]

But if the microenvironment is damaged or altered, the stem cells will not be as effective.

Various intrinsic programs and pathways facilitate the unique characteristics of stem cells, and these programs have to be tightly controlled by the microenvironment.

Osteoblasts: originating from fibroblasts, these cells, when mature, aid in bone production.

Dr. Kharazi, who spent eight years as chief scientist of the Immunotherapy Laboratory at St. Vincent Medical Center in Los Angeles, explains the concept of a faulty microenvironment-stem cell interaction with a simple metaphor:

Just as a social environment might affect a child, a microenvironment affects a stem cell. If you take well-behaved children and suddenly transplant them into a terrible school or a bad neighborhood, social science has taught us that this can have an effect. These environmental factors can stunt their full potential.[c]

Kharazi continues the metaphor by elaborating:

You need a good environment, you need good influences, in order to ensure that these kids reach their potential. In stem cell science, there's a similar idea as to the effect the microenvironment has on stem cells. If the environmental factors aren't right, the stem cells will be less effective.

Reciprocally, mesenchymal stem cells have the potential to bring a stem cell niche to full operating strength. Just as a good neighborhood requires good teachers, police officers, and paved roads, so does a microenvironment have several different types of cells that serve as regulatory components for stem cells. For example, hematopoietic stem cells have their primary niche in the bone marrow. The hematopietic stem cell niche, researchers have discovered, has several different components which affect the role that HSC cells will play in the body.[12] These components include **osteoblasts** and stromal cells, which result from MSC differentiation, illustrating how MSCs contribute to a positive microenvironment for hematopoietic stem cells.[13]

The ability of MSCs to work with HSCs is evidence of the mesenchymal stem cell's remarkable ability to work with other cells to help the body heal. It is evidence that stem cells are not just biological superstars; they are also team players.

Expanding the Field

While some scientists continued to explore the uses of MSCs and HSCs, others turned their attention to newer arrivals to the stem cell field, in the form of newly discovered stem cell types.

Exploring the potential of these new stem cell populations was not always a simple task. In several cases, a fundamental conceptual shift had to occur before scientists were able to realize these discoveries. This was certainly the case when it came to the discovery, isolation, and subsequent use of neural stem cells, the stem cells that are responsible for forming neurons. In the same way that Maximov would not have been able to conceive of hematopoietic stem cells without first becoming an adherent of the unitarian theory of hematopoiesis, researchers would probably not have considered using neural stem cells for clinical applications, if it were not for significant breakthroughs in the theory of neurogenesis.

Adult Neurogenesis

Can neurons in the brain regenerate themselves? Until the end of the last century, the answer was presumed to be "no." It was widely believed that we entered the world with approximately 100 billion neurons, and that the number simply dwindled from there, without any generation of new, functional neurons. Previous scientific research had suggested that this might not be true for all animals; Dr. Joseph Altman (PhD) of Massachusetts Institute of Technology (MIT) discovered neuron generation (**neurogenesis**) in rats in 1962.[14] Altman went on to hypothesize that the adult brain was capable of creating new neurons, a process called adult neurogenesis. Working with fellow scientist Dr. Gopal Das (PhD), Altman went on to discover adult neurogenesis in other species, further cementing his hypotheses.[15] In a drama familiar to students of medical history, his results were mostly dismissed by the scientific community. Many scientists refused to accept the idea of adult neurogenesis, which meant that very few research institutions were interested in studying the proliferative capacity of different brain cells.

This institutional complacency was shaken again in the 1980s, when Dr. Fernando Nottebohm (PhD), a professor at Rockefeller University in New York, found similar evidence of adult neurogenesis in birds. He admitted to *The New Yorker* journalist Michael Specter that his findings were "a real shock, because we had all been taught that an adult brain was supposed to stay the same size, with the same cells, forever."[16]

With the body of research amassed by Nottebohm, scientists were forced to revise one of their most commonly held assumptions; that the adult brain was incapable of regeneration. Altman, whose own studies were initially marginalized by the scientific community, was later seen as a scientific visionary when a new

Can neurons in the brain regenerate themselves? Until the end of the last century, the answer was presumed to be "no." It was widely believed that we entered the world with approximately 100 billion neurons, and that the number simply dwindled from there, without any generation of new, functional neurons.

Neurogenesis: the development of the nervous system, including nerves and nervous tissue.

generation of neurologists acquainted themselves with his work. But many argued that Altman and Nottebohm's results could not be applied to humans. Dr. Charles Gross (PhD), a Princeton professor, acknowledges, "People basically said, 'Even if this is true, big deal. It's just birds. All they do is fly around.'"[16] In contrast to the brain of a small animal, the human brain was viewed as far too complex to go through the process of adult neurogenesis.

Neurobiologist Dr. Fred Gage (PhD), of the Salk Institute for Biological Studies, elaborated in an interview the reasons why scientists held to these beliefs, even without evidence to support their theories:

First of all, neurons are very complex cells—long branches, receiving hundreds of thousands of connections. The idea that confused people is how something as complex as a neuron could undergo cell division. This idea was not well integrated with the emerging notion that maybe some primitive cells remained and that those were doing the dividing... The other roadblock was that there were several prominent statements in the literature contending that adult neurogenesis couldn't happen, because the brain and structures like the hippocampus need to be stable for memory to be stable. If new brain cells were added, that would make it hard to store long-term memories. It was a loose statement, but it resonated with many people.[17]

Gage was instrumental in proving these beliefs wrong. In 1998, Gage, with Swedish neuroscientist Dr. Peter Eriksson (PhD), published a paper in the scientific journal *Nature Medicine*. The paper, entitled "Neurogenesis in the Adult Human Hippocampus," established that the human hippocampus (the part of the brain responsible for much of our memory, as well as our spatial orientation) could generate new neurons.[18]

The hippocampus is the part of the brain responsible for memory and spacial orientation.

Neural Stem Cells

As the concept of adult neurogenesis evolved, researchers began further experimenting with an exciting new multipotent line of stem cells which had been discovered in the brain. Dr. Evan Snyder (MD, PhD), Director of the Program in Stem Cell and Regenerative Biology at the Burnham Institute for Medical Research, was one of the researchers whose work in the late 1980s and early 1990s was seminal in establishing the properties of these neural stem cells (NSCs).[19, 20]

Hippocampus

Snyder explains that his early experiments with these cells compelled him to accept the newly-developing theory of adult neurogenesis:

Initially, I was simply trying to build a brain; it was my original intention merely to place various cell types within a dish, and then mix-and-match them to see if I could build an in vitro brain structure for research purposes. But I never got to that point, because I would start with one cell that would differentiate into other cell types.[D]

Because the theory of adult neurogenesis had not been fully sketched out, Snyder and his colleagues were originally skeptical that they were watching a neural stem cell in action.

My colleagues believed that I had used a tissue culture artifact, that my results were a byproduct of trying to grow cells in a dish. After a while, I said, 'I don't think this is a mistake. I actually think this is how the brain is put together.'

Snyder's realization represented a serious breakthrough for stem cell research, but his were not the only results that boded well for the potential of neural stem cells. Other pioneers include Drs. Carlos Lois (MD, PhD) and Arturo Alvarez-Buylla (PhD), who tracked the migration of neural progenitor cells to different areas of the adult brain.[21] Lois and Alvarez-Buylla, who are now professors at Massachusetts Institute of Technology and University of California, San Francisco, respectively, acknowledged, "The generation, migration, and differentiation of neurons are generally thought to end soon after birth."[22] But their research demonstrated that neuronal cells may have the ability to migrate from one area of the brain to another well into adulthood.

Considering NSCs for Treatment

Before the new theory of adult neurogenesis had been articulated, the dominant paradigm was that the brain could not heal itself after an injury. The studies that demonstrated that the brain was able to produce new neurons during adulthood, as well as studies that demonstrated that neuronal precursors were capable of migration, had researchers asking, "Since it is now evident that new neurons are constantly being generated in the adult, why does the mature brain display only a very limited capacity to repair?"[21]

Scientists attempting to answer this very question quickly learned that there is a proliferation of neural precursors after an injury to

With every clinical study and bench-top breakthrough, the vision of stem cell treatment becomes more closely aligned with reality. More and more, people are beginning to accept that, with stem cells, we have the tools to counter an epidemic of degenerative and traumatic conditions.

the body's central nervous system. It is believed that the reaction of these precursors, which include neural stem cells as well as neural cells in their very first stage of differentiation, represent the body's attempt to repair the damage.

But an adult nervous system has significantly fewer stem cells than the nervous system of, say, a young child. Thus, "the small population of endogenous neural stem cells seem unable to reconstitute fully and restore function after damage."[21] There are not enough NSCs in place to make the repairs; more are needed.

With this realization came another important question: could introducing new NSCs into the brain affect brain injury, or even injury to the nervous system in general? Preliminary studies with fetal neural cells, and their effect on Parkinson's disease, left "little doubt that under appropriate conditions, cellular grafts can integrate and function in the brain."[21, 23] Scientists began conceiving of potential neural stem cell therapy treatments for a host of neurological conditions. This fueled the massive amount of pre-clinical and clinical research from which stem cell clinicians draw upon today. Later research revealed that the central nervous system (CNS), consisting of the brain and the spinal cord, possesses a level of immune-privilege: the cells of the immune system will not cross the blood brain barrier (BBB) that separates the brain from the rest of the body. This characteristic makes it possible to use allogeneic stem cell treatments for neurodegenerative diseases.[24] Admittedly, this situation becomes more complicated in the case of trauma to the CNS, which can rupture the BBB, a fact which argues for the use of fetal neural stem cells for treatments of traumatic injury to the central nervous system.

Although other organs do not share the brain's inherent immune-privileged status, many contain their own population of stem cells, which can be isolated and cultivated. Scientists have found stem cells for the lining of the nose, hair follicles, reproductive organs, the cardiac system, the skin, even for mammary glands. It stands to reason that these stem cells can be used to repair damage to the appropriate tissue. And if a body can use its own stem cells, it also has the potential to use donated stem cells of the same type, as long as those cells exhibit immune-privileged characteristics.

In science, a major discovery is often accompanied by a shift in thinking. Maximov's discovery of hematopoietic stem cells went hand in hand with the nascent unitarian theory of hematopoiesis; the Russian aristocrat's theory put him on the front lines of an intellectual debate which took decades to resolve. Similarly, the theory of adult neurogenesis represented a shift in scientific dogma without which clinicians would not have been able to grasp the implications of neural stem cell therapy. More generally, the idea that the human body contains many distinct populations of stem cells required scientists and doctors to re-evaluate several basic biological concepts. But today, what was once a far-out theory has become fact; stem cells have transitioned from a hypothetical concept to a biological truth.

A conceptual shift is occurring as policymakers and medical experts increasingly realize the potential of stem cell-based clinical treatment. With every clinical study and bench-top breakthrough, the vision of stem cell treatment becomes more closely aligned with reality. More and more, people are beginning to accept that, with stem cells, we may have the tools to counter an epidemic of degenerative and traumatic conditions.

The metaphor of stem cells as tools is, in fact, an apt one. If there is a problem with the heart, it stands to reason that cardiac stem cells will be the appropriate tool for the job. But if we advance our understanding of stem cells, we will see that, just as a complicated task may require several different tools, seriously compromised tissue may require several different stem cells in order to heal. This concept may sound both simple and logical, however, it also represents a shift in our understanding of how to use stem cells to achieve optimal clinical results.

Multi-cell Treatment

Consider the human brain as the body's engine. Composed of hundreds of billions of neurons, the brain requires intricate chemical and biological processes to maintain its full power. Like an engine, it is meant to be handled with the utmost care. So what if something goes wrong with your engine? If you use just a screwdriver, you can perhaps fix some of the problem. But you'll need several different tools, perhaps even a whole toolbox, in order to restore the engine's function.

The same concept applies to multi-cell treatment. If the brain suffers an injury, neural cells will most likely be required. Proponents

But if we advance our understanding of stem cells, we will see that, just as a complicated task may require several different tools, seriously compromised tissue may require several different stem cells in order to heal.

of multi-cell therapy argue, however, that neural stem cells are not enough. They point to mesenchymal stem cells, which can restore the microenvironment, and hematopoietic stem cells, which enrich the blood supply, as examples of other stem cell types that could play a useful supporting role in effecting repair for a neurological injury. Astroglia may also provide neuron support.

Previous studies have demonstrated that MSCs have an incredible ability to regulate and strengthen the stem cell niche, so that other stem cells can be used to their optimal ability. In his interview, Kharazi further explains this concept:

Take the situation of a stroke. In a stroke, significant numbers of neurons have died off. Logically, we need to apply neural stem cells to the area. These NSCs will differentiate into neurons, to replace the neurons that have died off. But if these neurons don't have the appropriate environment to proliferate and differentiate in, the overall effect will be diminished. The theory is that MSCs can create that kind of environment. The microenvironment of the brain is shifted to accommodate neural stem cells and promote differentiation.

People need food, clothes and shelter to operate. Stem cells, similarly, need a proper environment. They cannot differentiate in a vacuum.

The inter-relationship between different stem cells can grow beyond just creating optimal environmental factors. Research has shown that the relationship between two sets of stem cells is far more complicated than a simple linear connection. Instead, it is more like a dense, inter-connected web, where thousands of connections work synergistically.

Cells can produce growth factors, inhibitors, and stimulatory factors, proteins and enzymes. Kharazi gives one example:

Mesenchymal stem cells often produce VEGF, or vascular endothelial growth factor. The main purpose of VEGF is to stimulate the growth of new blood vessels. Mesenchymal stem cells can both produce and respond to VEGF. When one MSC emits this signal, other MSCs modulate their behavior upon detecting this growth factor. Now, there are 22 sub-populations of VEGF, different variations on the same signal. And some of these sub-populations are also expressed by other stem cells. So, if MSCs are emitting a certain VEGF-upregulating signal, other stem cells might respond.

And this, Kharazi continues, is just one of the growth factors that MSCs can stimulate. Currently, medical science has not yet fully mapped out the complicated inter-relationships between different cell factors. But Kharazi notes:

We know that cells can work not just by themselves, but synergistically with each other. One cell may produce some factor, a growth factor for example, to which another cell responds. So if you're just introducing one type of stem cell into the body, and you don't have that second cell type to produce that growth factor, you won't trigger the necessary response from the first cell type. You have to introduce both cells to the body in a conjunctive treatment regimen, so that one cell promotes the working mechanism of another.

The Realization of Dr. Nikolay Mironov

This basic idea, that different stem cells can constitute a whole that is more than the sum of the parts, is what originally drove Dr. Nikolay Mironov (MD, PhD), currently an associate professor of Neurology at the University of Post Graduation Education of the Kremlin's Presidents Hospital in Moscow, to begin crafting the concept of multi-cell treatment. Mironov began his involvement in the stem cell field in the 1970s, studying the ways that stem cells could be used to treat a range of disorders. Primarily working with neurological disorders such as stroke, Parkinson's and trauma to the spine, Mironov sought and eventually received permission to start treating patients approximately 20 years ago. His first patient was an American baseball player, whom Mironov treated for a neurological condition. Later, Mironov went on to treat prominent members of the Soviet establishment.[E] Provided with regulatory approval for small-scale clinical studies in Moscow, Mironov has continued to advance his clinical protocols, the most important of which is his pioneering use of multi-cell treatment.

For patients with CNS disorders, Mironov and his colleagues began by first using neural transplantation techniques. As his protocols evolved and as new developments occurred in the field, Mironov was able to use more sophisticated culturing techniques. His patients responded to neural stem cell treatment alone, but Mironov felt he could achieve better results. One problem, he realized, was that:

The administration of neural cells alone does not address the endothelialization that needs to occur in order to support the

Fate and Trophic Factors

What is the fate of the mesenchymal cells that are injected into the blood stream? Dr. Jeffrey Karp (PhD), of the Harvard Stem Cell Institute, and James Ankrum, a graduate student at Harvard-MIT Division of Health Sciences and Technology, note that only a small percentage of the cells reach the target tissue. Most are entrapped in the capillaries within the liver, spleen and lungs. The MSCs exert their primary action based on immunomodulatory properties as opposed to the ability to engraft and differentiate. This effect occurs through the secretion of many trophic factors. For example, micro-embolisms in the lungs create a local injury that activates the MSCs to secrete TSG-6, a powerful anti-inflammatory protein. The researchers note that the secretion of this protein from MSCs is 120-fold greater than that of fibroblasts obtained from the same donor.[27]

endogenous and transplanted cells with a blood supply. What is needed therefore is a treatment therapy that addresses both the regeneration of damaged or lost neurons, and the regeneration of the endothelial framework for the damaged area.[26]

In other words, the neural stem cells were reaching the afflicted area, but they did not have enough blood to operate. The neural stem cells were, as Kharazi put it, good kids suddenly thrust into a bad neighborhood.

Mironov realized that in order to effect more significant repair of neurological injuries or conditions, he also needed to boost the endothelial framework that would allow the injected NSC cells a chance to thrive. Realizing that mesenchymal stem cells had the ability to differentiate into connective tissue and thus re-energize the vascular system, Mironov tried a new procedure; he inserted NSCs into the central nervous system, as he had before, but this time he also administered MSCs through the patient's circulatory system. The results, he found, were better than when he had used neural stem cells alone.

Neurological disease is just one possible application of multi-cell therapy. Another example includes the treatment of diabetic retinopathy. While the obvious choice of cells for treating eye diseases would be retinal pigment epithelium (RPE) cells, mesenchymal stem cells can also be used to great effect. Dr. Paul Tornambe (MD), former president of the American Society of Retina Specialists, explains, "Diabetes is a disease of small blood vessels, and diabetics go blind because of poor profusion in the eye."[F] The clinical hypothesis is that the MSCs may be able to strengthen the underlying blood vessels.

In fact, Mironov's multi-cell treatment concept lends itself to many different therapies. When treating traumatic injury, it is almost always beneficial to clean up the microenvironment of the injured area and increase blood flow. In instances of organ failure such as heart failure, different populations of stem cells have been shown to achieve benefit.

Today, clinical studies involving multiple stem cell treatment are being performed outside the United States. Results of selected case studies can be found in the chapters ahead. In the United States, however, the FDA's policy has been to start with single-cell use for consideration in clinical trials. The FDA's position is to first fully understand all the properties of individual stem cells, before studying their properties in conjunction. But when these administrative hurdles are cleared, multi-cell therapy will offer a treatment option that would bring even greater results to those who have been afflicted by serious conditions.

From the Past to the Present

The development of multi-cell therapy, in conjunction with many other scientific breakthroughs, has brought us to where we are today. We are on the threshold of a medical revolution, one that stands to help millions in the future. In the next few chapters, we will offer you a scientific explanation of how and why stem cell treatments are able to achieve results, demonstrating these improvements with a collection of clinical case studies. In conjunction with our explanation of the science behind stem cell treatments, these patients' stories will bear powerful testament to this life-changing therapy.

These pages will reveal not only their stories, but the stories of their doctors, their caretakers, their family members and friends, revealing an emotional aspect of stem cell research that cannot be shown through facts and figures. The patients who have benefitted from stem cell therapy stand today not just as a representation of the power of science, but of the power of the human will to overcome significant challenges and to never accept "no" as an answer.

Placebos and Primary Endpoints

One of the confounding factors in understanding the results of both investigator-initiated clinical studies and more rigorously designed clinical trials is the placebo factor. It is well-known, though not well understood, that the control group often improves, to a degree, without treatment. Individual patients may also improve with treatments that do no harm, but have no effect.

With clinical trials there is also the challenge of study design and the selection of the primary endpoints, or outcome measures. It is possible for patients to have clinical improvement in a variety of areas, however, if this improvement is not the primary endpoint, then the trial is deemed unsuccessful. Careful inclusion criteria must also be applied to clinical trials. These factors complicate our understanding of stem cell treatment efficacy.

Chapter 6
Stroke

JB's Story

Life was going well for 66-year-old JB. A retired professional athlete in two sports, he was still fit, active and engaged in community events. But something happened that would change JB's life for the worse. It started with a small warning sign; he had gone to bed the night before with a feeling of numbness in his right hand. He assumed that it had something to do with his earlier session with the chiropractor. But at 4 AM, he woke up to an increased feeling of numbness and weakness. His right hand seemed unresponsive to his brain's commands. He drifted back to sleep, waking up again at 7:30 AM. His wife noticed that he was acting odd, responding incoherently to her questions and apparently unable to dress himself. Concerned, she called the paramedics, who rushed JB to the hospital.

In the emergency room, doctors established that JB had expressive **aphasia**, the clinical diagnosis of a patient's inability to speak.

Aphasia: an impairment or loss of ability to use language, either expression or comprehension, including writing, speech and signs. This generally occurs due to disease or injury to the brain, possibly stroke.

He was also found to be profoundly weak on the right side of his body. An MRI revealed a lack of perfusion down the left middle cerebral artery of JB's brain. In JB's case, the lack of perfusion was caused by a blood clot in the artery.

The results of this stroke were all-encompassing and devastating. Integral cells in JB's brain had died from lack of blood, leaving a lesion of dead tissue. Previously completely healthy, JB was struck with a series of cognitive and physical symptoms that greatly affected his quality of life. The most he could utter were a few words, and even that required substantial concentration. JB had previously been a world-class athlete, and even at his advanced age (65 at the time of the stroke), he had normal physical function. But after his stroke, he walked with a pronounced stoop, favoring his left side, while his right forearm had contracted against the chest in a permanent position.

Following his stroke, JB went through extensive therapy, working with physical rehabilitation experts and speech therapists. But after over five years of dedicated work, he was still unable to perform everyday tasks that others would take for granted. For JB, who was used to commanding his body to perform extreme feats, the lack of progress was frustrating. Therapy is a vital part of recovery after any traumatic neurological event, but there is only so much that it can accomplish in undoing massive damage to the brain. And in JB's case, the magnitude of his stroke meant that his gains in therapy would be minimal.

Seeking help with his condition, JB was referred to cardiologist Dr. Jackie See (MD) of the Laguna Cardiovascular Institute. Dr. See wondered whether improvements in clinical stem cell therapy might help JB. Aware of an existing human clinical stem cell study being conducted for stroke in Moscow, See worked with Russian researchers to have JB enrolled in the clinical study. In Moscow, JB was treated with mesenchymal stem cells (MSCs), delivered to his body intravenously; in addition, neural stem cells (NSCs) were administered through a lumbar puncture. The mesenchymal stem cells would course through the entire blood stream; the neural cells would directly enter the cerebrospinal fluid and make their way to the brain. As a precaution, the day before the therapy, JB received an immunosuppressant drug to reduce inflammation at the site of the lumbar puncture.

Doctors waited by his side, monitoring his condition. An hour after the procedure, the patient declared that he was resting comfortably and there were no observable side effects. After 24 hours, the attending doctors noted:

Patient states as if a cloud has been lifted from his brain. He has real clarity of thought. Contracture in the forearm has significantly relaxed and his gait is much steadier. Antalgic posture [limping] is reduced. There are no adverse events observed. At discharge patient was happy and whistling, something he has been unable to do since his stroke. Gait and balance visibly improved, no adverse side effects noted and no negative experienced [sic] by the patient.[1]

Follow-up with JB found that he was feeling fine, with no negative side effects. His therapist reported progress with his physical recovery. He was able to walk with much better balance. Physical strength had improved; he was working out two times a week with a personal trainer. JB admitted that the ability to renew a physical health routine was comforting to him; as a former athlete, he took pride in working out to ensure his physical health. While the right fingers in his hand had not shown much progress, his forearm was more relaxed than before. JB was more talkative, readily responding to questions, albeit with one–word answers.

JB was excited to see if a second stem cell treatment could offer further improvement. In March 2007 he returned to Moscow, where he received another stem cell treatment, again consisting of an intravenous injection of MSCs, and NSCs injected into the cerebrospinal fluid. JB again showed no negative reaction to the stem cell transfusion.

At 24 hours after the second procedure, an examination revealed that JB had better balance, and he again reported feeling a new sense of clarity. Follow-up found him making physical progress with his therapy. His speech therapist declared that his speech had further improved, to the point where he could say two– or three–word phrases. In addition, his mental acuity increased significantly. By January of 2009, he was able to actively participate in conversations that previously would have daunted him. Now he was able to pronounce short phrases and sentences. His balance and strength returned to the point where he could practice his pitching and putting golf skills. Furthermore, JB declared that he was walking farther than before, and that the pain he had previously felt in his hip and back had been dramatically reduced (although pain in his left shoulder still occasionally troubled him).

"The first time I saw him he could barely walk and needed assistance and couldn't talk. Actually, after I found out the extent of [the stroke], I didn't know that he would even survive it," said one of JB's friends.[2]

Encouraged, JB went to Moscow for his third treatment. Just as he had done twice before, he boarded a plane and made the long trip to the Moscow clinic. But there was one difference. Previously, JB had been accompanied by a caretaker, to assist him in his journey. This time, his family decided that he had regained enough independence to make the trip by himself. At the clinic, the same procedure was repeated, and no negative symptoms were reported. More improvements followed. JB's facial symmetry returned, and he reported that his mind was clearer. He was able to work harder at his physical therapy, with the eventual goal of getting back to the golf course.

JB's friends and family, but also his therapists and caretakers, noted improvement. His cognitive skills had improved, he had regained some of his physical abilities, and he was able to communicate again, using short sentences. Since the treatments, JB has even been able to renew his passion for golf.

JB was not "cured" of his stroke, but he was able to make meaningful progress with his condition, thanks to his treatments. JB's story is an inspiring one, yet he is just one example of stroke patients who have been treated with stem cells, through clinical studies across the globe. Unfortunately, he's just one among many Americans who suffer from stroke in an epidemic that claims more lives every year.

Stroke: The Numbers

Every year in the United States alone, almost 800,000 people suffer a stroke. Of that number, more than 137,000 will die from a stroke, making it the third highest cause of death in the United States.[3] African-Americans are at almost twice the risk of suffering a stroke, compared to Americans of European descent. While the risk of stroke may disproportionately affect different segments of society, once a stroke hits, the possible ramifications of such a debilitating event are all too predictable.

Stroke occurs when the brain is deprived of oxygen. This is due to a blood vessel being blocked or when a blood vessel breaks. If the blood vessel is blocked, usually through a blood clot, then the blood flow is halted. Imagine a golf ball stuck in a garden hose and you will have a fairly good visual image of what a blood clot can do to an artery. The stroke that results from a blocked blood vessel is called an ischemic stroke and it accounts for about 87% of stroke cases.

Another type of stroke is a hemorrhagic stroke, which occurs when the blood vessel ruptures. Blood leaks into the brain and builds up, putting pressure on the brain tissue and damaging it. A third type of stroke is called a transient ischemic attack (TIA). It is often referred to as a "mini-stroke" or a "warning stroke" because its effects are not permanent but can warn of a much greater likelihood of an actual stroke; about one third of those who suffer a TIA have another, more serious stroke within a year.

There is much that one can do to prevent a stroke. Exercise and nutrition, the staples of a healthy body, are an important start. Because a stroke is caused by a cardiovascular problem, anyone who is concerned about preventing a stroke should have a series of conversations with their doctor. Certain drugs, such as anti-platelet agents, can mitigate the blood's ability to create a clot and lessen the chance of stroke. In addition, certain surgical procedures can help clean out blockage from blood vessels. To learn about other ways to reduce your risk for stroke, we recommend a visit to the website of the American Stroke Association (www.strokeassociation.org).

But while there are many ways to lower your risk of a stroke, there is essentially no good option for undoing the damage caused once a stroke hits. Prompt medical care has saved millions of lives. But the brain damage that is caused by stroke cannot be repaired, or undone, with traditional medical techniques. There is no drug that rebuilds destroyed brain tissue. Americans alone pay over $73 billion a year to handle the medical and disability costs associated with stroke, but none of that money can erase a stroke's effects.[4]

The greater the magnitude of the stroke, the greater the damage a patient is likely to suffer. This is to say, the more blood vessels that are sealed off or constricted by an ischemic stroke, or the more blood that piles onto the brain as the result of a hemorrhagic stroke, the greater the size of the lesion. Every minute wasted in getting to the hospital worsens the effects of a stroke; as the American Stroke Association

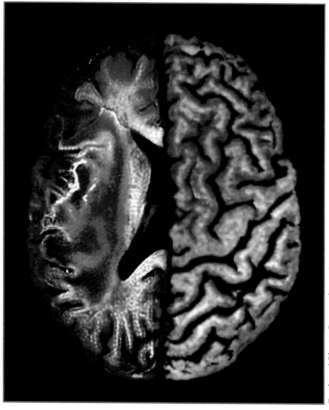

Zephyr / Photo Researchers, Inc.

A stroke occurs when the blood supply to part of the brain is disturbed, which deprives the brain of oxygen and nutrients, causing a decrease in brain function. A large infarct (area of dead tissue, red) is seen in the sylvian fissure of the right hemisphere (seen here on the left as the brain is viewed from below).

puts it, "time lost is brain lost."[4, 5] The effects of a stroke, then, are worse for some than for others.

Effects of a stroke can include involuntary contraction of the muscles, loss of balance, and even consistent and debilitating pain, known as central pain syndrome. Stroke sufferers can develop aphasia, as a result of damage to the language center in the brain. This can severely impact the ability to speak. Stroke victims can even lose their ability to swallow correctly. A stroke that affects one side of the brain can cause loss of contact with one side of the body, effectively causing partial paralysis.

Besides the physical changes, there is also what stroke survivor Dr. Arthur Gottlieb (MD) calls "the psychological and emotional setbacks of a stroke."[6] Stroke survivors can become severely depressed when, because of this one event, they lose the ability to perform basic tasks. After a stroke, survivors can lose interest in things that used to excite them or become frustrated by their inability to participate in activities they previously enjoyed. These feelings of helplessness and disconnection can spread and affect the loved ones of the stroke victim as well. Gottlieb, author of a book on stroke, explains that "the forced identity change from loved one to caregiver can be as stressful as a stroke itself."[6]

CT scan of a 66-year-old female's brain, showing a hemorrhage in the left posterior temporal area of the brain

Back

Front

Scott Camazine / Photo Researchers, Inc.

Recovery from these effects is slow, drawn-out, and painful. Patients can participate in years of physical therapy and voice therapy, and only experience minimal gains. Having lost the brain cells responsible for sometimes-crucial functions, physical therapy patients must relearn how to perform tasks that were previously mundane, such as eating or bathing. Depending on the extent of the damaged brain tissue, survivors may not be able to live without assistance, even with rehabilitation.

And, in a cruel twist of fate, many stroke sufferers trying to recover find themselves in a race against time. "With Medicare, there's a calculation based on certain benchmarks for healing," explains physical therapist Dr. Manuel Soto (DPT, GCS):

Although we know that every body heals differently, and at a different rate, these recovery benchmarks are based on averages. After a stroke, insurance companies will use these benchmarks to

measure a patient's progress. If a patient does not hit a certain benchmark by a certain time, the insurance company may decide that the patient's body has healed as much as it can.[A]

The unfortunate result of this formula is that some stroke sufferers, whose bodies are trying to repair the neurological damage but cannot do so in time, receive no more insurance money for physical therapy, even when continued physical therapy would continue to help them. "With the system we have in place, if physical therapy doesn't achieve results fast enough, or if someone's recovery plateaus for a while, insurance will be able to stop payments" says Soto.

Dr. Pamela Duncan (PT, PhD), a doctor in the Physical Therapy Division of Duke University School of Medicine, agrees. "Reimbursement for stroke therapy is not consistent with what we know about the neurophysiologic basis of recovery [after a stroke]," she declares.[B]

This problem demonstrates the need for an efficacious and safe treatment that could accelerate the painstaking gains that stroke survivors must work for in physical therapy. Soto explains that such a treatment would not only ease the substantial physical suffering of the stroke victims, and the emotional toll on the patient and the patient's caregiver, but also would lift a financial burden on the patient's family:

From the vantage point of a physical therapist, these stem cell treatments help accelerate the process of recovery. That means less time spent in physical therapy for a recovery breakthrough. This offers a more cost-effective series of treatments for the patient.

But stem cell therapy may be able to offer even more. By building new neural cells in the afflicted patient's brain and saving injured or nutrient-starved cells, stem cells could enable stroke patients to reach new heights of recovery.

Stem Cells and their Mechanism of Action

Let us return to the case of JB. Since stem cells have an array of mechanisms by which they catalyze healing in the body, it is impossible to accurately depict everything that the neural cells accomplished when they were introduced to JB's nervous system. While not all the actions of neural stem cells (NSCs) on the central nervous system are completely understood, it is possible that some of the following actions took place. The NSCs, upon

But stem cell therapy may be able to offer even more. By building new neural cells in the afflicted patient's brain and saving injured or nutrient-starved cells, stem cells could enable stroke patients to reach new heights of recovery.

Factor: an element or substance that actively contributes to the functioning of a particular physiological process or biological system.

reaching the affected area:

1. Grafted onto the injured area to form working neurons.

2. Accepted, transmitted, produced and released signals that helped the body's own (endogenous) stem cells better respond to the injury.

3. Differentiated into neurons and a variety of glial cells, a type of brain cell that produced a beneficial effect on damaged but salvageable tissue operating in the penumbra of the dead-tissue area.

4. Secreted biochemical **factors** that worked to rebalance the cell microenvironment.

The first action, forming working neurons, is perhaps the most straight-forward. The lasting effects of a stroke result from the death of brain cells, including neurons (the brain cells that both receive and process information and send signals to the rest of the body), and glial cells, which provide a variety of support functions for the neurons. The human brain contains approximately 100 billion neurons, and many more glial cells. But a stroke can dramatically lessen the number of working cells in the brain; every minute a stroke goes untreated, approximately two million brain cells will die.[7] Some of these brain cells will be the all-important neurons.

Transplanted stem cells, upon reaching the area most affected by the stroke, will encounter the brain lesion, a sphere of dead brain tissue where the stroke has hit hardest. In order to effect any meaningful healing, the tissue will need to be completely replaced. Stem cells have the capability of affecting this replacement, and transplanted neural cells offer the exciting possibility of beating back the effects of a stroke.

It is important to note that, while there has been a reduction in the amount of dead tissue, this patient has not been restored to pre-stroke status; a stem-cell injection cannot erase the effects of a stroke or other significant neurological events. But there is promising evidence that further developments in stem cell research will allow us to effect even greater repair to the brain in the future.

Recently, for example, researchers in the United Kingdom performed a study using stem cells to repair brain damage in stroke-afflicted rats. They added one step, however, by placing the stem cells on a "cell scaffolding," a polymer-based structure that the stem cells cling to. With this added layer of control over the stem cell's behavior, the researchers, led by Dr. Mike Modo (PhD) of the Institute of Psychiatry of King's College in London, hoped to prevent transplanted stem cells from migrating to surrounding tissue, thus assuring a better result.

Their hypothesis was confirmed when they found the rats' affected brain tissue fully repaired after stem cell treatment, in just seven days.[8] In a press statement, Modo laid out the implications of his discovery. "We would expect to see a much better improvement in the outcome after a stroke if we can fully replace the lost brain tissue, and that is what we have been able to do with our technique."[9]

Joe Korner, Director of Communications at The Stroke Association, based in the United Kingdom, was one of those who hailed the study as a promising development for the future of stem cell treatments, saying:

> *This research is another step towards using stem cell therapy in treating and reversing the brain damage caused by stroke. It is exciting because researchers have shown they are able to overcome some of the many challenges in translating the potential of using stem cells into reality. The potential to reverse the disabling effects of stroke seems to have been proved.[10]*

However, there is a big difference between a successful animal trial and a successful human trial. It is possible that what leads to clinical success in rats could have side effects in humans. We still have a ways to go before advancing stem cell treatments to the point where they can completely replace dead tissue, but the promise of such a treatment is very encouraging.

While transplanted stem cells have proven capable of replacing destroyed tissue, they do much more than that. Neural stem cell transplants can set off a healing cascade within the brain, working with the stem cells that are already present.

The Chaperone Effect

Dr. Fred Gage explained in a 2005 interview:

> *Everything I have done so far in the CNS leads me to believe that the nervous system tries to repair itself after an injury. It does this at one level or another, and usually it accomplishes some moderate level of recovery.[11]*

After a neurological injury, our body's own stem cells do respond to the damage. So why does the body not replace its damaged neurons after a stroke?

For one thing, the damage is just too great. As we age, the number and quality of our stem cells decline as the cells become more senescent. With strokes occurring mainly in older people, the stem cells that are tasked with repairing the damage are far beyond their prime, resulting in a woefully inadequate response to a major trauma. A stroke can kill off millions of brain cells; meanwhile, Gage and Eriksson found that neurogenesis in elderly patients created only hundreds of new neurons.[12] These hundreds of neurons are a drop in a bucket, compared to the tidal wave of damage the stroke has caused.

There remains some concern that the body's neural stem cells stay dormant, not responding effectively to significant neurological injury. If all the cells in a certain area are completely killed off, it affects which signals reach the endogenous neural stem cells. Receiving few signals, not all the stem cells respond to the injury.

Transplanted stem cells are able to spur the endogenous stem cells to action. It is a phenomenon called the Chaperone Effect.

In his interview, Gage affirmed that the existence of endogenous stem cells does not guarantee their effective response:

Our conclusion is that there are neural stem cells all over the brain and in the spinal cord, but they don't give rise to neurons under normal conditions because the local environment doesn't provide them with the appropriate cues.[11]

If the microenvironment of the injured site does not send out the appropriate signals, the stem cells will not know anything is wrong.

Scientists have noted that a brain's stem cell response to an injury seems inherently limited.[13] Endogenous NSCs are lying dormant, seemingly not responding to the injured signals sent out by affected brain tissue. Some scientists wonder if "such limitations may simply be a progressive muting of responsiveness in the aging brain rather than an inherent 'deafness' to injury cues on the

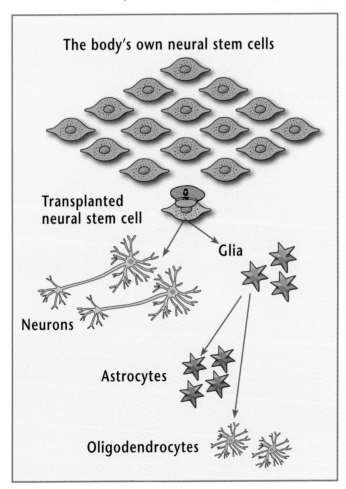

The body's own neural stem cells

Transplanted neural stem cell

Glia

Neurons

Astrocytes

Oligodendrocytes

part of the neural stem/progenitor cells."[13, 14, 15] The brain's **progenitor cells**, it is alleged, are either lazy or deaf; either way, they fail to adequately respond to a major trauma.

But transplanted stem cells are able to spur the endogenous stem cells to action. It is a phenomenon called the Chaperone Effect; a term coined by a group of researchers in 2002. The researchers, investigating whether NSCs could rescue dysfunctional neurons, learned that the transplanted NSCs were able to rescue host cells that previously were lying dormant. The group declared, "These observations suggest that host structures may benefit not only from NSC-derived replacement of lost neurons but also from the 'chaperone' effect of some NSC-derived progeny."[16]

Dr. Evan Snyder, one of the authors of the 2002 study, believes that the Chaperone Effect illustrates an important truth about the power of stem cells: ability to coordinate and catalyze the effects of other cells is perhaps even more important than the direct effect they can have on damaged or aging tissue. "That may actually be the low-hanging fruit in the stem-cell field—taking advantage of this [the Chaperone Effect], and not the cell-replacement aspect that we always thought would be the key to stem-cell biology in regenerative medicine."[17]

By forming new neurons themselves, transplanted NSCs are like the cavalry reinforcements for the brain, rushing to the site of injury to effect immediate repair. But with the Chaperone Effect, these stem cells also function like generals, leading the previously inactive endogenous cells into battle. Their effect does not extend only to other stem cells, however; instead, they can spur different sets of cells to "carry out normal organ maintenance and initiate damage control."[17] Transplanted stem cells, then, do not just catalyze the endogenous cells' formation of new neurons, but also help stabilize the environment.

We have previously stressed the importance of a working microenvironment and its relationship to the healthy functioning of cells in a given area. After a stroke, however, this microenvironment is terribly damaged. Dr. Snyder explains, "Toxic processes that can destabilize a system following stroke include free radicals, inflammatory cytokines, excitotoxins, lipases, peroxidases, etc."[13] Essentially, the microenvironment's chemical balance has been skewed. But stem cells engage in "neurotrophic, neuroprotective, and anti-inflammatory actions" to rebalance the microenvironment

By forming new neurons themselves, transplanted NSCs are like the cavalry reinforcements for the brain, rushing to the site of injury to effect immediate repair. But with the Chaperone Effect, these stem cells also function like generals, leading the previously inactive endogenous cells into battle.

Progenitor cells: a variation of the stem cell, that is partially predetermined as to what cell it will differentiate into. Another distinction, progenitor cells are more senescent than stem cells.

Stem cells engage in "neurotrophic, neuroprotective, and anti-inflammatory actions" to rebalance the microenvironment and allow clear signals to flow to the requisite cells. By releasing their own set of signals, they can stabilize the system.

and allow clear signals to flow to the requisite cells.[13] By releasing their own set of signals, they can stabilize the system.

To use a metaphor, a stroke can cause a major traffic jam in the biochemical environment of the brain. Chemical factors are no longer flowing effectively, and cells are either not receiving their signals or not responding to them. By regulating the microenvironment, stem cells are both the traffic officers, getting traffic moving again, and the engineers that work to correct any damage to the road itself.

Through the Chaperone Effect, stem cells function in a directive capacity, clearing the way for other cells to do their work and catalyzing the reactions that will lead to a stable system. In their third mechanism of action (differentiating into glial cells), transplanted stem cells function in a supportive capacity.

Saving the Penumbra

When we focus on neurons and their integral contributions to brain function, it is easy to forget the role of other brain cell types. **Glial** cells (or glia), for example, account for around 90% of all brain tissue. The glial cells are often referred to as the "glue" of the nervous system (glia means "glue" in Greek), and the metaphor is fairly accurate. Glial cells work to hold neurons in place and insulate neurons from one another. They are also responsible for supplying nutrients and oxygen to the neurons, destroying pathogens in the nervous system, removing debris from dead neurons, and regulating cross-synaptic communication across neurons. Other glial cells, such as oligodendrocytes and Schwann Cells, surround the neuronal axons with myelin sheaths, a protective material that ensures that the CNS is functioning properly. Damage to these myelin sheaths results in multiple sclerosis.

These are several examples of how glial cells, the unsung heroes of the central nervous system, regulate the health of the entire system by modulating neuronal behavior. A healthy set of glial cells enables the neurons to do their job correctly.

A stroke affects all brain cells, however, not just neurons. During a stroke, glial cells die off, depriving neuronal cells, which might otherwise function normally, of crucial nutrients. This is not a problem for the cells within the lesion of the stroke itself; dead neurons do not need nutrients. But surrounding the lesion is an area of brain tissue that is not dead, but severely weakened. This area is called the

Glia: the supporting formations of nervous tissue.

The blue area represents the pneumbra at the edge of the dead brain tissue in orange.

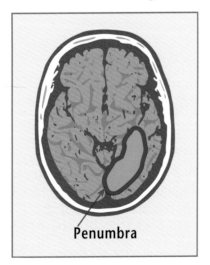

Penumbra

penumbra of a stroke, or the ischemic boundary zone (IBZ), and it is a serious concern for stroke patients. As a result of the damaging effects of the stroke, the tissue in the penumbra is struck by circulatory hypoxia, meaning that the cells are receiving an inadequate oxygen supply. With insufficient oxygen, neurons within the penumbra of the stroke are struggling to survive. A new set of glial cells could create a healthier infrastructure for these neurons, helping the penumbra repair itself. New glial cells may also reduce the risk of a future stroke; many strokes occur when blood vessels in the IBZ of an old stroke shut down or become congested with dead tissue.

Transplanted NSCs can differentiate into these glial cells, providing the support structure that the penumbra needs to recover after a stroke. In this situation, neuronal cells get the nutrients and oxygen they need to operate more effectively, and the danger of another stroke is lessened.

Mesenchymal Cells and the Nervous System

JB and other patients within the Moscow clinical study received both neural stem cells and mesenchymal stem cells. We have explained the mechanisms of action for NSCs, but what about the mesenchymal cells? Just like neural cells, mesenchymal cells play varied roles. Their own mechanisms of action include:

- Restoring homeostasis,

- Repairing the vascular structure,

- Repairing and regulating neural stem cell differentiation, forming gap junctions with neurons and releasing repair proteins and important genes, and

- Repairing damaged neurons.

We know that a stroke unbalances the microenvironment of the brain. Transplanted neural cells are able to release a set of biochemical factors that can help get endogenous brain cells back on track. Mesenchymal stem cells are able to release their own set of factors that re-establish the correct proportions of biochemical signals in the brain.

After a stroke there is a profusion of hypoxia-inducible factor 1 (HiF1). This factor, released in response to the hypoxia in the brain, helps reduce the brain's response to lessened blood flow. HiF1 will **up-regulate**, or encourage the expression of certain factors while down-regulating or discouraging others. One group of factors it up-regulates is **VEGF**, vascular endothelial growth factor.

Up/down-regulation: the change in behavior or structure in order to adapt to changed conditions. In particular, the control of the type and ratio of a cellular process by manipulating the activity of specific and individual genes. Up-regulation meaning an increase in cellular process, down-regulation meaning decrease.

Vascular endothelial growth factor (VEGF): a protein factor that contributes to, and stimulates the growth of blood vessels. VEGF also helps in tissue vascularization.

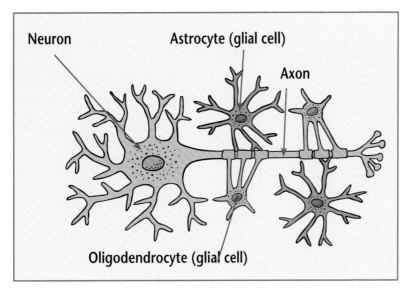

Neuron

Astrocyte (glial cell)

Axon

Oligodendrocyte (glial cell)

This factor increases the profusion of blood vessels, builds new blood vessels, and increases vascular permeability. At certain times, it is necessary to increase the amount of VEGF in the brain (as we will see in a later chapter). An up-regulation of VEGF, while promoting the increase of new blood vessels, can also lead to leaky blood vessels that will further worsen the effects of a stroke. In an acute hemmorhagic stroke situation, the up-regulation of VEGF can cause some harm.

By increasing vascular permeability after a hemmorhagic stroke, VEGF induces blood to pour into the affected area, causing edema that can damage cell tissues and cause swelling which puts pressure on the brain, killing even more brain cells. This side effect of VEGF is just one example of how the body's attempt to heal itself after this neurological insult can end up causing more harm; through its immunological response, the body may be destroying more of the brain in an effort to repair it.

Mesenchymal stem cells, through their immunomodulatory properties (see Chapter 4), could possibly mitigate the over-reaction of the body's immune response. They release another set of factors that protect the vasculature from the VEGF–induced plasma leaking. The main growth factor that prevents this effect appears to be angiopoetin-1, while other protagonists include the growth factor endostatin, which prevents blood vessels from overdeveloping.[18] Through the secretion of their own set of signals, MSCs can up-regulate or down-regulate other growth factors back to optimal proportions. Targeting the ischemic zone of a stroke, mesenchymal stem cells can induce more blood to the affected tissue. They can increase the percent of oxygen in the brain, lessening the degree of hypoxia. With so many chemical factors at their disposal, MSCs seem to be able to develop a nuanced response to a complex neurological situation.

The MSCs may also be able to catalyze the growth of new blood vessels from existing vessels in the brain. The growth of new vessels from pre-existing ones (a process called **angio-**

Angiogenesis: the creation and differentiation of new blood vessels. This process is also known as angiopoiesis and vasculogenesis.

genesis) allows for better blood profusion and helps the brain recover from a stroke.[19] A stroke damages blood cells, which may be starved for blood after an ischemic instance, or broken after a hemorrhagic stroke.

Moreover, macrophages trying to repair the damage may attack blood vessels in the IBZ. Macrophages, a type of immune cell, are like the police officers of the body's cellular system. They are designed to attack foreign invaders, like bacteria or viruses. They also clean up cellular debris, consuming dead cells so that new cells can grow in their place. Normally, they recognize that healthy endogenous cells should not be targeted. Because of damage to the blood brain barrier during a stroke, macrophages can penetrate into the brain. In a toxic post-stroke environment, these police cells are thrown into a volatile situation with no clear orders, and their discriminating nature is lost, causing attacks on cells that may otherwise survive an acute stroke. This is another example of how the immune system's over-reaction to a neurological injury can causeincreased harm.

Even though the brain undergoes angiogenesis on its own, it is not enough to affect significant revascularization. A 2009 paper by a team of American researchers, led by Dr. Jieli Chen (MD) of the Henry Ford Health Sciences Center in Detroit, explains, "Under normal circumstances after stroke, the contribution of angio-genesis to the brain capillary network is insufficient to support the brain plasticity required for functional recovery."[20]

Chen and her team set out to explore how MSCs could increase angiogenesis. In their animal study using human MSCs to treat stroke-afflicted rats, they found that MSCs promoted certain growth factors, including VEGF, therefore contributing to the revascularization of the ischemic boundary zone.[20] Their report also uncovered "significant increases in numbers of enlarged and thin walled blood vessels and numbers of newly formed capillaries at the boundary of the ischemic lesion in rats treated with hMSCs."[20] That is to say, new blood vessels had formed around the brain tissue that had been killed off by the stroke.

These results suggested that MSC treatments for stroke may offer meaningful healing to the injured area, and not just in terms of rehabilitation: "Stroke patients with a higher cerebral blood vessel density make better progress and survive longer than patients with lower vascular density."[20]

"MSCs have a direct and pronounced effect on the genesis of neurons and oligodendrocytes from NSCs in vitro."

Migration, Regulation, and Transdifferentiation

In 2006, researchers from Case Western Reserve University set up an *in vitro* study designed to explore why MSCs were able to stimulate enhanced NSC response to a CNS injury. To shed some light on the subject, they placed MSCs in the same cultured medium as a set of NSCs. In a cultured medium, NSCs will often form what is called a neurosphere, a spherical structure in which all the NSCs cluster together. The Case Western researchers hypothesized that the MSCs, through a process of cell-signaling, would stimulate the NSCs to migrate from the neurosphere and spread out across the medium. They were right; after several hours, the neural cells began to drift away from the neurosphere and spread themselves across the entire culture.[21]

The researchers declared that this stimulated migration explained how MSCs "provide one type of critical trophic support to neurosphere derived cells."[21] If the same process occurs *in vivo* as it does *in vitro*, then this study helps delineate the process by which MSCs encourage NSCs to spread out and find the site of injury in the central nervous system, and subsequently act to repair the damage.

The researchers also found evidence of increased development of different brain cell types in the mediums co-cultured with MSCs, as opposed to the mediums that just had NSCs. The scientists looked for two cell types in particular: neurons, which gather and transmit information, and oligodendrocytes, a type of glial cell which insulate and protects the axons of the neuron by forming the protective myelin sheath. The researchers found that, in comparison to the control group of just NSCs, the co-cultured mediums had extensive development of neurons and oligodendrocytes.[21]

The study authors concluded, "MSCs have a direct and pronounced effect on the genesis of neurons and oligodendrocytes from NSCs in vitro."[21] They further concluded that the MSCs 'communicated' with the NSCs through the release of soluble factors, not through cell surface interactions. That is to say, the mesenchymal stem cells released biochemical signals that prompted the neural stem cells to respond; they did not need to be in direct contact with the neural cells.

The above examples clearly demonstrate the potential for MSCs to promote neurological wound healing in conjunction with NSCs, through a variety of tactics. There is evidence of another way the MSCs may help heal neurological wounds: by turning into neuronal-type cells.[22, 23] *In vitro* studies of MSCs have resulted in these mesenchymal cells differentiating into neural derivatives, while other studies have suggested that MSCs can differentiate into Schwann cells, the glial cells responsible for insulating the axons of the peripheral nervous system.[24, 25] The phenomenon of one cell type turning into a cell that is not within its path of differentiation is called transdifferentiation, or plasticity. These studies and others suggest that MSCs have a certain degree of plasticity and that they can thus form cells that normally would be differentiated only from neural progenitors.

Through their multiplicity of actions, neural stem cells and mesenchymal stem cells both seem to be able to repair the brain on many different levels after a stroke. Together their effects are even more pronounced.

While this may occur in stroke patients treated with MSCs, its effect is probably not that pronounced. In their 2006 study, the Case Western scientists explain that "the proportion of MSCs that can be directed towards a neural fate appears to be relatively small."[21]

Dr. Chen's research team came to similar conclusions in their own study of how MSCs could be used to treat stroke. They wrote:

> *Bone marrow stromal cells also likely contain a subpopulation of stem-like cells, which can differentiate into brain cells. However, these cells are a minor subpopulation of the hMSCs we use and do not contribute to the restoration of function, and only a very small percentage of the hMSCs assume parenchymal [a term used to denote functional tissue, as opposed to structural tissue] cell type.*[19]

The level of plasticity that MSCs may have is currently being debated by scientific circles around the world, and it is likely that it is other mechanisms of action by which MSCs affect the greatest degree of change in the CNS.[26, 27]

Through their multiplicity of actions, neural stem cells and mesenchymal stem cells both seem to be able to repair the brain on many different levels after a stroke. Together their effects are even more pronounced. But this stem cell combination is not limited to dealing with stroke alone; there are many other neurological conditions that can be treated with multi-cell treatment therapy.

Chapter 7
Spinal Cord Injuries

It could be the result of a fall down the stairs, or an automobile accident. It could have been initiated by a sports-related injury, or violence, or even a birth defect. There are many causes of a spinal cord injury (SCI), but regardless of the cause, the effects can be devastating. Over one million people in the United States currently have a spinal cord injury. These injuries will almost always include some form of paralysis, often severe. Thirty-five percent of Americans suffering from spinal cord injury report significant difficulty moving; another 13% report being unable to make any movements whatsoever.[1]

The resulting paralysis can be a jarring transition. In contrast to stroke, where lifestyle factors can reduce the risk of occurrence, there are very few preventive measures one can take in order to reduce the risk of spinal cord injury. While those who engage in extreme sports are at higher risk for injuries to the central nervous system, any traumatic blow to the spinal cord may be sufficient to cause permanent nerve damage. In a single moment, a person can

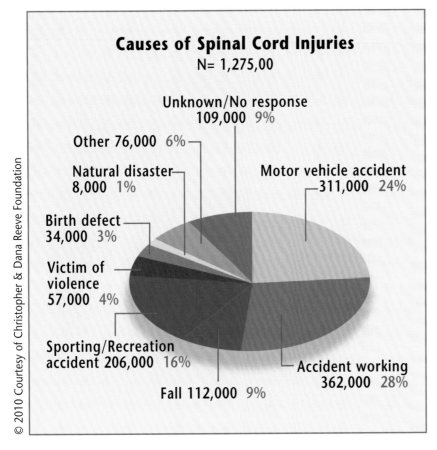

Causes of Spinal Cord Injuries
N= 1,275,00

Unknown/No response
109,000 9%

Other 76,000 6%

Natural disaster
8,000 1%

Motor vehicle accident
311,000 24%

Birth defect
34,000 3%

Victim of
violence
57,000 4%

Sporting/Recreation
accident 206,000 16%

Accident working
362,000 28%

Fall 112,000 9%

lose the ability to walk, to play sports—to move at all.

And the toll is not just physical. The Christopher & Dana Reeve Foundation, an organization created on behalf of SCI patients and others affected by paralysis, was created by the late actor and stem cell research advocate, Christopher Reeve, and his wife. Today, the Foundation declares that the amount an SCI patient will end up paying for healthcare can easily run to millions of dollars. For those afflicted with quadriplegia, healthcare costs for the first year alone can range from $500,000 to over $750,000. Those afflicted with paraplegia can be expected to pay over $280,000 in the first year. These costs saddle the family of an SCI patient with a tremendous financial burden.

But family members and caregivers of SCI patients take on a set of responsibilities that are more than financial. A *Time* magazine article featured the story of Eddie Canales, whose son Chris received a paralyzing spinal cord injury while playing football:

Eddie, the director of operations at the University of Texas at San Antonio bookstore, quit his job to tend to his son. He turned him over every two hours to prevent bedsores because the insurance company initially refused to pay for a pressure-supported mattress. He inserted a catheter every three hours. He gave Chris medications every six hours. He slept on the floor next to Chris. His care commenced at 7:30 AM and did not end until 3:30 the following morning.[2]

While many family members will take on these responsibilities without complaint, they should not have to. A meaningful treatment option for spinal cord injury would not only help SCI patients themselves, but help relieve the demands placed on their loved ones.

What is a Spinal Cord Injury?

A spinal cord injury is far more serious than an injury to the spinal bone structure itself. A person can receive a fracture to the spine, for example, and not have a spinal cord injury. That is because the backbone, composed of rings of vertebrae, is actually in place not only to support the trunk of the body but also to protect the spinal cord. The spinal cord is a major grouping of nerves that perform two primary tasks: they transmit sensory perception from the body to the brain, and transmit orders from the brain to the body.

The spinal cord is part of the central nervous system (CNS), along with the brain. It is an electrical highway, the only means of communication between the body and the brain. There are twelve cranial nerves that connect parts of the head (such as the eyes and nose) directly to the brain; otherwise, the spinal cord is the primary way of sending nerve transmissions.

Putting your hand on a hot stove illustrates the importance of the spinal cord. The nerves in the hand immediately signal that something is wrong. This signal travels from the peripheral nervous system to the spinal cord, which then relays the signal directly to the brain. The brain processes this information, devises a reaction, and sends a signal down the spinal cord, which relays it on to the arm. Your arm jerks away from the stove, and you are protected from further damage to your hand.

If the spinal cord is injured to the point where it can no longer transmit nervous signals, the brain no longer receives sensations from the body, and the body no longer receives information from the brain. At the point where the spinal cord has sustained injury, any motor and sensory function below that point can be impaired. An SCI patient can no longer feel sensation in these parts of the body, or even command those parts to move at all. This loss of function can even include bowel and bladder control.

With a complete spinal cord injury, a patient will lose all function below the injured area. In contrast, an incomplete spinal cord injury will usually leave a patient with some function, but that person's ability to move and to feel will still be compromised.

The closer the injury is to the base of the skull, the worse the functional deficit will be. For example, an injury to the thoracic region, located in the upper back, may leave someone paraplegic. A paraplegic is typically unable to move his or her lower body.

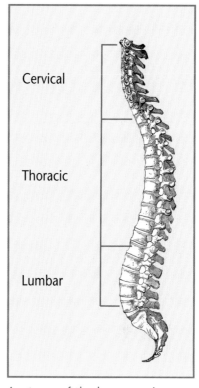

Anatomy of the human spine.

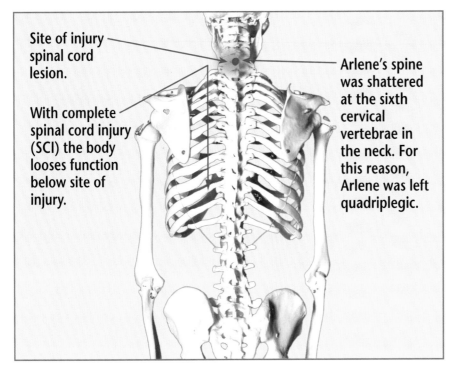

Site of injury spinal cord lesion.

With complete spinal cord injury (SCI) the body looses function below site of injury.

Arlene's spine was shattered at the sixth cervical vertebrae in the neck. For this reason, Arlene was left quadriplegic.

However, an injury to the cervical region, within the neck, will often leave an SCI patient quadriplegic. With quadriplegia, a patient traditionally loses function from the neck down, including the arms and legs.

The actual site where the SCI occurred is referred to as the spinal cord lesion. The segments of the spinal cord below the lesion are affected as well. Although they still receive their nutrients from the circulatory system, their lack of contact with the brain causes them to degenerate; the medical term for these isolated segments is "degenerating tracts." But it is not just the rest of the spinal cord that suffers. The rest of the body, no longer receiving signals from the brain, begins to wither. This is part of the reason that a paraplegic's legs will appear wasted; the degeneration of the affected body part, combined with lack of use, impacts the body's overall health.

In our introduction, we shared with you the story of our sister-in-law, Arlene. As a result of her automobile accident, Arlene's spine was shattered. The force of the car crash had caused damage that went past her vertebrae, past the cerebrospinal fluid that might have absorbed the shock of a lesser blow, and straight to the bundle of nerves itself. It was this injury to the nervous system that left her unable to move, with an all-but-complete SCI. The uppermost damaged spinal cord segment was at the sixth cervical vertebrae in the neck. For this reason, Arlene was left quadriplegic. Fortunately for her and for us, stem cells offered a meaningful treatment therapy.

The Human Face of SCI — Arlene's Story

There are millions of families worldwide with their own stories of a loved one suffering from this debilitating injury. For us, it was our sister-in-law, Arlene Howe. After her accident, Arlene underwent fifteen months of intensive physical therapy. Despite all these efforts, she could do little more than move her thumb and forefinger. Arlene relied on a motorized wheelchair, and needed constant assistance from caretakers. When in bed, she had to be turned every two hours, so that the pressure of her body against the bed did not cut off circulation to her underside (a condition known as pressure sores, or more colloquially as bedsores). She lacked the ability to perform basic physical functions including bowel and bladder control. She had also repeatedly expressed

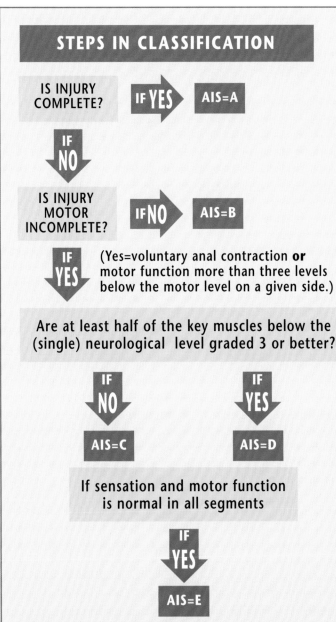

STEPS IN CLASSIFICATION

IS INJURY COMPLETE? — IF YES → AIS=A

IF NO ↓

IS INJURY MOTOR INCOMPLETE? — IF NO → AIS=B

IF YES ↓ (Yes=voluntary anal contraction **or** motor function more than three levels below the motor level on a given side.)

Are at least half of the key muscles below the (single) neurological level graded 3 or better?

IF NO ↓ AIS=C   IF YES ↓ AIS=D

If sensation and motor function is normal in all segments

IF YES ↓ AIS=E

ASIA IMPAIRMENT SCALE

A Complete: No motor or sensory function is preserved in the sacral segments S4-S5.

B Incomplete: Sensory but not motor function is preserved below the neurological level and includes the sacral segments S4-S5.

C Incomplete: Motor function is preserved below the neurological level, and more than half of key muscles below the neurological level have a muscle grade less than 3.

D Incomplete: Motor function is preserved below the neurological level, and at least half of key muscles below the neurological level have a muscle grade of 3 or more, up to 5* (muscles able to exert, in examiner's judgement, sufficient resistance to be considered normal if identifiable inhibiting factors were not present).

E Normal: Motor and sensory function are normal.

Note: AIS-E is used in follow up testing when an individual with a documented SCI has recovered normal function. If at initial testing no deficits are found, the individual is neurologically intact; the ASIA Impairment Scale does not apply.

American Spinal Injury Association: International Standards for Neurological Classification of Spinal Cord Injury, revised 2000; Atlanta GA. Reprinted 2008.

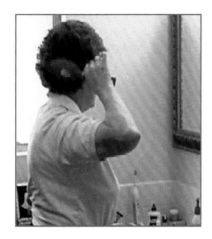

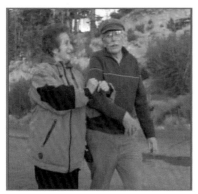

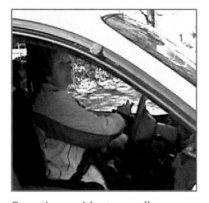

Over time, with stem cell treatment and physical therapy, Arlene was able to perform many of the tasks of daily living. She was able to comb her hair, walk with assistance, and drive a specially outfitted car.

frustration with her lack of improvement despite her most sincere efforts in physical therapy.

Arlene's first treatment was in April, 2006, sixteen months after her accident. Three months following her treatment, in which she received both mesenchymal stem cells and neural stem cells, Arlene began to feel sensations in her back and lower extremities. In fact, she called her physician to complain of lower back pain. She was surprised when he explained that this was actually a good sign; quadriplegics are typically unable to feel lower back pain, as the sensations that would transmit this information must go through the spinal cord. Arlene also informed her family that her therapy was progressing more smoothly, and that it was easier to transfer from her bed to her wheelchair.

Enthusiastic about Arlene's success, her family and friends impatiently waited to see the results of her second treatment, which she received in March of 2007. A month later, she brought home a note from her physiatrist Dr. John Jahan (MD):

She can now walk approx. 150 feet with aided balance transitions to turn around. She can now walk with a high rolling walker but still needs assistance getting in and out of bed and in and out of her wheelchair. Bowel function continues to improve with both bladder and bowel.[3]

Dr. Jahan also reported that, using the American Spinal Cord Injury Association (ASIA) rules of classification, Arlene was now in category ASIA-C. This category, which signifies "some sensory and motor preservation," was an improvement from her previous classification of ASIA-B, a more pronounced category of impairment used to denote a sensory-only level of function below the spinal cord lesion.[4] This was a measurable step up for Arlene, and a strong sign that her treatment program was having an effect.

A couple of months after Dr. Jahan's observations, Arlene's recovery had progressed to the point where she could pull herself out of her wheelchair unassisted, as well as transition from the bed to the wheelchair by herself, a development which meant one less responsibility for her husband. Arlene reported that she had regained bladder and bowel sensations; something that rarely occurs through physical therapy alone. The family noted that Arlene seemed happier, more satisfied with the progress of her recovery and more at peace with her physical situation. The incremental changes in Arlene's physical condition seemed to fuel her motivation; she became determined to succeed in her physical therapy regimen.

Arlene regained her ability to perform many everyday tasks, such as fixing herself a meal, pouring a cup of coffee, and even putting in her own contact lenses. She drove a specially outfitted automobile, and was able to walk brief distances with assistance. Using her index fingers, Arlene was able to type on a computer. For Arlene, these everyday tasks represented a great change from her previous months of helplessness.

The Human Face of SCI — CT's Story

The Russian clinical study team that treated Arlene has used the neural/mesenchymal stem cell combination to treat several other patients from around the world. One such patient, whom we will call CT, was a 25-year-old man from Florida who suffered a spinal cord injury in October 2006. CT was in a car crash that left him with drastically reduced function from his C4 vertebrae down. The C4 vertebra is in the neck, and a spinal cord injury at that location usually results in quadriplegia; he was no exception.

Before receiving a treatment in April of 2008, CT could not perform any basic tasks without assistance. He used the computer and phone through a voice-activated control program; he was mainly confined to his bed or his electric wheelchair. For his wheelchair, he relied on a chin-control mechanism to move. Although CT did have some function below his neck, it was extremely limited.

For many quadriplegics, physical therapy is a long and difficult program that offers minimal gains. However, it is one of the few ways in which SCI patients can attempt to recover some function after their debilitating injury. For CT, the spinal cord injury had interfered with his brain's ability to regulate his blood pressure. If he was placed in an upright position for more than 30 seconds, his blood pressure would drop, and he would pass out. This vasovagal response made it impossible for CT to enroll in any comprehensive physical therapy sessions. Faced with a lack of traditional treatment options, CT enrolled in a stem cell study like the one in which Arlene participated.

After his stem cell transplantation, CT reported an increase in sensation, being able to feel someone holding his hand. He sat straighter; before, his head was slumped to the side, affecting his breathing. With a simple change in posture, he was able to breathe easier, a change that positively affected his oxygen intake. His family and caretakers reported that his stamina, sensory perception, and body awareness had improved. Before the treatment, CT stated that everything below his neck felt "dead." After the treatment, he reported that his body felt alive again. Eventually, he was able to stay in an upright position for up to six to seven hours at a time, a substantial difference from before.

Arlene and CT both received their first stem cell transfers more than a year after their original injury. Although no two patients are alike, it is important to note that they had similar injuries, and both improved as a result of a stem cell treatment using a combination of neural and mesenchymal stem cells. A review of recent scientific breakthroughs regarding our understanding of SCI will explain why.

The Evolving Science of SCI

When scientific researcher Dr. Noelle Huskey's (PhD) brother became paraplegic in 2001, she began studying the uses of stem cells to treat spinal cord injuries. Huskey, who currently conducts studies at University of California, San Francisco, discovered that "Spinal cord injury research represents a new and rising field—more progress has been made in the last five years then in the previous fifty. This sudden success resulted from the new understanding of stem cell technology."[5]

Amazing leaps have been made within the past couple decades. It was in 1995 that a team of Swedish researchers led by Dr. Jonas Frisén (MD, PhD) discovered expression of nestin in rats that had received significant injuries to the central nervous system (CNS), including spinal cord injuries. Nestin, a protein that induces axon growth, is associated with neural stem cells. In fact, nestin's association with neural stem cells is so pronounced that it is often utilized by scientists as a marker to follow the migration of neural progenitor cells. If nestin is present in the CNS, it is usually because neural stem cells are producing the protein. The increased presence of nestin in the CNS after a spinal cord injury, then, is evidence of activation and proliferation of neural stem cells trying to heal the spinal cord. As Frisén's team put it:

Although by no means proven, our data taken together, may suggest the existence of a cell population endowed with progenitor or stem cell qualities which can be identified by virtue of nestin expression and which is recruited to the area of injury.[6]

This cell population, Frisén's evidence suggested, was trying to repair the damage in the spinal cord. His discoveries contributed to

Johansson and Momma's discovery that NSCs were only producing astrocytes after a spinal injury strongly implied that the spinal cord's stem cells are mostly interested in performing "clean-up" operations after a spinal insult.

the mounting evidence against the widespread scientific belief (as noted in chapter 5) that the CNS was incapable of repair.

As with other CNS injuries, the endogenous stem cell response is not strong enough to effect meaningful healing on its own. A later study by Swedish scientists Drs. Carina Johansson (PhD) and Stefan Momma (PhD) provided an explanation for why this is the case in spinal cord injuries. Johansson and Momma were investigating ependymal cells, cells that line the central canal of the spinal cord and are involved in producing spinal fluid. Johansson and Momma discovered that these cells were neural stem cells, but their conclusions did not stop there. Their studies led them "to observe that only astrocytes and not neurons are formed from stem cells in response to injury."[7] Astrocytes are the glial cells whose functions involve producing scar tissue and disposing of the debris of dead cells. Johansson and Momma's discovery that NSCs were only producing astrocytes after a spinal injury strongly implied that the spinal cord's stem cells are mostly interested in performing "clean-up" operations after a spinal insult. What is really needed after a spinal cord injury, however, is neurogenesis, the rebuilding of the neurons in the spinal cord.

In their paper, Johansson and Momma speculated that "the utilization of endogenous stem cells to generate new neurons or glial cells in the treatment of nervous system diseases is therefore a tantalizing possibility."[7] Their hope, that neural stem cells could be coached into producing greater numbers of the correct cell types, has since been realized, but not with endogenous stem cells. Instead, it is *in vitro*-grown stem cells that can be primed into various paths of differentiation.

In most clinical situations, it behooves the patient to have a transplant with as undifferentiated a set of stem cells as possible. That way, it is the patient's own body that gives the stem cells their orders, optimizing the results of their operations in the affected area. And the stem cells already have an understanding of what they are supposed to do. Dr. Joseph Yanai (PhD), a medical scientist at Jerusalem's Hebrew University-Hadassah Medical School, has pointed out that, for example, "stem cell therapies are ideal for treating birth defects where the mechanism of damage is multifaceted and poorly understood."[8] Yanai illustrates that stem cells themselves are very capable in their own right: "they are your little doctors. They're looking for the defect, they're diagnosing it, and they're differentiating into what's needed to repair the defect."[8]

Stem cells themselves are very capable in their own right: "they are your little doctors. They're looking for the defect, they're diagnosing it, and they're differentiating into what's needed to repair the defect."

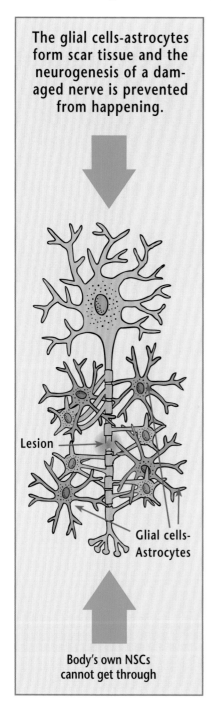

The glial cells-astrocytes form scar tissue and the neurogenesis of a damaged nerve is prevented from happening.

Lesion

Glial cells-Astrocytes

Body's own NSCs cannot get through

In most cases then, stem cells are more than capable of directing themselves, and do not need to be primed into specific differentiation pathways beforehand. A spinal cord injury, however, is not one of those cases. After an SCI, the body's response of producing more astrocytes actually ensures that there will be limited prospects for neurogenesis.

Astrocytes essentially surround the injury site with thick walls of scar tissue, called glial scars. While this protects the injured area from another accident and infection, it essentially walls off the spinal cord lesion from the rest of the body. The axons that were previously connected to the injured area attempt to reach across the site of injury and reestablish the connections of the central nervous system, but they cannot get through the scar tissue. Later in the healing process, neural stem cells that could build new neurons within the injury site are unable to reach the lesion.

In addition, astrocytes express several molecules such as tenascin C and proteoglycans, molecules suspected to be growth inhibitors.[9] These growth inhibitors further ensure a lack of axonal activity around the lesion site, stifling efforts to regenerate the spinal cord's neuronal connections. These factors all help explain why glial scars block neural regeneration.

The increased proliferation of astrocytes after a spinal cord injury, combined with other biological processes designed to prevent the spread of damage from a wound, ends up hurting the body's prospects of recovering neurological function.[9] In order to effect meaningful repair, some researchers believe that stem cells need to get to the spinal cord lesion before it is walled off by glial scar tissue. But the CNS's endogenous stem cells are too busy differentiating into the same astrocytes that are making that scar tissue in the first place, in a somewhat misguided attempt to limit the extent of injury.

A stem cell treatment, with neural stem cells already primed to differentiate into neurons and oligodendrocytes, is what many believe the CNS needs. And through the process of priming, it is possible to cultivate this specific set of stem cells. For this reason, a stem cell treatment might achieve its best results when delivered closer to the time of injury. This may help to restore neuronal connections before significant muscle atrophy sets in.

On the other hand, it is during the acute phase of a spinal cord injury that the affected area experiences extreme inflammation. This inflammatory environment could kill off the transplanted stem cells before they have a chance to engraft themselves within the treated area. Some scientists believe that the optimal treatment window would occur in the sub-acute phase of the spinal cord injury, after the cellular environment has been somewhat stabilized.

The fact that scientists and physicians have not yet determined the exact parameters of the optimal treatment window for spinal cord injury illustrates that there is still much to be learned about stem cells. Educational and research institutions around the world work daily to expand our body of knowledge, so that we may have the answers to these and other unresolved questions. And once these questions are answered, stem cell treatments will have taken one step further along the pathway of translational medicine.

Regenerative Strategies

Arlene and CT received their stem cell treatments more than a year after their original injuries, demonstrating that even with substantial amounts of glial scarring, stem cell transplants may still offer significant improvement to SCI patients. There is encouraging but preliminary evidence that stem cell transplants may induce axons to either circle around the scarred area to re-establish neuronal connections, or "push through" the glial scars and into the spinal cord lesion, apparently through the up-regulation of neurotrophic growth factors. Separate studies have shown that neurotrophic growth factors, such as neurotrophin-3, can cause axons to grow around the site of a spinal cord lesion, and even penetrate several millimeters into the lesion itself, illustrating repair at the very site of injury.[10, 11] Another study, published in *The Journal of Neuroscience*, demonstrated that a similar list of neurotrophic growth factors can promote the proliferation of endogenous oligodendrocytes, the glial cells that are responsible for myelination.[12] Myelination involves the creation of a type of insulation for electrical conduction involving the axons. Without appropriate myelination, these newly formed axons would only be able to transmit electrical impulses at a fraction of their original speed. (Myelination will be discussed further in Chapter 9.)

Stem cells can effect a significant amount of repair to the spinal cord partly because, after an SCI, there is a lot that needs repairing. According to Dr. Fred Gage (mentioned previously) and Dr. Philip Horner (PhD) of the University of Washington's Institute for Stem

Glial Scars

The fact that glial scars interfere with neuroregeneration was noticed as far back as 1928, when Spanish neuroscientist (and Nobel laureate) Santiago Ramón y Cajal noted: "Neither is it rare to see conductors that turn back on encountering the scar, near which they accumulate, forming complicated plexuses, as though the edge of the nerve presented an obstacle that the cones find it very difficult to cross."[10]

Cell and Regenerative Medicine, a CNS injury will set off:

A cascade of events that can lead to neuronal degeneration and cell death... Following a specific traumatic or chemotoxic event, or as a result of ongoing degenerative processes, long-term structural and functional deficits occur in the adult CNS. In severe cases, these insults are not repaired or compensated for by surviving systems. On a cellular level, these deficits include demyelination, degeneration, abortive or aberrant sprouting, and cell death.[14]

Part of the reason all these deficits occur is due to the nature of the injury itself. Any traumatic event to the CNS, such as an SCI, will have a large impact on the afflicted tissue and the surrounding area. Just as in a stroke, the microenvironment of the spinal cord is put into a severe state of imbalance and the injured area of the spinal cord often suffers from cell-killing hypoxia (oxygen deprivation). Also comparable to a stroke, the body's natural immune response after an SCI can worsen the situation. Besides building scar tissue that limits the extent of axonal regeneration, the body's immune response includes an over-mobilization of **phagocytic cells** that end up attacking neuronal cells which would otherwise recover from their damage, and promoting inflammation of the injured area. While inflammation is often a beneficial immune response, swelling of an affected area within the CNS will often put pressure on nearby cells, damaging them.

Multi-Cell Therapy for Spinal Cord Injury

Dr. Ivan Cheng (MD), Assistant Professor at Stanford University School of Medicine, believes that an MSC/NSC combination therapy could potentially be useful in bringing a functional improvement to chronic spinal cord injuries that may not respond as well to single-cell therapy.

The environment where a spinal cord injury occurs becomes a very toxic environment. It is inhibitory towards the survival of pre-existing cells, as well as applied cells. This is an environment which is not ideally conducive to the re-establishment of neural pathways.

The thinking is that mesenchymal stem cells could foster a more favorable environment for healing. If we can apply the mesenchymal stem cells, even intravenously, they could find their way to the site of injury and create a better milieu.

Phagocytic cells: a cell that surrounds and consumes microorganisms and debris, e.g. white blood cells. The consumption process is known as phagocytosis.

We would subsequently apply neural stem cells directly to the site of injury, and these cells would benefit from a better microenvironment.[A]

In the same way that one must remove weeds for a garden to grow properly, the MSCs would clean up the toxic injury site so that the NSCs could better take root. Cheng, a spine surgeon, illustrates some potential clinical situations where multi-cell treatment would be most beneficial:

Patients who come in with multiple injuries, as well as a spinal cord injury, may be unstable from a medical standpoint. We may need to reduce the number of surgeries we perform in the sub-acute or acute phase. It would be fairly straightforward to inject cells intravenously, but then we could bring these patients back at a later time for the surgical application of stem cells directly at the site of the spinal cord injury. Another example would be military personnel who are wounded on the battlefield. It may be impossible to treat them on an acute basis, but once we had them at the right medical facility, then we could proceed with treatment.

Cheng envisions performing multi-stem cell studies in his Stanford laboratory in the near future. He and other scientists hope to uncover more definitive answers regarding the effectiveness of stem cells at different points in the chronology of spinal cord injury. So far, it seems that there may be a window within which administration of stem cells would be best for patient outcomes.

Walking Again?

Horner and Gage explain that the list of regeneration strategies for a CNS injury include "cellular replacement, neurotrophic factor delivery, axon guidance and removal of growth inhibition, manipulation of intracellular signaling, bridging and artificial substrates, and modulation of the immune response."[14] Stem cells have the potential to achieve all of these actions.

Through their effects on the microenvironment, transplanted stem cells can rewire the intracellular signaling mechanisms of the affected area, remove growth inhibition factors and secrete their own set of growth factors. Stem cells also can modulate the immune response, and neural cell-derived oligodendrocytes can help ensure that new axon growth bridges the gap caused by SCI. But the first regeneration strategy, cellular replacement, is perhaps the most

Stem cells have the potential to achieve all of these strategies— "cellular replacement, neurotrophic factor delivery, axon guidance and removal of growth inhibition, manipulation of intracellular signaling, bridging and artificial substrates, and modulation of the immune response."

"The first regeneration strategy, cellular replacement, is perhaps the most exciting use of stem cells for treating SCI, partly because no other type of treatment can create new neurons."

exciting use of stem cells for treating SCI, partly because no other type of treatment can create new neurons.

After an SCI, even if injured axons are repaired and the gap caused by the spinal cord lesion is successfully bridged, there are still dead cells that need to be replaced. As Horner and Gage put it, "No matter how well the lesion is bridged or re-innervated, the target motor neurons that project to the muscles are irrevocably lost."[14]

Stem cells are perhaps the only way to replace dead cells within the CNS. Cheng says, "Stem cells really have a unique ability, not only to home into sites of injury and aid in the survival of injured tissues and cells, but also to differentiate into the necessary tissue in that area."[B]

Cheng was part of a Stanford research team whose results were recently recognized by the Orthopedic Research and Education Foundation, as well as the Orthopedic Research Society, which jointly awarded the team First Place in Basic Science Research at a 2010 research symposium. Cheng and others presented the results of their recent study, entitled "The Acute Transplantation of Human Neuronal Stem Cells Following Spinal Cord Injury."

Cheng explains that the study was designed to apply stem cells to different locations in a rat model of spinal cord injury: "We used an acute rat model, and we were testing to see if we could improve function. We injected Stemedica Technologies' stem cells locally at the site of the injury, and we also applied stem cells intrathecally, distal to the site of the injury." In applying the stem cells distally, in this case towards the lower part of the spine as opposed to directly within the injured portion of the spine, the researchers hoped to learn whether the cells could migrate to the site of the injury and effect repair. "It's been established that these cells have an innate ability to migrate through the cerebrospinal fluid and engraft themselves to sites of injury," Dr. Cheng elaborates, "but previous studies had never attempted to measure functional changes."

By measuring the rat's function, Cheng and his fellow researchers were hoping to discover if distally-applied stem cells would actually help the rats regain sensation and movement. The results? "We saw significant improvement." Dr. Cheng says:

Many of [the rats] were walking again by the end of the six week testing period. We also saw significant improvement for the distal application of cells. Statistically, there was no significant difference. Both sets of rats had a significant functional recovery.

Cheng acknowledges that his own results offer meaning that goes beyond the laboratory: "These are devastating injuries in patients, and it's a situation where they otherwise have little hope of functional recovery. We have promising results that these stem cells will restore these patients' function, and even give them the ability to walk again." And Stanford is just one of the many institutions around the world that is investigating how to better unlock the full potential of stem cell therapy's promise for spinal cord injury patients.

Chapter 8
Traumatic Brain Injury

"I was on a table just flopping around like a fish," former NFL player Kyle Turley confided to sportswriter Michael Silver. "I was fully conscious and knew what I wanted to say, but I couldn't speak... it was definitely the scariest experience of my life."[1]

Turley was referring to his experience in August 2009, when he was rushed to the hospital after passing out and later vomiting uncontrollably. Doctors believed that Turley's condition was a result of the multiple concussions he had received while playing professional football. Turley, faced with the ever-present fear that his mental faculties could degenerate, has become one of the increasingly louder chorus of ex-football players speaking out against the NFL's culture of apathy towards brain injury.

Turley and others have legitimate cause for grievance. The chance that an average 30- to 49- year-old man will develop a memory related disease is 1 in 1,000. For ex-football players of the same age, the chances are 1 in 53.[2] Researchers at the Center for the Study of Traumatic Encephalopathy at Boston University, studying the brains

Tau proteins: found in all cells, however particularly prevalent in axons and neurons, these proteins aid in microtubule construction and stability.

TBI Legislation

The call for new legislation aimed at protecting soldiers from the effects of TBIs echoes the support for a recent bill that hopes to protect youth athletes. The Lystedt Law, which is in effect in Washington state, requires that youth athletes with a concussion or head injury during a game or practice must refrain from participation in the sport until they are cleared by a medical expert.[5]

The bill is named after young athlete Zackery Lystedt, who received a concussion during a 2006 football play. After continuing to play, Zackery suffered a brain hemorrhage and went into a month-long coma. Zackery lived through his experience, but remains partially paralyzed today.

of deceased football players, have noticed that the brains contain irregular build ups of **tau protein** similar to those in Alzheimer's patients (see Chapter 9).

Dr. Ann McKee (MD), the co-director of the Center, explained to CNN in a 2009 interview that the brains she has examined resemble those of an elderly dementia patient. But many of the players who donated their brains were only in their 30s or 40s when they died. One football player was only eighteen. "I knew what traumatic brain disease looked like in the very end stages, in the most severe cases," admitted McKee, "to see the kind of changes we're seeing in 45-year-olds is basically unheard of."[3]

Researchers have a name for the condition that is presumably causing this damage: chronic traumatic encephalopathy, or CTE, a condition that can induce memory loss, reasoning problems, and severe emotional disturbance. Andre Waters, whose brain was donated to Boston University's Center for the Study of Traumatic Encephalopathy, was an NFL defensive back for the Philidelphia Eagles and the Arizona Cardinals. Waters committed suicide in 2006; a neuropathologist from the University of Pittsburgh examined his brain and reasoned that Waters was combating depression brought on by CTE.[4] His is just one case of ex-NFL players struggling with emotional stress attributed to CTE.[3]

Although the study of traumatic encephalopathy is still in its infancy, experts are fairly uniform in their agreement that the major cause of CTE appears to be serial instances of head trauma, a fact that explains why boxers are another segment of the population at risk for the disease. For football players, this head trauma usually occurs in the form of a traumatic brain injury (TBI).

It is not uncommon for an athlete who participates in football or other contact sports to receive a concussion from a blow to the head during a game. A concussion is another name for a mild traumatic brain injury, and it was previously commonly believed that the effects were temporary.

But recent research from the Center for the Study of Traumatic Encephalopathy and others has called this belief into question. Doctors now acknowledge that even a mild TBI may cause symptoms that can last for over a year, symptoms such as memory loss, concentration problems, and even significant emotional problems. A severe traumatic brain injury will often manifest itself in far worse symptoms, including aphasia, loss of perception, seizures, and a host of other physical and cognitive deficits. Traumatic brain injuries can also cause emotional changes, such as aggression or depression. Even if one traumatic brain injury manifests none of these symptoms, TBIs can lead to neurological conditions like CTE farther down the road.

Once one understands how a TBI can occur, it becomes clear why football players are in such danger of receiving these injuries. In the same way that a blow which passes through the bones of the spine can cause a spinal cord injury, a force which passes through the skull will cause damage to the brain. This damage can result in a traumatic brain injury, whether or not the skull actually fractures. The Center for Disease Control and Prevention estimates that 1.5 million people in the United States receive a traumatic brain injury each year. This number includes 50,000 people who will die from such an injury, and 85,000 who will suffer long-term disabilities.[6]

The Brain Goes to War

The top three causes of traumatic brain injury are car accidents, firearm-related injuries and falls. For American servicemen and women currently fighting overseas, there are other potential causes of TBI, including bomb blasts from improvised explosive devices. "Traumatic brain injury," says a 2008 *New England Journal of Medicine* paper, "has been labeled a signature injury of the wars in Iraq and Afghanistan."[7] The paper details the results of a study conducted among over 2,500 soldiers returning from combat. Among their results:

- Approximately 15% of soldiers reported an injury during deployment with loss of consciousness or altered mental status, clinical signs of a traumatic brain injury.

- Mild TBI is strongly associated with **Post-Traumatic Stress Disorder** (**PTSD**) and physical health problems three to four months after injured soldiers return home.

- Soldiers with mild TBI reported significantly higher rates of physical and mental health problems than did soldiers with other injuries.[7]

This study aimed to measure the effects of mild traumatic brain injury. The mental and emotional toll on soldiers with severe TBI is presumably much higher. The numbers of soldiers returning home

Post Traumatic Stress Disorder (PTSD): a psychological, anxiety disorder which may develop after encountering a deeply traumatic event; examples include, but are not limited to, assault, rape, military combat, natural disasters, accidents and illness. The onset of PTSD may not appear for months or even years after the event has occurred. PTSD manifestations may include reexperiencing the traumatic event (nightmares, flashbacks, or other), avoiding stimuli that are or have been associated with the trauma, an overall anesthetizing of emotional response, and a state of hypervigilance.

Traumatic brain injury is the "signature injury" for servicemen and women in the Iraq and Afghanistan wars.

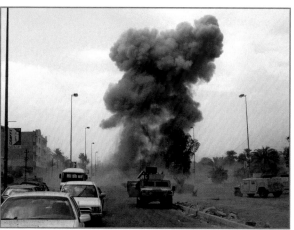

Courtesy of the U.S. Army, SPC Ronald Shaw, Jr.

Nucleus Medical Art/Visuals Unlimited, Inc.

Normal brain

Frontal region
of brain impacts
inner surface
of skull

Head and
neck in
hyper-
extension

A

Occipital region of
brain impacts
inner surface
of skull

Head and
neck in
hyper-
flexion

B

C

Coup contra coup stages
of injury:
A. Head and neck in hyper-
extension with frontal region
impacting the inner surface of
the skull.
B. Head and neck in hyper-
flexion with the occipital
region impacting the skull.
C. Resulting brain damage
to the frontal and occipital
regions of the brain.

with traumatic brain injuries are staggering; the military estimates that over one hundred thousand service members have suffered a TBI since 2002.[8]

American military leadership has been increasingly compelled to acknowledge the serious impact that TBI has on the country's armed forces. In June of 2010, General Peter W. Chiarelli, Army Vice Chief of Staff, appeared before the Senate Armed Services Committee to discuss how the armed forces are dealing with brain injuries and mental health problems. General Chiarelli acknowledged that traumatic brain injury and PTSD have a high rate of co-morbidity. He also mentioned that, of the Army's most severely wounded soldiers, at least 60% are diagnosed with PTSD or TBI.[9]

Statistics like these have led some legislators and journalists to question if the military needs to take a more active approach to dealing with combat-related TBIs. Days before the Armed Services Committee hearing in June, House Representatives Tom Rooney (R-Florida) and Michael McMahon (D-New York) called upon the military to implement legislation that would improve detection of TBI and related injuries, declaring in a joint press release, "our troops and veterans deserve action to improve screening and detection of traumatic brain injuries."[10] Similarly, National Public Radio and *ProPublica* have produced a series of articles alleging that the military has failed to diagnose brain injuries in troops returning from combat, under-representing the severity of the problem.[11] The articles also quoted soldiers who felt their problems were "swept under the carpet," and that the military system is indifferent to their injuries.[12]

The images that these articles depict, of soldiers struggling to return to normalcy after combat-related brain injuries, are poignant: "a sergeant who once commanded 60 men in battle got lost in a supermarket," "a soldier who once plotted sniper attacks could no longer assemble a bird house." The reporters go on to point out that all of the soldiers they spoke to perceived their treatment as inadequate for the severity of their condition.[12]

Given the seriousness of the problem, Representatives Rooney and McMahon are right in calling for better detection efforts for TBI. Soldiers returning home with traumatic brain injury also deserve better treatment options. Stem cell medicine has the potential to be one such option.

An important proof-of-principle study for stem cells and TBI was completed in Russia in 2005.[13] There, doctors used fetal neural and liver-derived hematopoietic (blood) cells to treat 38 patients who had received severe traumatic brain injuries. As a result of their injuries, these patients had fallen into a coma. Traditional therapeutic intervention had done nothing to restore consciousness, and by the time the fetal cells were administered, the patients had been comatose for between five to eight weeks, with no signs of improvement. In fact, the researchers explained, "The probability of the development of a long-term vegetative status was high for all patients."[14]

The doctors treated these patients with the mixture of fetal neural and hematopoietic cells, delivering the cell mixture via lumbar puncture, and then compared the results to a control group of 38 untreated TBI patients who had gone into a similar comatose state. The results were momentous. Among the study's conclusions:

- The death rate in the treated group was 5%, while the death rate in the control group was 45%.

- Using the **Glasgow Outcome Scale (GOS)**, researchers found that 87% of the treated patients had a favorable outcome, as opposed to 39% in the control group.

- Statistical analysis showed improvement of the treated patients compared to the control patients.[13]

The researchers noted that 33 of the 38 comatose patients had received a favorable outcome. What that means, they explained, was that these patients all regained consciousness between three and seven days after the stem cell procedure. Within the next five days after regaining consciousness, the patients were able to contact medical personnel and their families. Functional restoration occurred within two to three weeks of treatment.[13] For the two patients who died, the researchers attributed the cause of death to be "extracranial complications," presumably unrelated to their brain injuries. This is in juxtaposition to the results of the control group, where 17 of the 38 patients died and only 15 had a favorable result.[13]

The researchers, led by Dr. Victor Seledtsov (MD, DSc) of the Institute of Clinical Immunology at the Russian Academy of Medical Sciences, published their results in 2005 and 2006. They expanded on their previous results by conducting a follow-up review of both treated and control patients for four to six years after the stem cell procedure. They found that, for 20 of the 25 treated patients included in the follow-up review, mental status was completely restored one year after the original traumatic brain injury. The researchers

Glasgow Outcome Scale(GOS): a 5-point scale that was used for the general assessment of individuals who had suffered from a TBI. The five classes were: good recovery, moderately disabled, severely disabled, vegetative and dead. There is also an extended version of the scale. GOS, as a succinct description of the patient, has been replaced by the Disability Rating Scale (DRS). However, it is still used in some literature and studies.

33 of the 38 comatose patients regained consciousness between three and seven days after the stem cell procedure.

Karnofsky Performance Status Scale: a performance scale designed by Dr. David A. Karnofsky and Dr. Joseph H. Burchenal in 1949. The system assesses on a scale of 0 to 100 the normal functions of a patient, where 0 is death and 100 is entirely normal functioning.

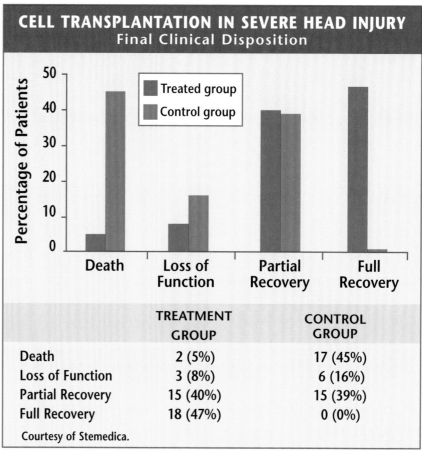

CELL TRANSPLANTATION IN SEVERE HEAD INJURY
Final Clinical Disposition

	TREATMENT GROUP	CONTROL GROUP
Death	2 (5%)	17 (45%)
Loss of Function	3 (8%)	6 (16%)
Partial Recovery	15 (40%)	15 (39%)
Full Recovery	18 (47%)	0 (0%)

Courtesy of Stemedica.

also found that treated patients appeared to have a significantly higher quality of life than control patients, with a difference of 80% to 55% on the **Karnofsky Performance Status Scale**.[14]

Dr. Seledtsov's team studied the results and hypothesized why the cell transplants had been so successful. They surmised that, "since apparent [signs] of recovering of patient's consciousness typically occurred as early as within 7 days after CT [cell transplantation] treatment, the effects of a CT therapy on brain functionality are most likely due to a release by grafted cells of mediators stimulating coordinative work of various brain structures." The researchers continue, "This suggestion is consistent with the published data indicating an ability of neural progenitor cells to elaborate essential neurotrophic factors and promote, thereby, both survival and functionality of degenerating neurons after traumatic brain injury."[13]

The researchers also hypothesized that their treatment was particularly effective because it had utilized cells of both neural and hematopoietic cell lineage. They were thus led to conclude that:

In general, to our opinion, the cell [transplant] composed of various types of stem and progenitor cells may be much more effective in repairing an injured tissue in comparison with the [transplant] consisting only of one type of stem or progenitor cells.[13]

It is an opinion which supports the idea that multi-cell therapy is the most effective mechanism for treating neurological diseases with stem cells.

Seledtsov et al.'s 2005 study helped establish proof-of-principle for clinical studies with stem cells; at the same time, other researchers have been performing pre-clinical studies on animals with TBI. The Neurosurgery Department at the Henry Ford Health Sciences Center in Detroit, for example, has been conducting studies of MSC transplantation in TBI-afflicted rats since 2001. Their animal study, led by neurosurgeon Dr. Asim Mahmood (MD), found that the transplantation led to "a statistically significant improvement in the outcome of MSC-treated rats compared to control rats."[15] Mahmood's research team found that, after the MSCs had been delivered to the brain, the injured rats showed higher expression of three key trophic factors: **nerve growth factor** (NGF), **brain-derived neurotrophic factor** (BDNF), and **basic fibroblast growth factor** (bFGF).

In their paper on the subject, the researchers point out, "These compounds have shown neuroprotective and beneficial effects on the functional outcome in animal studies of ischemia and traumatic brain injury," with NGF being linked to spatial memory retention, BDNF to increased motor function, and bFGF to improved cognitive function.[15] All three trophic factors have also been shown to have histological effects on the brain, helping prevent apoptosis (cell death), reduce the size of lesions, and promote regeneration.[15]

Mahmood et al. (2004) point out that previous studies have consistently acknowledged that bone marrow-derived MSCs have shown functional improvement in rats.[15] It is a paradigm of science that later scientific studies often confirm the results of their predecessors. For Mahmood, whose research spans almost a decade, this is no different. His hypothesis that MSCs are able to induce functional recovery in a TBI model by up-regulating certain growth factors was given additional support by a more recent study.

In 2010, doctors at the Ajou University School of Medicine in Korea published a paper detailing the results of their own animal study, using MSCs to treat a rat model of traumatic brain injury.

Nerve growth factor (NGF): a small protein that is secreted and supports the development of the sensory and sympathetic nervous systems. It is required for the preservation and maintenance of sympathetic neurons.

Brain-derived neurotrophic factor (BDNF): a neurotrophin factor that impacts many neuronal systems by aiding in growth, development and maintenance. It is purported that BDNF may also play a role in cognitive and emotional functioning.

Basic fibroblast growth factor (bFGF): one of several growth factors that promote the proliferation of endothelial cells and angiogenesis.

Endothelial progenitor cells: a rare type of progenitor cell that circulates in the blood and has the ability to differentiate into endothelial cells (the cells that make up the lining of blood vessels.)

They also found that MSC treatment induces expression of neurotrophic growth factors, results which "strongly suggest that the therapeutic effects of hMSC transplantation may involve promotion of anti-apoptotic activity as a result of secreted growth factors."[16] While the Korean team's results disagreed slightly with Mahmood's findings—mostly in concluding that bFGF was not one of the up-regulated neurotrophic factors—the two studies agree that MSCs appear able to provide a therapeutic effect for TBI.[16]

Another study at the Southern Medical University in China was recently completed using **endothelial progenitor cells**, or EPCs, to treat a rat model of traumatic brain injury. EPCs are the cells that differentiate into endothelial cells, the cells that comprise the inner lining of blood vessels. The term progenitor cell is used to refer to EPCs because they have less differentiation capacity than stem cells, being already committed along the endothelial pathway. However, they are similar to other stem cell types not only in their potency but in their ability to secrete growth factors and manifest reparative effects on injured tissue.

Attempting to see if EPCs could promote functional recovery for TBI patients, the Southern Medical team treated rats with EPCs cultivated from adipose (fat) tissue. They found that "these cells participated in adult brain neovascularization, and promoted tissue reconstruction. Transplantation of EPCs resulted in improvement in behavioral performance and reduction of volume of injury cavity."[17]

While pre-clinical trials have gone well, stem cell solutions for TBI have been slow to advance to the clinical stage. In 2005, the University of Texas Health Science Center in Houston began a clinical study of autologous (from same patient) stem cell treatment for traumatic brain injury in children. The trial was completed July 2010; the results have not yet been published. To our knowledge, there are no other clinical studies being conducted for allogenic stem cell-based treatment of traumatic brain injury.

Traumatic brain injury can affect professional athletes, military members, and everyday citizens, alike. Organizations like TraumaticBrainInjury.com exist to help those who are affected by TBI. Meanwhile, legislators, journalists and TBI patients continue to courageously advocate for reform, in professional sports and the military, which would more seriously protect against the effects of traumatic brain injury.

While these efforts are laudable and should unquestionably be supported, there is more that can be done to ease the burden that TBI places on families around the world. Stem cell therapy has impressive proof-of-principle and pre-clinical trial results, indicating that it could provide therapeutic relief for current and future patients. If this country is serious about protecting the mental and physical health of those who serve overseas, among others, then scientific research into traumatic brain injury, including stem cell research, should be made a major priority.

CH's Story

"For CH, the perfect day was a few hours of work, then tennis, a couple rounds of golf, and a game of polo," his wife acknowledges. "He was always very active."

She was referring to her husband, a retired business owner in his early 70s. CH was a self-starter, a successful businessman who loved nothing more than to be out in the sun playing sports. Above all else, his true passion was horses; CH was an expert polo player who had been riding most of his life.

It was on the polo field that he received his traumatic brain injury. In August of 2005, CH was on summer vacation with his family. He was playing a polo match, as he had done hundreds of times before. This time, his horse stumbled and fell, and CH was thrown.

CH was rushed to the nearest hospital, where he stayed for several days, rendered comatose by his fall. The doctors did not need to hear the bystanders' accounts to know that CH had received a serious traumatic brain injury, one that would permanently and significantly affect his brain function. They monitored him closely, waiting for him to wake from his coma. After his condition was stabilized and he regained consciousness, CH was flown to a hospital near his home, where he began the process of rehabilitation.

Originally, CH was unable to admit that anything was wrong. Doctor's reports make it clear that his responses were "quite impoverished and vague," and his memories of his fall were hazy at best. CH insisted that "he was having no problems other than a slight change in his balance."[A] The doctors found themselves speaking to the family, having to ask them what CH's symptoms were. His wife admitted that CH was not participating in conversation, seemingly disengaged from family events. Furthermore, CH was found to be constantly off balance, and his cognition was suffering.

He experienced long-term memory deficits (forgetting his children's ages) and short-term memory problems (being unable to recall what he had eaten for dinner). He spoke less and less, withdrawing from the outside world, partly because he had trouble forming sentences but also as an emotional consequence of his injury.

CH was put on a strict regimen of rehabilitative therapy, but its effect seemed limited. "Dad hated working out," explains his son. "Before the fall, he hadn't worked out a day in his life. He played sports every day! So for him, the idea of staying in one room and lifting weights for an hour was torture."

Realizing that CH was not responding well to traditional therapy, his family looked for other treatment options. They changed CH's therapy regimen while setting up different opportunities to keep him more active. After hearing from friends about stem cell therapy, they began looking into whether it could help CH.

Three months after his treatment, his family noticed the changes. His wife said:

At first he was angrier, because he was more cognizant of all the things he couldn't do. But he later became much more manageable. He was speaking closer to full sentences. He was hearing us shout questions from thirty feet away, in another room, and he was answering. For him this was previously a fairly difficult task.

Building on these improvements, CH's family decided to put him back in the saddle in October of 2009, working with a physical rehabilitation group that uses horseback riding as a mechanism to stimulate their patients. "People couldn't believe the change," his wife declares. "His attitude becomes completely different when he rides." Riding again helped CH manifest improvements in his coordination and focus, and his attitude brightened.

Months later, CH went for another treatment. "His balance is better, he's walking better, and he seems to feel better," his son points out today.

CH's wife agrees. "We've seen him talk more at length, and he's more aware of his surroundings. One of the biggest things, for me, is that he is looking people in the eye again when they speak to him." She also points out that they have stepped up his physical therapy regimen. CH's physical therapist reinforces the importance of aggressive rehabilitative therapy following stem cell treatment.

"The important thing about stem cell therapy is to build on the results with rehabilitation afterwards."

For CH's wife, her only regret was that they did not begin the stem cell regimen sooner. As for CH himself, he is back where he belongs: on the back of a horse. His rehabilitation is still progressing, but with each riding session, CH becomes a little more assertive and self-reliant. Recently, he has started hitting the polo ball again, though it often takes him a few swings to connect. It is possible that the stem cell treatments and aggressive physical therapy have helped CH reconnect with his old passions: a passion for sports, a passion for horses, and a passion for life.

Chapter 9
Parkinson's, Alzheimer's & Other Neurological Conditions

The previous neurological examples—stroke, spinal cord injury and traumatic brain injury—are the result of a trauma to the central nervous system (CNS). In such a situation, stem cells hold the potential to repair injured cells, restore homeostasis to the wounded area, and differentiate into new cells. But stem cells can also be used to treat conditions that do not result from traumatic injury. Conditions such as Parkinson's disease (PD) and Alzheimer's disease (AD) are not the result of a life-altering neurological insult; instead, the body's own cells have an inherent malfunction, resulting in a problem within the CNS.

Parkinson's and Alzheimer's are two well-known examples of this type of condition; they are both prevalent within the general population. Parkinson's disease affects over one million people in the United States alone, with over 50,000 new cases diagnosed each year. The international number is much higher; four to six million people suffer from PD worldwide.[1] Alzheimer's is an even more statistically daunting disease. Approximately 5.3 million Americans have AD.

Researchers Drs. Lamya Shihabuddin (PhD) and Isabelle Aubert (PhD) explain that the two diseases "share a number of characteristics, the most obvious being neuronal loss. Neuronal degeneration eventually leads to devastating cognitive and motor deficits in AD and PD, respectively."[2]

Parkinson's strips people of their ability to move, while Alzheimer's destroys memory and cognition. Parkinson's sufferers have a mortality rate that is two to five times higher than non-PD-affected individuals.[3] Alzheimer's is a fatal disease and is the sixth leading cause of death in the United States.[4]

The toll of destruction from both these conditions goes beyond the mental and physical effects on the patient. In the United States, medical bills for Alzheimer's patients amount to $172 billion a year.[4] This does not include the financial costs of an estimated 9.9 million unpaid caregivers. Meanwhile, PD costs the United States over $26 billion a year in disability costs and lost productivity.[5] These conditions are a serious societal problem, and they are getting worse. The prevalence of Alzheimer's is expected to more than double within forty years, while the societal costs of Parkinson's is expected to increase as the Baby Boomer Generation ages.[4, 5]

The exact cause of both diseases has not yet been determined, but they appear to have a strong genetic component. This makes it difficult for people to protect themselves from the disease through deliberate lifestyle choices. There is currently no effective medical cure for Parkinson's or Alzheimer's, although medications can help control the symptoms and slow the spread of the diseases. Once patients are diagnosed with either PD or AD, they will struggle with the disease for the rest of their lives.

Before we look at how stem cell treatments may offer PD or AD patients the tools to better fight these diseases, let us take a look at how these conditions affect the brain.

Parkinson's disease (PD) is a neurodegenerative condition where neurons within the striatum and the substantia nigra, the parts of the brain responsible for motion and other functions, begin to die off.

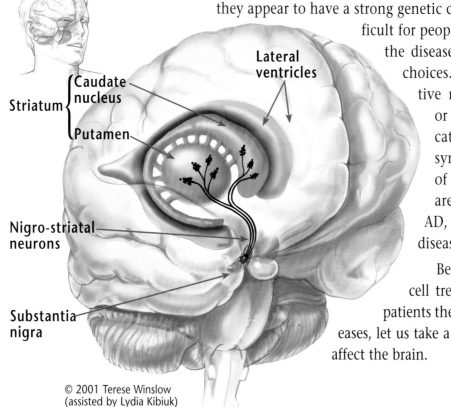

Striatum
Caudate nucleus
Putamen
Lateral ventricles
Nigro-striatal neurons
Substantia nigra

© 2001 Terese Winslow
(assisted by Lydia Kibiuk)

Parkinson's/Alzheimer's: What Goes Wrong

Parkinson's disease (PD) is a neurodegenerative condition where neurons within the striatum and the substantia nigra, the parts of the brain responsible for motion and other functions, begin to die off. The afflicted neurons are usually dopaminergic neurons; they produce the neurotransmitter dopamine.

Dopamine is one of the many neurotransmitters necessary to regulate the proper functioning of the brain. It plays several roles in the brain, but perhaps the greatest involves movement coordination. Other roles include cognition, regulation of the pituitary gland, and focus. If the production of this neurotransmitter is severely depressed, all these behaviors may be affected.

Without dopamine to control movement coordination, the PD-affected brain will lose its ability to control the motions of the body. PD patients will typically suffer from four motor symptoms:

- *Tremor* – Involuntary shaking of the limbs,

- *Rigidity* – Abnormal stiffness in the limbs,

- *Bradykinesia* – The slowing down of voluntary movements, and

- *Postural instability* – The loss of balance.

In addition to these effects, there may be other physical, cognitive, or even emotional symptoms. While the motor symptoms of Parkinson's can be partially controlled through drugs or other therapies, there are currently no options for treating the non-physical manifestations of PD, or counteracting the progression of the disease.[6]

Alzheimer's disease also causes the atrophy of brain cells, but its impact is not focused on the substantia nigra. Instead, AD causes cell death and tissue loss throughout the brain. Over time, this tissue loss becomes even more pronounced, manifesting increasingly more severe symptoms. This cerebral tissue loss is believed to be a result of two issues: the build-up of the protein called beta-amyloid, which causes large plaques that interfere with cell signaling, and the formation of neuronal tangles, which block brain cells from receiving nutrients. Although it is not known what triggers these two processes to occur, they appear to be the prime culprits for the causes of Alzheimer's disease.

As the plaques and tangles spread through the brain, so does the disease. First, cells start dying off in the parts of the brain

Autologous stem cell transfusions "may not be optimal for genetically based diseases—one may be reimplanting adult stem cells that contain the same genetic defect present in the target tissue and with the same susceptibility to degeneration."

responsible for learning, memory, and long-term cognition. As the disease progresses, the damage to affected areas gets worse, and spreads to other parts of the brain. Memory and cognition are further damaged, and speech and spatial awareness may also be affected. By the time the disease draws to its fatal conclusion, the brain has suffered widespread damage. The effects of Alzheimer's are so pronounced that physical changes can be seen in the brain of AD patients. The comparative illustration on page 150 shows how destructive Alzheimer's can be.

Since PD and AD kill off brain cells, researchers are attempting to learn whether infusion of new cells could halt, slow down or even reverse the spread of the disease. For this reason, stem cell therapy has been seen as a promising candidate to treat these debilitating neurodegenerative diseases. But the ultimate goal of stem cell therapy is not merely to add new cells for these diseases to eventually consume; it is to introduce a healthy source of new cells that recognize the faulty neurodegenerative processes and work to combat them. For Parkinson's, producing new dopaminergic neurons might stave off the disease. The best result may come from cells that also can save the endogenous neurons which are in danger of dying. For Alzheimer's, new cells should stop the neurodegenerative processes, not just add an extra layer of cells to be destroyed.

The cells that offer the greatest potential are allogeneic cells. In neurodegenerative diseases, the patient's own brain is somehow malfunctioning and allowing a harmful condition to arise. An autologous stem cell transplant may perpetuate the problem. As American neurologists, Drs. Jeffrey Rothstein (PhD) and Evan Snyder (previously noted), pointed out in their research, autologous stem cell transfusions "may not be optimal for genetically based diseases—one may be reimplanting adult stem cells that contain the same genetic defect present in the target tissue and with the same susceptibility to degeneration."[7] Rothstein and Snyder continue by pointing out that:

An alternative to autografts is the use of established, somatic stem or progenitor cell lines that might serve as 'universal donor cells'. These have the appeal of being homogeneous, stable off-the-shelf reagents, well characterized and maintained under good manufacturing practices, readily available in limitless quantities for the acute phases of an injury or disease and documented to be safe.[7]

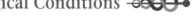

The scientists go on to warn about the issue of immune incompatibility with adult allogeneic cells, a warning that reinforces the importance of proper cultivation and testing techniques for any allogeneic stem cell line.

The principle behind using stem cells to treat PD has been understood as far back as the late 1970s, when researchers used fetal human brain tissue to treat rats with Parkinson's-like conditions. The rats were given induced lesions in their nigrostriatal tissue, so that their brains would take on the same qualities as a human afflicted with PD. In these and subsequent animal studies, the transplants were shown to "reverse or ameliorate impairments" in behaviors caused by PD-like brain damage.[8]

Based on these and other animal studies, fetal cell grafts were used to treat patients in 1987.[8] Most of the grafts were placed within the putamen, a part of the striatum which is also greatly interconnected with the substantia nigra; in Parkinson's, the putamen is one of the areas where dopamine-producing neurons die off in great numbers.

Several studies reported that the patients benefitted from the grafts, with some patients even withdrawing from their **L-dopa** regimen.[9] L-dopa is a drug used to supplement the naturally-occurring dopamine production of PD patients; a patient withdrawing from L-dopa marks a superb clinical result.

Swedish neuroscientists Drs. Olle Lindvall (PhD) and Anders Björklund (MD, PhD) reviewed the results of several of these studies. They concluded that the fetal grafts were inducing symptomatic relief for PD patients, although clinical outcomes varied. They wrote, "Human fetal mesencephalic DA (dopamine) neurons survive transplantation into the brain of PD patients. Significant increases of FD uptake in the grafted striatum have been observed in several studies, and in one patient, uptake was normalized after transplantation."[9] By FD uptake, the neuroscientists are referring to fluorodopa, dopamine that is "tagged" with fluorine so that it will show up on brain scans.

What does FD mean?

Lindvall and Björklund went on to explain that:

Histopathological analyses have confirmed survival of the dopaminergic grafts and demonstrated their ability to reinnervate the striatum… The grafts can also restore regulated release of DA in the striatum… [and] the fetal DA neuron grafts can become functionally integrated into neural circuitries in the PD patient's brain.[9]

Levodopa (L-dopa or L-DOPA): an isomer of dopa (a compound generated by the oxidation of tyrosine) that has been used in the treatment of Parkinson's disease for approximately 30 years. It is administered orally and converted into dopamine by dopaminergic neurons using dopa-decarboxylase.

These various positive results, drawn from approximately 350 patients who received fetal cell grafts, were considered "proof-of-principle," evidence that cell therapy as a concept offered a meaningful treatment option for Parkinson's. But fetal brain tissue is not a realistic wide-spread treatment option, whereas neural stem cells can be primed to be dopaminergic. These neural cells have the potential to restore dopamine production and slow the progression of Parkinson's.

But, the best Parkinson's treatments will require more than just neuronal replacement. The hope is that allogeneic stem cell transplants will not just create new cells, but through their immunomodulatory properties and trophic growth factors, also stop the neurodegenerative disease from progressing. Olle Lindvall explains in a paper with fellow Swedish neuroscientist, Dr. Zaal Kokaia (PhD), that with PD:

Stem cell-based approaches could be used to provide therapeutic benefits in two ways: first, by implanting stem cells modified to release growth factors, which would protect existing neurons and/or neurons derived from other stem cell treatments; and second, by transplanting stem cell-derived DA neuron precursors/neuroblasts in the putamen, where they would generate new neurons to ameliorate disease-induced motor impairments.[6]

GR's Story

A 56-year-old man, whom we will refer to as GR, had retired from the real-estate business and maintained an active lifestyle. He rode horses, skied in the winter, and often went on long hikes across the Montana countryside. With his active lifestyle, GR was used to waking up with sore muscles and perhaps even a headache. But in August of 2003, he woke up with something else: a tremor in his left hand. GR was quickly diagnosed as being in the early stages of Parkinson's disease.

Before his first treatment in November of 2006, GR's condition had progressed, and he was manifesting several classic PD symptoms, including bradykinesia, as well as rigidity and tremors along his left side. GR was not taking traditional medication for his PD; he feared that the side effects would further impinge upon his quality of life. Instead, he was taking a second-tier medication that, while still offering some symptom relief, was less effective than many other medication options.

GR underwent a stem cell treatment, and for a month, his tremors essentially disappeared. But there were setbacks unrelated to the stem cell treatment; GR contracted pneumonia and was hospitalized for several weeks. Soon after, GR was thrown off a mule he was riding and was hospitalized for a second time. The attending surgeon said that GR was lucky to be alive.

After recovering from this last setback, GR had his second stem cell transfusion seven months later. He received another injection of neural and mesenchymal stem cells. A week after his second treatment, GR reported the disappearance of his tremor and rigidity, and continued to state that his tremors were stabilized for several months thereafter.

Nine months later, however, he informed his physicians that his tremors had started to recur. Over the next three months, his tremors progressively increased. He confided to his friends that he felt he should have had another treatment three months before, to maintain his asymptomatic status. His tremors and rigidity, although not as severe as before, were still bothering him.

GR received a third treatment. A week later, he indicated that his tremors had again disappeared, along with the rigidity. And again, for several months after, he described his PD symptoms as being significantly diminished.

GR's fourth treatment differed from his previous treatments in one important respect. Parkinson's primarily affects dopaminergic neurons, which meant that GR might benefit more from a set of these particular cells. GR's previous treatments consisted of undifferentiated NSCs; this time, half of the NSCs were primed to differentiate into dopaminergic neurons, while the other half remained completely undifferentiated.

For approximately a month and a half after his fourth treatment, GR was entirely asymptomatic. In late February of 2009, he reported that his tremors had gradually returned, but he could stop them at will. His shaking was also much less intense, and he had reduced the amount of drugs he was taking to control his symptoms. He and his wife stated that these were the best results thus far, and that this treatment seemed to take effect faster than the previous two.

In June of 2009, GR received a deep brain stimulation (DBS) procedure, where surgeons placed a medical device within his brain.

GR believes that the stem cell treatments were a major part of his ability to control the advancement of this degenerating disease.

The medical device, called a "brain pacemaker," sends electrical impulses to the affected parts of the patient's brain and has had success in mitigating the symptoms of PD. GR reports that he is receiving half the voltage levels of other patients with comparable results. He has also exclaimed his amazement at feeling "as good as I did pre-diagnosis 7 years ago," while watching others from his Parkinson's support group further degenerate in their condition.[A, 10]

GR believes that the stem cell treatments were a major part of his ability to control the advancement of this degenerating disease. Admittedly, GR was also on a pharmaceutical regimen, as well as deep brain stimulation; therefore, it is impossible to attribute a specific percentage of GR's success to his stem cell regimen. However, the ability for GR to continue his active athletic lifestyle, seven years after being diagnosed with Parkinson's, illustrates a result not often achieved with traditional medical approaches alone. GR's pattern of asymptomatic expression of PD for an amount of time after each stem cell transfusion strongly suggests a causal link.

This clinical result rests on top of decades of scientific studies that demonstrate the "proof of principle that neuronal replacement can work in PD patients."[6] If more patients participate in clinical studies, advances can be made in our understanding of:

- What mechanisms of action stem cells use to combat PD,
- What level of efficacy we can expect from stem cell treatments,
- How specialized the NSC cells used to treat PD should be, and
- What treatment intervals will ensure an optimal result.

These are questions that subsequent scientific and clinical research has yet to fully answer. But years of groundwork have already been laid, and isolated Parkinson's patients have already benefited from approved clinical study treatments.

Parkinson's: An Argument for Periodic Treatment

GR noticed that an interval of eight to nine months between treatments was best for controlling his tremors and rigidity. GR's results mirror those of patients in a clinical study performed at the neurology departments of three different hospitals within Russia in the 1990s.

Eighty-six patients with Parkinson's participated in this study, which aimed to treat PD with fetal brain cells. Of these patients, twenty received stem cells introduced into the spinal fluid by lumbar injection.

In the Russian study, "the follow-up of patients showed that there was a decrease in illness severity in all patients, as well as in motor disturbances to different extents."[11] This is consistent with GR's results. Also in accordance with GR's results was the interesting fact that "improvement was seen in these patients for 6-9 months after the procedure, and then an increase in severity [of the condition] was observed."[11] The doctors concluded, "The follow-up of patients after the intralumbar transplantation showed that [improvement was noted] in all patients from the first month after the procedure on average for 6-10 months. This was evident in a decline in disease severity."[11]

The cell transplants seemed to reduce the severity of disease for a while, but then patients slowly lost their neurological gains over a period of time. This is consistent with our understanding of neurodegenerative diseases, which continue to progress over time. In these cases, the stem cell transplants appear to successfully effect neurological change for a matter of months. But these transplants are not a cure; Parkinson's continues its degenerative influence even after the cells have fully engrafted. And while the cells release neurotrophic factors to slow the disease's progression, Parkinson's is a fearsome adversary.

Part of the problem may be that PD spreads its pathology to the engrafted neurons, so that even new brain cells eventually succumb to it. Fortunately, this takes time to occur; several independent studies have shown that, while PD can spread into new neurons, "propagation of pathology would take time to develop in graft."[12] The concern that PD might affect transplanted cells is greater in an autologous transplant, which "carries the risk of developing pathology after transplantation due to any genetic deficiency that is carried by PD patients."[12]

It may be that NSC transplants keep patients' dopaminergic cells above a certain threshold of cells needed to function. We know that "clinical symptoms of PD do not manifest until 60-80% of dopamine neurons degenerate."[12] Part of the stem cell therapy's apparent success could be explained by an ability to keep the number of degenerated neurons below that percentage.

Preliminary results suggest an optimal model of stem cell therapy for PD; a treatment every nine months might effectively stave

"Clinical symptoms of PD do not manifest until 60-80% of DA neurons degenerate."

off progression. For GR, it was a matter of several months before his tremors manifested at levels approaching his pre-treatment state. PD patients, then, could benefit from a continuing treatment regimen. In the same way that a cancer patient is tested periodically in order to make sure the cancer does not resurge, a PD patient could hypothetically receive an infusion on a periodic basis to maintain a symptom-free or symptom-lessened state. Similarly, those who are at genetic risk for Parkinson's could receive stem cell treatments before manifesting symptoms, keeping dopaminergic neurons at functional levels and preventing their genetic tendency for Parkinson's from ever developing into active disease.

Alzheimer's

Alzheimer's (AD) is another disease in which the use of stem cell technology still poses many scientific challenges. Alzheimer's is the most common form of **dementia** (a blanket term for loss of cognitive function). Since different forms of dementia manifest the same symptoms, it is often difficult to determine whether a patient is suffering from Alzheimer's, or a different form of dementia.

The problem is compounded by the fact that the cause of AD is still debated. The predominant hypothesis involves tangles and plaques in and around the neurons, which are caused by protein abnormalities.[13] The plaque build-up is composed of beta-amyloid (A-beta, amyloid-ß or Aß) proteins, while the tangles result from a malfunction in the tau protein. To date, medical science has been unable to accurately explain how these malfunctions ultimately cause AD.

Recent scientific studies have pointed to the role that stem cells may play in treatment of AD. A 2008 study led by Drs. Jong Kil Lee (PhD), Hee Kyung Jin (DVM, PhD) and Jae-sung Bae (DVM, PhD) of the Stem Cell Neuroplasticity Research Group at Kyungpook National University in South Korea, found that

The brain of a normal person shown above. Note the shrinkage and destruction of an Alzheimer's brain below.

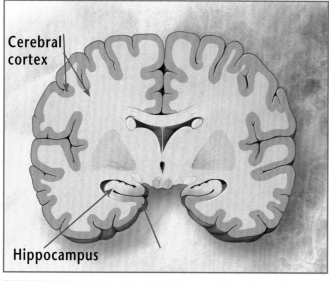

Cerebral cortex

Hippocampus

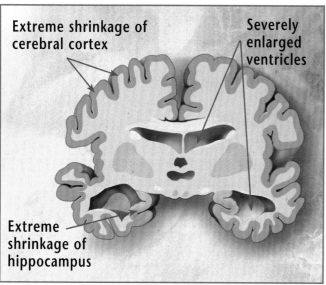

Extreme shrinkage of cerebral cortex

Severely enlarged ventricles

Extreme shrinkage of hippocampus

intra-cerebrally delivered MSCs can reduce the amount of A-beta in the brain. In order to test the effect of MSCs on Alzheimer's, the researchers injected A-beta into the brain of several mice, artificially inducing an AD-like condition. Later, they injected bone marrow-derived MSCs (BM-MSCs) into the injured area. They compared their results to a control group that received only peripheral blood (PBS) or dead cells:

> *The levels of Aß deposition could not be detected [emphasis added] at 7 days BM-MSCs post-transplantation in an acutely induced AD model, but the levels of A-beta deposition in PBS or dead-cell treated mice remained high.[14]*

Examining their results, the researchers concluded that the MSCs had reduced the A-beta deposits in the brain. It is a promising result, but how did it work? The researchers noticed their findings "demonstrated that BM-MSCs transplantation seems to strongly induce endogenous microglia/macrophage activation rather than differentiation of microglia/macrophages from BM-MSCs."[14] The researchers concluded that this was most likely the effective mechanism of action; the MSCs had stimulated the microglia within the brain to act against the malfunctioning A-beta plaques.

This is another example of the Chaperone Effect at work; transplanted stem cells induce endogenous cells to "wake up" and respond more forcefully to the body's condition. Microglia, the immune cells of the central nervous system, are able to devour broken or malfunctioning material and clean up the brain. With AD, microglia appear to be uniquely able to eliminate the plaques, formed by broken fragments of A-beta, which clog inter-neuronal pathways.[15]

In the 2008 study, the MSCs were introduced directly into the brain, bypassing the blood brain barrier (BBB), which keeps outside cells from entering the central nervous system. But other studies have shown that MSCs can cross the BBB and even differentiate into perivascular microglia, one of the three types of microglia.[15] Other studies have demonstrated the brain's microglial reaction can be stimulated by immune cells that surround the BBB, or that cytokines in the blood stream can activate a CNS immune response.[15] Furthermore, bone marrow-derived cells, upon crossing into the CNS, "are preferentially attracted to regions afflicted by neurodegeneration or neurological insults."[15] These studies illustrate that MSCs do not have to be placed directly within the brain in order to affect a clinical result for AD patients.

Dementia: with a variety of forms and types, dementia is a generally progressive condition which is noted with a loss in mental abilities, including, but not limited to, impairment of memory, aphasia, and an inability to perform or initiate complex tasks.

Testing for Alzheimer's
On January 20, 2011, an advisory committee to the Food and Drug Administration (FDA) unanimously approved a brain scan test created by Avid Radiopharmaceuticals.

This brain scan is the first test that is capable of showing plaques in live Alzheimer's patients. Prior to this technology, the only way to know if plaques were present was during autopsy.[16]

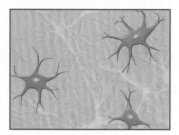

Normal

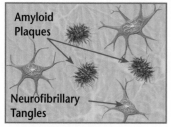

Alzheimer's

Amyloid Plaques- accumulation of amyloid plaques between nerve cells (neurons) in the brain. Amyloid is a general term for protein fragments that the body produces normally. In a healthy brain, these protein fragments are broken down and eliminated. In Alzheimer's disease, the fragments accumulate to form hard, insoluble plaques.

Neurofibrillary tangles are insoluble twisted fibers found inside the brain's cells. These tangles consist primarily of a protein called tau, which forms part of a structure called a microtubule. The microtubule helps transport nutrients and other important substances from one part of the nerve cell to another. In Alzheimer's disease, however, the tau protein is abnormal and the microtubule structures collapse.

MSCs are able to both stimulate endogenous microglial cells and differentiate into microglial cells as well, and "in the case of AD, increasing the infiltration of blood-derived microglial cells seems to be a good therapeutic approach since they are able to eliminate or prevent the formulation of ß-amyloid deposits."[15]

The scientific consensus on the role of microglial cells in AD pathology is far from uniform. We have already explained that sometimes these cells can make a neurological condition worse; in the case of a stroke, for instance, their effects need to be modulated. Similarly, some studies have "demonstrated that Aß can activate microglia to produce cytokines and neurotoxins, hence promoting degeneration."[17] Other studies "have suggested that microglia are actually beneficial by secreting neurotrophic agents and eliminating toxic Aß by phagocytosis."[17] It is not surprising to any neuroscientist that the same cell type can have wildly different and sometimes contradictory effects when dealing with a neurological condition. Some researchers have even hypothesized that different types of microglia may play various beneficial or detrimental roles at different points in the pathology of AD.[15]

With such a diversity of viewpoints, it was vitally important to confirm that MSC transplantation, which seemed to stimulate endogenous microglial cells, was actually benefiting an AD-afflicted brain. For this reason, the Korean team of researchers who studied BM-MSCs effect on beta-amyloids in 2008 released a follow-up report in 2010. The researchers explained that "based on this somewhat contradictory literature, we decided to examine the relationship of elevated microglia BM-MSC-transplanted AD mice and decreased Aß deposits in more detail."[17]

In this subsequent report, the researchers confirmed their previous findings:

Our results suggest that BM-MSCs enhance Aß clearance by increasing the levels of Aß-degrading enzymes secreted by microglia... In agreement with other reports, our results demonstrate that plaque-associated alternative activated microglia produced following BM-MSC transplantation could reduce Aß toxicity.[17]

Beyond confirming that MSCs induced microglia to protect the brain against Aß-buildup, the new report found that MSC transplantation also helped with the other suspected causal factor of Alzheimer's (neuronal tangles caused by malfunctioning tau proteins). The study found that "compared with PBS-treated mice [control group injected with dead blood cells], both the cortex and hippocampus exhibited a significant decrease of 35% and 39%, respectively" of malfunctioning tau proteins.[17]

The discoveries did not stop there. By conducting memory and learning exercises on the treated mice, the researchers also proclaimed that "the results indicated that BM-MSC transplantation is able to reduce the cognitive impairment of spatial memory associated with the accumulation of Aß peptide."[17]

While MSC transplantation can mitigate the advancement of Alzheimer's in an animal model, neural stem cell transplants can be used to replace the neurons that have already been lost. A 2009 study conducted by scientists at the University of California, Irvine declared, "NSC transplants in the hippocampus of animals with Aß plaques and neurofibrillary tangles survive (at least for 1 month) and rescued spatial learning and memory deficits via brain-derived neurotrophic factor (BDNF) related mechanisms."[18, 19] BDNF, a neurotrophic factor, has been shown to rescue neurons and improve compromised cognitive function.[20] By up-regulating BDNF, transplanted neural stem cells can help save dying endogenous neurons. This is in addition to their own abilities to differentiate into new neurons, to replace those that have died off.

Unfortunately, it seems that the NSCs themselves cannot undo the tangles and plaques that are causing neurons to die; the same research that demonstrates the possibility of NSCs affecting rescue of dying neurons also "suggest[s] that increasing BDNF's levels is unlikely to reverse Aß pathology."[19] A 2010 review of previous studies concluded, "For short-term treatments, BDNF-based therapies could be beneficial to rescue neurons and cognitive functions. For longer treatments over the course of the disease with increasing Aß pathology, BDNF and anti-Aß therapies may need to be combined for optimal efficacy."[19]

These results add support to the therapeutic potential of multi-cell therapy. In the case of AD, a combined regimen of NSCs and MSCs may deliver a more beneficial result than a single-cell treatment. The NSCs work to replace dead neurons and rescue dying ones through differentiation and up-regulation of neurotrophic factors, while MSCs fight Aß and tau pathology, slowing the progression of the disease.

In the case of AD, a combined regimen of NSCs and MSCs may deliver a more beneficial result than single-cell treatment. The NSCs work to replace dead neurons and rescue dying ones through differentiation and up-regulation of neurotrophic factors, while MSCs fight Aß and tau pathology, slowing the progression of the disease itself.

RH's and KM's Stories

RH started losing his memory at 73. His Alzheimer's disease advanced for almost two decades before he received stem cell treatment. RH was extremely forgetful, constantly disoriented, and could not accurately answer questions about his past. He slept

Looking Good Versus Doing Well

One of the reasons that may explain the failure of early studies treating neurological conditions with NSCs has to do with the dilutive effect of multiple stem cell passes. The cells look good, acquire markers, but they do not function properly.

A Stemedica funded study, conducted at the Institute of Developmental Biology in Moscow and independently reviewed at the University of Lausanne has demonstrated the potentcy of fetal stem cell-derived neurons produced by Stemedica. It was shown that the cells: 1. produced electrical potential, 2. transferred this potential to another cell and, most importantly, 3. released the appropriate neurotransmitters. The after photo below shows florescence transfer as a result of these three steps.[21]

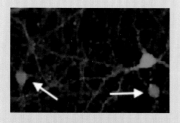

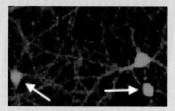

Image courtesy of Stemedica.

for much of the day, he was disengaged from daily living, and he required constant supervision. RH received his first and only stem cell treatment at the age of 89.

The day after his first treatment, RH reported a renewed clarity in his brain. Other patients, treated for different neurological disorders, have reported the same feeling of a "fog lifting."

After the treatment, RH's balance improved, and his attention span also showed great improvement. RH began completing daily crossword puzzles, an activity usually precluded by AD patients' decreased attention spans. His sleeping schedule stabilized, and his daughter could now leave the house for a few hours at a time without worrying about him. His improvements included an enhanced ability to perform daily tasks. He was more focused on his surroundings, and manifested improved balance.

An amusing anecdote on RH's part demonstrates the fact that, although his memory had not materially changed, his ability to function normally had improved. RH had previously lived in a town 180 miles from his daughter's home. One day, he decided to visit his old home, driving his car without his daughter's knowledge. RH made the 180-mile trip without incident, despite the fact that he had not driven in several years.

While the incident was a scare for RH's daughter, it is remarkable that someone who had suffered from Alzheimer's for almost two decades could drive three hours, from one specific location to another, successfully.

RH's road trip also helps illustrate the fact that the family of a neurodegenerative patient is often profoundly affected by the disease. This was evident, in a far more serious manner, with KM, a 75-year-old woman whose dementia caused her to lash out at her loved ones. KM's family had noted for a while that her memory was slipping. She began forgetting where she was born, where she lived, even who she was. As the years went by, KM's dementia worsened. She began neglecting her appearance, exhibiting aggressive behavior, and becoming unresponsive to requests by family and friends.

Dementia is often linked with behavioral disorders; in fact, it is estimated that noncognitive mental and behavioral issues affect approximately three-fourths of dementia sufferers.[22] Aggression, in particular, has been estimated to affect 15-20% of all dementia patients.[23, 24] Other behavioral symptoms include depression and apathy. In KM's case, it was clear that her dementia was wreaking havoc not only on her cognition, but her emotions, and her relationship with her loved ones.

In 2006, KM received her first stem cell treatment. KM's case was a complicated one; she was officially diagnosed with Alzheimer's, but her doctors suspected that she also had vascular dementia. Vascular dementia, the second most common type of dementia behind Alzheimer's, is caused when blood flow to parts of the brain is impaired, depriving brain cells of oxygen.

Experts have increasingly begun to realize that vascular dementia and Alzheimer's often occur in the same patient. The evidence comes from brain autopsies which have shown that up to 45% of people with dementia have signs of both Alzheimer's and vascular disease.[25] To describe a patient with vascular dementia and Alzheimer's, doctors use the term **mixed dementia**. The Alzheimer's Association urges doctors to suspect mixed dementia if an Alzheimer's patient has cardiovascular issues, since the causes of vascular dementia can almost always be traced back to a problem with blood flow to the brain. In KM's case, her physicians noted that she had underlying cardiac disease.

Many of the drugs approved to treat Alzheimer's have shown a similar benefit in addressing vascular dementia. Likewise, a stem cell treatment for KM's Alzheimer's may hold the potential to treat her vascular dementia. In the same way that stem cells can improve the cellular microenvironment after a stroke and prevent cell apoptosis through the Chaperone Effect, KM's cell treatment could strengthen blood flow and undo hypoxia in oxygen-starved areas of the brain, while also treating her Alzheimer's. At least, that was what her doctors hoped would occur. That June, KM received her stem cell treatment, and her family waited to see the results.

The results of her two different PET scans are shown on page 156. Color denotes metabolic activity; blue and green areas of the brain are inactive, while red and orange areas of the brain are active. Essentially, the more blue/green a PET scan shows, the less brain activity is occurring. Conversely, the more orange/red seen, the more evidence there is that the brain has increased activity.

Before her treatment, KM's PET scans revealed a pronounced lack of metabolic activity; the dementia had essentially shut off some portions of the brain. The second set of PET scan images, taken two months after KM's treatment, showed significantly more activity, even in areas of the brain that previously were unable to function.

Mixed dementia: a form of dementia that involves both Alzheimer's and vascular dementia. Mixed dementia becomes more common with advanced age.

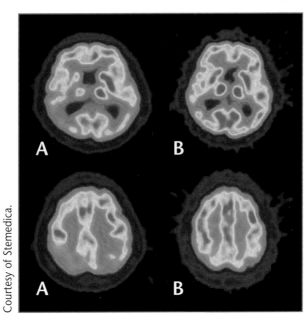

KM's PET images before (A) and two months after (B) stem cell treatment. The increase in orange/red shows more brain activity.

If the results of the PET scan were remarkable, the changes in KM's behavior were even more striking. Speaking to the doctors, KM's granddaughter exclaimed, "It's like night and day... her memory has been restored and she's self-sufficient. Now she's cooking, washing clothes and doing household chores." KM's memory improved soon after her treatment. After the treatment, KM required significantly less supervision and regained a greater degree of independence and well-being. Her unresponsive and sometimes aggressive behavior towards others ceased. She was able to completely recognize her family, friends and caretakers, and she no longer required their assistance full-time.

Today, KM's family is able to enjoy more quality time with her, thanks to the cognitive and behavioral gains she achieved after her stem cell treatment. As for RH, he passed away three years after one treatment, from natural causes. He was 92. RH went from requiring constant supervision to regaining many of his activities of daily living, from being unengaged in the outside world to more fully participating in events with his loved ones. As our understanding of Alzheimer's (and other dementia types) advances, and as we learn more about how stem cells interact with the AD-afflicted brain, we hope to have a better understanding of how stem cells can effect even more repair. But even so, current clinical results indicate that patients may be able to increase their quality of life after these treatments.

Other Neurological Conditions

Cerebral Palsy (CP)

"My mother was in labor for at least 27 hours," explains GA, speaking to us from her home in Southern California. "This was before fetal monitoring. I was born eight weeks early while my mom was sick with a staph infection."

For GA, the circumstances of her birth help explain why she has cerebral palsy, a condition with which she has struggled for her entire life. Cerebral palsy is an umbrella term for a group of symptoms and syndromes that affect the brain and nervous system, causing a series of physical and cognitive disabilities. The condition is characterized by abnormal brain development within the first two years of life. Cerebral palsy is not progressive, but it is life-long, and there is no known cure.

There is no typical cerebral palsy patient; each person may suffer from a host of disorders. GA, for example, had suffered from cerebral palsy all her life, and at 49, she manifested the following symptoms:

- Nystagmus, or involuntary eye movements,
- Swollen ankles,
- Uncontrolled muscle spasms, including flailing arms,
- Dizziness,
- Headaches,
- Chronic joint pain,
- Leg cramps, and
- Lower extremity paralysis.

For GA, the worst symptoms of her cerebral palsy were the spasms; the muscles of her body would suddenly contract uncontrollably, robbing her temporarily of control of her movements and leaving her in pain. "I was told to count my spasms," GA explains. "After 15 minutes, when I got past 20 spasms I would quit counting."

GA's cerebral palsy was so severe that she had surgery to release her tendons and ease the pressure on her joints. Many CP patients look into surgery to relieve some of the pain and to increase movement, but, as a result of her CP, GA went through more than the average number of operations. All in all, GA had undergone 38 surgical procedures in order to reduce the symptoms of her condition. A few years ago, GA decided "I was getting too old to go through all those surgeries any more. It was too much stress on my body."

GA started making some changes to her life in 2008. She began a medically supervised diet that would lead her to lose over 60 pounds. In August of that same year, GA received a stem cell treatment. She reported a significant decrease in her muscle spasms, and also improved her balance and the fluidity of her movements. Before her treatment, she was having approximately 25-30 spasms every 40 minutes. After her treatment she demonstrated long-term improvement with her spasms; more than a year later, she was having only 3-4 spasms an hour. "It's huge for me," GA explains, "that I can go places and not have my legs jerk uncontrollably and have people see that. It's been fantastic."

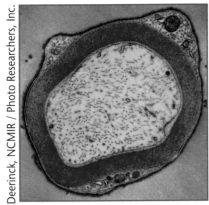

Myelinated nerve. Colored transmission electron micrograph (TEM) of myelinated nerve fibers and Schwann cells. Myelin (red) is an insulating fatty layer that surrounds nerve fibers (axons, yellow), increasing the speed at which nerve impulses travel. It is formed when Schwann cells wrap around the fiber, depositing layers of myelin between each coil. The outermost layer consists of the Schwann cell's cytoplasm (green) and is known as the neurolemma or sheath of Schwann.

Thomas Deerinck, NCMIR / Photo Researchers, Inc.

GA also reported a decrease in overall muscle pain, from 6/10 to 4/10 in a subjective pain rating scale. Her leg strength improved, as did her balance and her aerobic conditioning. Another unexpected benefit, GA mentions, was that "I'm now an inch and a half taller than before. That's not because I've grown. My muscles have relaxed to the point where I can pull myself up into a straighter position."

GA attributes her ability to "still walk, drive, and ferry my two boys around" to the combined results of her new health regimen and her stem cell treatment.[B] She points out, "I'm 50 years old. In the cerebral palsy world, I'm a senior citizen. Most people my age right now, with my condition, are in assisted living." For GA, stem cell treatments may have helped keep her from that outcome.

Huntington's Disease (HD)

Huntington's disease, a genetic neurodegenerative disorder, is caused by abnormalities in the "Huntingtin" gene which eventually results in damage to specific regions of the brain. Although the genetic component of Huntington's means that stem cell treatments would be more effective in mitigating the disease than in treating it, some researchers believe that Huntington's is an especially compelling candidate for stem cell therapy. Neuroscientist Dr. Steven Goldman (MD, PhD), of the University of Rochester Medical Center, has argued "While the promise of stem cells is broadly discussed for many diseases, it's actually conditions like Huntington's—where a very specific type of brain cell in a particular region of the brain is vulnerable— that are most likely to benefit from stem cell-based therapy."[26]

Goldman is one of the researchers who has looked into using brain derived-neurotrophic factor (BDNF) to treat Huntington's. His team received promising results in a 2007 animal study that used BDNF and a neural induction protein to activate new neuron growth in the brain.[27] BDNF, notably, is one of the neurotrophic factors that can be up-regulated through stem cell therapy.

Another study conducted with five Huntington's disease patients showed improvement with fetal neural grafts. Three of the five patients treated showed a "striking recovery observed at 2 years in frontal and prefrontal cortices [which] persisted over time."[28] In another clinical trial where fetal neural cells were used, the patient's brain was autopsied after death and it was noted that "the disease [did] not appear to induce HD-like neurodegeneration within the cell implant."[29] These results may suggest that the transferred fetal brain tissue remained free of the effects of Huntington's disease. These clinical studies hint at a therapeutic result that could be achieved with stem cells.

Multiple Sclerosis & ALS

Multiple sclerosis (MS), the most common of the demyelinating diseases, affects approximately 400,000 individuals in the United States and about 85,000 in the United Kingdom.[30] It is estimated that the annual U.S. healthcare costs for this disease are $6.8 billion; European costs run almost twice this amount.[31]

The pathology of MS is complex and not well understood. The condition results when the immune system attacks the protective myelin sheath around the nerve fibers of the central nervous system. Myelin and Schwann cells are` responsible for the rapid transmission of the neural impulses; in MS, the myelin eventually becomes destroyed and is replaced by scar-like tissue.

The optimal stem cell-based clinical treatment would presumably aim to repair the myelin sheath, while modulating the deviant immune response. Dr. Divya Chari (PhD), lecturer for the School of Medicine at Keele University in England, pointed out that several stem cells and other precursor cells are able to achieve significant remyelination, including **oligodendrocyte precursor cells, olfactory ensheathing cells** (progenitor cells found within the inside of the nose), neural stem cells, and bone marrow-derived stem cells.[25] Furthermore, NSCs and MSCs are known to induce anti-inflammatory effects, and stem cell treatments can also reduce glial scarring around the injured tissue which would prevent subsequent repair. For demyelinating diseases, it is hoped that transplanted NSCs could differentiate into new oligodendrocytes, the cells which work to produce new myelin, in order to repair previous damage.

Most recently, a research team led by Dr. Neil Scolding (MD, PhD), of the University of Bristol, presented promising Phase I safety data with a small group of six MS patients. The group members were treated with autologous bone marrow cells without previous immunosuppressive preconditioning. Each of the six patients had relapsing-progressive MS. Over the 12 months that the patients were followed, clinical disability scores showed either no change or improvement. Other tests showed neurophysiological improvements. Furthermore, MRI scans did not show any disease progression over a three month period.[31]

Oligodendrocyte precursor cell: a cell from which oligodendrocyte cells develop. An oligodendrocyte is a glial cell which is similar to an astrocyte, however it is smaller and has fewer branches than its larger counterpart.

Olfactory ensheathing glia (OG): a type of glia cell which is present in the olfactory bulb and mucosa (the area of the brain which allows us to perceive smells). Also nicknamed olfactory Schwann cells, olfactory ensheathing glia assist in the regeneration of the axon. These glia express Lyz proteins that play a role in immunoprotection; these cells are exposed directly to the external environment.

Amyotrophic lateral sclerosis, also known as ALS or Lou Gehrig's Disease, is a fatal neuromuscular condition where the motor neurons of the central nervous system die off. The result is muscle atrophy, which eventually results in important muscle groups shutting down. ALS is associated with a genetic defect, but the cause of the disease is still not clearly understood.

In 2009, a group of Italian researchers, led by Dr. Letizia Mazzini (MD) of Eastern Piedmont University, convened to discuss the prospects of stem cell therapy for ALS. Their opinion, published in the journal *Expert Opinion on Biological Therapy*, was that stem cells had therapeutic potential for ALS. They reasoned that transplanted stem cells could produce neurotrophic and growth factors to enhance the survival and function of endogenous brain cells, differentiate into neurons and supporting glial cells, and also protect against neurotoxicity and harmful immune response.[33]

Mazzini et al. also pointed out that several animal studies have achieved positive results. Some of these are summarized on page 164. Furthermore, some clinical trials such as a 2009 hematopoietic stem cell transplantation study have shown promise, although results from other clinical trials are conflicting.[34, 35]

Mazzini and her colleagues ended their opinion piece by declaring that there are still questions that need to be answered before stem cell therapy fully crosses the translational medicine gap. These questions, they argue, can be answered by "develop[ing] new small meaningful Phase I clinical trial[s]," which would "represent a hope and an answer for these patients" who suffer from ALS.[33] The same argument can be made for multiple sclerosis or Huntington's disease, or indeed, for any of the neurological diseases currently being investigated. Well-conducted clinical trials advance the scientific understanding of how stem cells interact with different pathological states, and hasten the day that a large-scale stem cell product can be available for patients around the world. While it is impossible to predict which condition will have a stem cell-based treatment soonest, it is inarguable that patients suffering from any of these conditions deserve better treatment options than what is currently available. This is why it is morally imperative that continual efforts are made to push forward with scientific research and clinical trials that may unlock the answers to handling this epidemic of neurological diseases. And, stem cells may well be the key to doing so.

The causes for different neurological conditions are diverse. Conditions like Alzheimer's disease, for example, appear to contain a strong genetic component, while other conditions such as spinal cord injury occur due to trauma. Other neurological problems may be triggered by environmental conditions, abnormal fetal development, drug abuse or infection.

Because the causes and pathologies of neurological conditions are so diverse, researchers and clinicians know that stem cells may not work for all neurological diseases. The neurological diseases detailed above, and in previous chapters, are those which may be most receptive to allogeneic stem cell treatment.

In degenerative diseases like ALS, a disturbance of the balance between glial cells and neurons occurs, leading to the death of motor neurons. The chart below shows how stem cells can be neuroprotective in SOD1 mice, delaying onset and progression of disease and extending survival.

EXAMPLES OF PRECLINICAL TRANSPLANTATION STUDIES OF STEM CELLS IN ANIMAL MODELS OF ALS

Cell source	Disease model	Route of delivery	Number of cells	Proposed therapeutic mechanism	Outcomes	Ref
Human UCBs (pooled donors)	Presymptomatic, irradiated sod 1 (G93A) mice	Intravenous (retro-ocular)	$34.2 - 35 \times 10^6$	Immunomodulation/ providing non mutant (functional) sod1 enzyme	Delay in disease onset (22 days) and increased lifespan (21 days)	[36]
Wild-type mice BMCs	Presymptomatic, irradiated sod1 (G93A) mice	Intravenous (retro-ocular)	5×10^6	Immunomodulation/ providing non mutant(functional) sod1 enzyme	Delay in disease onset (7 days) and increased lifespan (12 -13 days)	[36]
Human UCBs	Presymptomatic, SOD1 (G93A) mice	Intravenous	10^6	Neuroprotection by modulation of autoimmune processes	Delayed disease progression (at least 2 - 3 weeks) and modestly increased lifespan	[37]
Human UCBs	Presymptomatic, SOD1 (G93A) mice	Intravenous	10×10^6 25×10^6 50×10^6	Modulating the host immune inflammatory system response	Dose of 25×10^6 cells increased lifespan by 20 - 25% and delayed disease progression by 15%	[38]
Wild-type mice versus SOD1 (G93A) BMCs (mesenchymal)	Presymptomatic, irradiated SOD 1 (G93A) mice	Intraperitoneal	3×10^6	Positive 'non-neuronal environmental' effects	Delay in onset (14 days) and increased lifespan (12 -13 days) on wild-type BMCs, no effect of SOD1 mice BMCs	[39]
Human bone marrow MSCs from adult donors	Presymptomatic, SOD1 (G93A) mice	Bilateral lumbar spinal cord injection, different levels	Total amount 10^5	Increasing neuron survival and preventing astrogliosis and microglia activation	Increased motor neuron count, decreased astrogliosis and microglia activation, increased lifespan in males, amelioration of motor performances	[40]
NSCs from spinal cord of human embryo (8 weeks old)	Presymptomatic, immunosuppressed SOD1(G93A) mice	Bilateral lumbar spinal cord injections	Four sites, 5×10^4 cells/site	Differentiation of NSCs into neurons, initial networks with host nerve cells, release of growth factors	Delay in onset (7 days) and increased average lifespan (11 days)	[41]
Wild-type mice embryonic stem cells	Adult rats with chronic diffused motor neuron deficiency (sindbis virus)	Bilateral lumbar spinal cord injections, one site	6×10^4	Motor neurons differentiation, forming junctions with host muscle	Partial recovery from paralysis	[42]
Wild-type adult mice NSCs (purified from adult brain and primed into a motor neuron phenotype)	Presymptomatic, immunosuppressed SOD1(G93A) mice	Bilateral lumbar spinal cord injections, one site	10^4	Neuronal and glial differentiation, release of growth factors (trophic support)	Delay in onset (21 days) and increased average lifespan (22 - 23 days) (unchanged progression), delayed loss of lumbar motor neurons	[43]
Wild-type mice NSCs from embryonic spinal cord	Presymptomatic nmd mice (animal model of SMARD1)	Intrathecal delivery	2×10^4	Neuronal and glial differentiation, release of growth factors (trophic support)	Delayed onset and increased average lifespan (18 - 19 days), decreased loss of motor neurons	[44]

BMC: Bone marrow cell; GRP: Glial-restricted precursor; h: Human; MSC: Mesenchymal stem cell; MSC (GDNF): MSC engineered to secrete glial cell line-derived neurotrophic factor; NSC: Neural stem cell; NSC (GDNF): NSC genetically modified to release GDNF; SMARD1: Spinal muscular atrophy with respiratory distress type 1; UCB cell: Umbilical cord blood cell. Mazzini, *Expert Opinion on Biological Therapy*, 9: 1245-1258, © 2009, with permission from Informa Healthcare Communications.

Chapter 10
Cardiovascular Conditions

"He was relatively young for heart problems," recalls Dr. Nabil Dib (MD). "He was only 55."[A] Dr. Dib, director of Cardiovascular Cell therapy at the University of California, San Diego, is speaking of CS, a patient from Arizona who learned firsthand the potential life-saving effects of stem cell therapy. CS, Dib remembers, "had suffered a heart attack in the past, and one day he came to the hospital with heart failure. His blood pressure was between 70 and 80." A systolic measurement of less than 90 millimeters, Dr. Dib explains, indicates hypotension. Low systolic blood pressure cannot profuse the heart and brain tissue, resulting in ischemia and cell death. CS's blood pressure was too low, and he was in danger of going into shock. "We immediately admitted him," Dib says, "and put him on a support device, an intra-aortic balloon pump, in order to get him through."

Dib and his team performed bypass surgery on the ailing patient. They also performed a stem cell transplant in the area of the heart attack.

Months later, Dib compared CS's PET scans to the new scans after the procedure. "At six months," Dib explains, "you can see evidence of new viable tissue, in the area of transplantation. This is tissue that was previously scar tissue and now is viable." The transplant had created new, living cells in the area of the heart attack, and replaced scar tissue with new muscle, all of which helped treat CS's heart failure. "Today," Dib says, "this patient is not only still alive, the guy is playing basketball."

CS is just one of the many people in the United States who have received stem cell treatments for cardiac conditions. From animal studies, potential stem cell treatments for diseases such as heart failure have already progressed to clinical trials. At present, most of the treatment efforts are focused on autologous (same patient) stem cells. The lower regulatory barrier and ease of stem cell acquisition facilitates these treatments. Cardiovascular conditions have a major effect on a significant percentage of American society.

The Prevalence of CVD in Society

Over 81 million Americans suffer from one or more types of cardiovascular disease (CVD). More than eight million people in the United States are struggling with the consequences of a heart attack, and over five million have heart failure. Cardiovascular disease (including stroke, which is caused by a problem in the blood vessels of the brain), accounts for more than one-third of all deaths in the United States. In fact, cardiovascular disease has been the main cause of death in the United States for over a century.[B]

As a society, we are paying the price for this epidemic. The total costs of CVD for 2010 are estimated to be $500 billion, for the United States alone. This includes hospital fees, nursing homes, and drug expenditures. Heart disease can create a severe financial hardship for a family. A pacemaker, for example, costs over $50,000, while coronary bypass surgery is at least $100,000. These procedures are not just costly, they also have associated medical risks. The in-hospital death rate of a coronary bypass, for example, is over 3 percent.[1]

Many lifestyle choices can prevent or reduce the effects of cardiovascular disease, such as smoking cessation, regular exercise, and a healthy diet. There are also pharmacological options; for example, millions of people take drugs to control their blood pressure or modify their cholesterol levels. But as a recent article in the popular press candidly acknowledges, the limitations of current medical and lifestyle techniques for repairing a heart that has already been damaged are quite limited:

> [You can] downshift your daily life so that watering the garden ranks as your most strenuous activity, or get in line with the other 3,000 Americans waiting for one of the 2,200 donor hearts available annually. The human heart may be one of our most mechanically sophisticated organs, but it's just not a good healer. With its own electrical system and unique muscle tissue beating 100,000 times a day, the heart is just too complex and too busy to repair itself significantly.
>
> Deprive critical cardiac tissue of oxygen, even for just a few minutes, and it dies. Weaken a single chamber or a single valve, and pumping efficiency plummets. Allow the damaged parts to dip below a certain baseline level of functioning, and they only become worse, never better.[2]

So, how do you repair the damage to a heart injured by cardiovascular disease? How do you significantly increase perfusion to areas where the vascular system is too weak to convey blood flow? How do you build new blood vessels, or strengthen essential heart muscles? These questions are not easily answered. Even surgery, a costly and invasive option, cannot solve all cardiovascular problems. And while there are many ways to lower the risk of a subsequent heart problem after a heart attack, it is not as simple to undo the damage once it has been done. Stem cells hold a promise of filling in the gaps where medical science has not yet found a solution to cardiovascular problems.

Acute Myocardial Infarction (AMI) and Heart Failure

Everyone knows that a heart attack (known clinically as a myocardial infarction, or MI) can often be fatal. On the other hand, few people are completely aware of the extent to which a myocardial infarction, if survived, profoundly affects the health of the person who had the attack. It is estimated that a heart attack reduces life expectancy by up to fifteen years.[1] Part of the reason is due to the damaging effect on the muscles of the heart.

During a myocardial infarction, the vessels supplying blood to the heart become blocked. Much as a blocked blood vessel in the brain will cause brain cells to die, the blockage of a major blood

So, how do you repair the damage to a heart injured by cardiovascular disease? How do you significantly increase perfusion to areas where the vascular system is too weak to convey blood flow? How do you build new blood vessels, or strengthen essential heart muscles?

Stem cells hold a promise of filling in the gaps where medical science has not yet found a solution to cardio vascular problems.

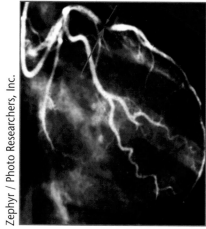

Narrowed coronary artery. Colored coronary angiogram (X-ray) of a 54 year old patient with severe stenosis (narrowing, arrowed) in the left anterior interventricular coronary artery. The coronary arteries are found on the surface of the heart, and supply blood to the heart muscle.

vessel to the heart causes the cardiac muscles to die, due to a lack of oxygen. If blood flow to the heart is not quickly re-established, the heart will often stop beating, a condition referred to as cardiac arrest.

Many people believe that the terms "heart attack" and "heart failure" refer to the same event, which is incorrect. Heart failure is a condition where the heart is unable to pump adequate amounts of blood to the body. A person with heart failure is like an engine perpetually running on low battery; a heart failure patient may feel perpetually weak and run down, and his or her quality and even longevity of life suffers as a result.

While there are many contributing factors to heart failure, the most prominent is a heart attack, when the muscles of the heart are irrevocably damaged and unable to adequately circulate the blood throughout the body. Surviving a heart attack, then, usually leaves the cardiovascular system severely compromised. "The typical progression of the disease after heart attack," explains Dib, "is that the inflammatory process ends up damaging many of the heart cells. Simultaneously, the cells of the heart go through continuous apoptosis—cellular death—even years after the original heart attack. The heart goes through a remodeling process and enlarges itself. It enlarges until it finally fails, at which point you have heart failure." Dib further says: "Out of all patients who survive a myocardial infarction, only one-third will have a full recovery. The remaining two-thirds of all patients will have to deal with the consequences of their heart attack, and those consequences primarily include heart failure."

After heart failure, a heart attack, or other types of heart disease, the body attempts to repair the damage on its own. Cardiomyocytes, the muscle cells of the heart, begin proliferating at a vastly increased rate. For example, "in patients with end-stage ischemic heart disease, the rate [of proliferation] rises 10-fold."[3] The problem is that there are not enough cardiomyocytes present in the heart to begin with. According to a paper published by the National Academy of Sciences, it is estimated that the rate of proliferation of cardiomyocytes in the human heart is fourteen cells per million.[4] Even with a ten-fold increase, the amount of endogenously regenerated muscle tissue is underwhelming. The number of endogenous cardiac stem cells (CSC), the stem cells best able to differentiate into new cardiomyocytes, is even less impressive: "Cardiac stem cells are rare with an average of one cardiac stem cell per 18,000 cardiomyo-cytes."[5] Without enough endogenous cells to do the job of repairing the heart muscles, a failing heart could use some outside help, in the form of a stem cell transplantation.

While autologous stem cells have been used in an attempt to repair cardiac damage, they have significant limitations, as dicussed in Chapter 1. Heart problems usually strike those of more advanced age; the older the patient is, the older his stem cells are. We know that as we age, our stem cells suffer from senescence (see Chapter 1), and thus become less effective. Dr. Victoria Ballard (PhD), principal scientist at healthcare company GlaxoSmithKline, explains:

> *Human EPCs from older individuals have impaired prolif-erative and survival capacity compared to those from young subjects. The cardiac differentiation capacity of bone marrow cells from old versus young mice is also impaired, suggesting that aging stem cells have a more limited capacity for repair via cardiac regeneration.[3]*

As a result of this reduced capability of autologous stem cells, some in the medical field believe that allogeneic stem cells hold the promise of a more potent treatment alternative. Even after deter-mining the optimal cell source, however, clinicians have the option of selecting several different stem cell types to choose from.

Endothelial Progenitor Cells (EPCs)

The endothelial progenitor cells (EPCs) mentioned by Dr. Ballard can differentiate into various types of endothelial cells, with endo-thelial cells comprising the lining of several blood vessels, and offer great promise for cardiac conditions.

A German study led by Dr. Nikos Werner (MD) suggested a cor-relation between EPCs and cardiac repair: "During the observational period of 12 months, a significantly higher incidence of death from cardiovascular causes was observed in patients with low baseline levels of endothelial progenitor cells."[6] The basis for this hypoth-esis was first conceived after an earlier study demonstrated that EPCs were mobilized in response to ischemic insult in humans.[7] In another published study, Dr. Lael Werner, of the Department of Cardiology at Tel-Aviv Sourasky Medical Center, used EPCs to treat rats with dilated cardiomyopathy (a common form of heart failure). Dr. L. Werner found that the EPCs "partially attenuated myocardial damage induced by experimental myocarditis."[8] The

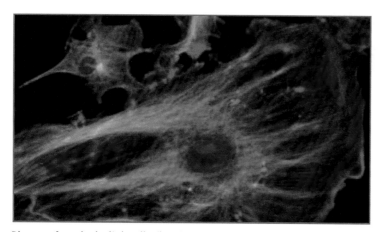

Photo of endothelial cells (bovine pulmonary artery) under a microscope. Nuclei are stained blue, microtubles are marked green by an antibody, and actin filaments are stained red.

results demonstrated that EPCs might be useful in the treatment of various heart conditions. These and other early studies created a body of scientific literature which suggested that EPCs, administered hours after a heart attack, "have a favorable impact on the preservation of left ventricular function."[9]

In 2008, Dr. Takayuki Asahara (MD, PhD) of Japan's Riken Center for Developmental Biology published a review of the literature, examining the potential of EPCs for use in "strategies for vascular regeneration and the future direction of vascular regeneration including cardiac regeneration."[10] He noted that the biggest challenge with using endothelial progenitor cells was that there simply were not enough of them in the body:

In order to provide enough EPCs to affect [sic] a good clinical result, the cells need to be cultured and put through several rounds of division. With some stem cell types such as hematopoietic stem cells, there is a large enough population of stem cells within the body, and thus few rounds of division are needed to gain enough cells for a transfusion. With EPCs, however, it is difficult to have enough of the cells for therapeutic purposes, without going through many rounds of division. And generally with each division, the stem cells lose some of their potency and efficacy. In the same way that old stem cells become senescent within the body, stem cells that have gone through too many divisions become less effective.

Asahara and his Riken Center colleague Dr. Satoshi Murasawa (MD) concluded in their review that, "the primary scarcity of a viable and functional EPC population constitutes a potential limitation of therapeutic vasculogenesis based on the use of ex vivo expansion alone."[10] But research has shown that one of the most significant ways in which stem cells effect repair is by releasing trophic and protective growth factors. What if, instead of using large numbers of weak EPCs, clinicians used smaller numbers of EPCs that were engineered to release more growth factors?

Scientists who have attempted to answer this question have found promising results. One animal study used EPCs to treat limb ischemia, a condition where a blood vessel in the limb is blocked.

These EPCs were genetically modified to produce significantly more VEGF than they would normally make. Drs. Murasawa and Asahara call VEGF (a growth factor that catalyzes the production of new blood vessels) "the most critical factor for vasculogenesis and angiogenesis."[10]

The results were encouraging: limb necrosis and auto-amputation were reduced by 63.7% in comparison with controls. The interesting part of the study, however, is that the researchers had used one-thirtieth the amount of EPCs they would normally use to get the same result. Thus, EPCs modified to produce more growth factors can be far more effective than EPCs without these modifications, allowing EPC transplantation to remain "one of the promising therapies in clinical situations regarding vasculogenic properties."[10]

Mesenchymal Stem Cells (MSCs)

It appears that EPCs are able to effect significant change by secreting growth factors, which is consistent with what much of modern science has taught us about the stem cell's mechanisms of action. In terms of differentiation, however, EPCs are designed to become endothelial cells, the cells that line the inner surface of the blood vessels. Endothelial progenitor cells cannot differentiate effectively if blood vessels are not already in place, and the stem cells responsible for building the blood vessels are mesenchymal stem cells. Dr. Dib explains the rationale behind MSC therapy:

The idea of stem cell transplantation for acute myocardial infarction is to delay or halt the inflammatory process that happens immediately after a heart attack. Currently, the idea is to use stem cells within 4-7 days of the heart attack. We know that bone marrow-derived stem cells can delay or even halt the inflammatory process. Through this mechanism, they would potentially be able to affect the remodeling of the heart and avoid, or at least delay, heart failure as a consequence of heart attack.

For these and other reasons, MSCs are another good candidate for treating cardiovascular disease. A review article, written by an established team of researchers led by Dr. Ahmed Abdel-Laftif (MD) of the University of Louisville, examined eighteen different clinical studies using bone marrow-derived cells for cardiac repair after acute myocardial infarction. These eighteen studies, with almost one thousand patients between them, used a variety of cells, including MSCs. Other cell types included EPCs, peripheral blood stem cells, and mononuclear cells (which derive from HSCs). The results were encouraging:

Compared with controls, BMC transplantation improved left ventricular ejection fraction (pooled difference, 3.66%; 95% confidence interval [CI], 1.93 to 5.40%; P<.001); reduced infarct scar size (-5.49%; 95% CI, -9.10% to -1.88%; _=.003); and reduced left ventricular end-systolic volume (-4.80 mL; 95% CI, -8.20 to -1.41 mL; P=.006).[11]

The hearts of patients in all eighteen studies showed improvement in three key areas.

1. *Improved left ventricular ejection fraction (LVEF).* Ejection fraction is the amount of blood pumped out with each heartbeat. After a heart attack, the muscles of the left ventricle are weakened, and the LVEF is lower than normal. A normal LVEF should be somewhere between 50% and 70%; the heart is able to pump out more than half the blood stored within it with each heartbeat. After a heart attack, this percentage can plummet, easily losing an additional 20% of output. The more heartbeats it takes to pump blood out of the heart, the more the patient's tissues suffer from delayed reception of oxygen and vital nutrients. Thus, a clinical result of almost 4% improved LVEF is significant.

2. *Reduced infarct scar size.* The scar tissue that forms in response to an AMI needs to be replaced with healthy cardiomyocytes (properly working muscle tissue that will help the heart regain its function). In some studies, the transplanted cells delivered an almost 10% reduction of scar tissue.

3. *Reduced left ventricular end-systolic volume (LV-ESV).* The LV-ESV is the amount of blood still in the left ventricle after it has just finished contracting. A high LV-ESV indicated that the ventricle is weak, as it was not able to pump out more blood. The cell transplants reduced this number by almost five milliliters, on average.

Two years later, several of the same researchers conducted a follow-up review, including studies that had occurred since the previous review was published. The follow-up confirmed that "analysis of pooled data indicates that BMC therapy in patients with acute

MI and chronic IHD [ischemic heart disease] results in modest improvements in left ventricular function and infarct scar size without any increase in untoward effects."[12]

The reviews demonstrate that bone marrow-derived cell therapy shows clinical benefit, but the studies utilized a variety of different cells. In order to reach any significant conclusions regarding MSCs alone, it is necessary to examine studies that only used mesenchymal stem cells. A study published in the *American Journal of Cardiology*, for example, discussed 34 patients who received autologous bone marrow-derived MSCs after a myocardial infarction. After their heart attack but before their stem cell treatment, their LVEF was at an average of 49 percent. Three months after receiving MSCs, their LVEF was at an average of 67 percent. The control group, three months after receiving saline solution, was only at an average of 53 percent.[13]

A later study led by Dr. Qun Li (PhD) of the University of Wyoming found that "MSCs transplantation can indeed restore MI-induced heart dysfunction."[5] This is not surprising; the researchers acknowledged that their findings were in line with other similar research. The Wyoming team, however, went on to explain why MSCs are able to help heal the heart. "Our work revealed for the first time that the improved myocardial contractile function following MSC transplantation may be due to, at least in part, the beneficial effect of cell transplantation in individual cardiomyocytes from the area at risk."[5] In other words, the MSCs had a beneficial effect on the heart muscle cells that were in danger of dying—the Chaperone Effect in action. The researchers argued that MSCs were making "possible contributions of anti-apoptosis and angiogenesis in MSCs-exerted myocardial effect following MI." The transplanted mesenchymal cells were preventing cell death and creating better vascularization, helping to rescue injured cells.

Li et al. found that, in addition to improving the LVEF and **LVEDV** parameters, the MSCs also improved fractional shortening, a mathematical measure of how well the left ventricle is functioning. Their results were further proof that stem cells may be most effective as a treatment option not because of their own ability to differentiate, but because of the various means of support they provide to other cells. Dib points to an animal study: "The mesenchymal precursor cell, as shown in a sheep model, can stimulate the division of the cardiac stem cells themselves, in the heart.

Left ventricular end-diastolic volume (LVEDV): the volume of blood left in the left ventricle of the heart directly preceding a contraction.

We call this 'endogenous cardiac stem cell stimulation.'" In this case, the mesenchymal stem cells are providing the signals that the endogenous stem cells need in order to reproduce. If part of the MSCs' effects are achieved by stimulating an endogenous cardiac stem cell population, therapeutic improvements could perhaps be achieved by transplanting these cardiac stem cells themselves into the heart of an AMI patient.

Cardiac Stem Cells (CSCs)

Both mesenchymal stem cells and endothelial progenitor cells have demonstrated clinical efficacy in helping to repair the heart after an AMI. But the heart has its own population of stem cells, known as cardiac stem cells (CSCs). The hypothesis is that a transfusion of CSCs themselves could be a useful therapeutic tool for treating cardiac diseases.

These cardiac stem cells have a few drawbacks, however. Dib explains:

It's not easy to get a sample of cardiac stem cells, and once you have a sample, you still have a very limited number of cells. There are significant limitations in terms of obtaining the number of the cells that are required for cell transplantation. A myocardial infarction can destroy around 800 million cells. So it's necessary to have a large number of stem cells to replace that amount.

Cardiac stem cells alone are not numerous enough. Cardiac stem cells are a recently discovered addition to the stem cell family; they were first uncovered in 2004, meaning that CSC researchers have some catching up to do.[14]

But cardiac stem cells have one powerful advantage over other stem cell types; they can differentiate into cardiomyocytes, the cardiac muscle cells that become damaged by a heart attack. Technically, they are not the only stem cells that can form cardiomyocytes. There is evidence that different types of stem cells can transdifferentiate into cardiomyocytes, essentially jumping into a different cell lineage to produce the cells that the body truly needs. But the hypothesis of transdifferentiation is a contentious one, and most scientists will acknowledge that, if the process of transdifferentiation occurs, it does not take place in large numbers. Therefore, for direct replacement and renewal of cardiomyocytes, cardiac stem cells may be the optimal choice.

In 2007, a group of researchers led by Dr. Claudia Bearzi (PhD), now an instructor at Brigham and Women's Hospital, set out to prove that CSCs were really stem cells. After confirming that the cells were "self-renewing, clonogenic, and multipotent," and thus that they fit the definition of stem cells, the researchers continued by using human CSCs (hCSCs) to treat the infarcted myocardium of rats and mice.[15] They found that the hCSCs resulted in "an increase of ejection fraction, attenuation of chamber dilation, and improvement of ventricular function."[15] This research demonstrates both the potential of CSCs, and the work that the scientific establishment has yet to accomplish.

CSCs have since progressed from animal studies to clinical trials. In 2009, doctors at the Cedars-Sinai Heart Institute completed the first procedure to use CSCs for treatment of a post-AMI patient. They biopsied patients who had suffered a heart attack and, over the course of four weeks, cultured each patient's cells in order to gain a therapeutic dose of CSCs. The autologous cells were then used for treatment. The results of the study are not yet available, but much is expected. Dr. Eduardo Marbán (MD), director of the Cedars-Sinai Heart Institute, says of the trial, "Five years ago, we did not even know the heart had its own distinct type of stem cells. Now we are exploring how to harness such stem cells to help patients heal their own damaged hearts."[14]

More recently, the team at Cedars-Sinai has been using magnetic targeting to guide the CSCs to the site of infarction. Imbuing the CSCs with iron microparticles, the doctors use a magnet to help the cells home in on the injured area. This development represents a possible solution to one of the problems that still vexes stem cell researchers: how to make sure the stem cells stay within the area of injury. Marbán says, "This remarkably simple method could easily be coupled with current stem cell treatments to enhance their effectiveness."[14] This exciting concept could later be expanded to other cell types, as well as cardiac-derived cells.

Compared to other cell types, however, autologous CSCs may be less ideal for use in treatment. After all, "heart failure is most prevalent among older individuals, and a growing body of evidence suggests that with increasing age, cardiac stem and progenitor cells undergo senescent changes that impair their regenerative capabilities."[16] There is an advantage to using allogeneic, as opposed to autologous, stem cells, provided that the allogeneic CSCs are undifferentiated enough to not display significant HLA.

Ischemia: a restriction in blood supply, generally due to factors in the blood vessels, with resultant damage or dysfunction of tissue. It also means local anemia in a given part of a body sometimes resulting from vasoconstriction, thrombosis or embolism (as in limb ischemia).

Cardiac stem cells are a relatively new discovery, and there is much excitement in the scientific community regarding the combination of these cells with other cell types for potential AMI treatments. The hypothesis is that a multi-cell solution may offer the best treatment option for AMI patients. CSCs could rebuild the muscles of the heart, while MSCs and EPCs revascularize the injured tissue and provide a variety of trophic effects to increase the efficacy of the result. Using cell priming processes and new techniques for "guiding" the cells to the site of injury, such as the use of cell matrices to keep the stem cells within the area of the injury, the result could be magnified. With these new techniques, clinicians may be able to achieve a therapeutic result with a sub-therapeutic number of cells.

Peripheral Artery Disease (PAD) and Limb Ischemia

Stem cell treatments can be useful for more peripheral cardiovascular problems, as well, such as limb **ischemia**. In dealing with these conditions, cardiac stem cells are of limited utility; they are designed to reconstruct only the cells of the heart. But mesenchymal stem cells build new connective tissue, while endothelial progenitor cells are designed to differentiate into the cells that form the innermost part of the different circulatory pathways.

Dr. Nikos Werner's study established that the number of functioning EPCs within the body "predicts the occurrence of cardiovascular events and death from cardiovascular causes and may help to identify patients at increased cardiovascular risk."[6] This begs the question, if higher numbers of EPCs are associated with better cardiovascular health, then wouldn't an EPC injection improve the cardiovascular system?

That was the question that Dr. Christoph Kalka (MD), research leader at the University of Bern, and others set out to answer. They expanded a population of human EPCs and transplanted them in nude mice with hind limb ischemia. Kalka et al. found that the EPC-treated nude mice had a greater recovery in bloodflow and enhanced collateral density, which is to say that the blood vessels of the mice were strengthened in response to the ischemic insult. But perhaps most significantly, the research team found that, in 60% of the EPC-treated injuries, they were able to save the limb from being amputated. This is in comparison to just 7% limb salvage for the control group.[17]

This animal study was meant to mimic the conditions of limb ischemia in humans, with limb ischemia being one major consequence of peripheral artery disease (PAD). PAD occurs as a result of plaque build-up in the arteries, and reduces blood flow to the limbs. Peripheral artery disease often co-presents with coronary artery disease and other types of cardiovascular disease. In fact, a patient with cardiovascular disease is far more likely to die of cardiovascular issues if he or she has PAD as well.[18]

Peripheral artery disease is a killer itself, since it often leads to severe limb ischemia. In the same way that a heart attack can kill off muscle cells in the heart or a stroke can kill off brain cells, limb ischemia shuts off the blood flow to a limb, leading to cell death and debilitating pain. Thirty percent of all cases of limb ischemia end in amputation. In the United States, that means approximately 120,000 major leg amputations a year. In Europe, the number is slightly smaller, with 100,000 major leg amputations a year. Of that number, 30% will die as a direct or indirect result of the operation, while another 40% will die within the next five years.[19]

With limb ischemia proving to be such a huge challenge for modern medicine, Kalka et al.'s animal study raises hope that EPCs can save lives by instituting vascular repair in ischemic limbs. Other animal studies involving hind limb ischemia have used MSCs, EPCs, and other cell sources on murine and rabbit models. A review of twenty such studies has found that each experiment reported an improved outcome.[19]

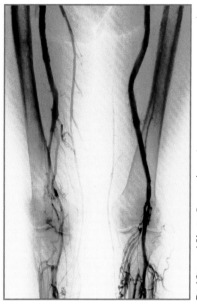

Thrombosis of the superfical femoral vein and popliteal vein. Colorised arteriography.

Dr. Vitoux / Photo Researchers, Inc.

Clinical Trials for PAD

From this pre-clinical data, researchers have moved to small-number clinical trials, using a mixed population of bone marrow-derived cells as proof-of-concept for larger trials aiming to treat PAD. This cell population, known as bone marrow-derived mononuclear cells (BM-MNCs or BMCs), represents a cross-section of the cells that are normally found in the bone marrow, including hematapoietic stem cells, mesenchymal stem cells, and endothelial progenitor cells.

The first pilot study, performed by Dr. Eriko Tateishi-Yuyama (MD), a professor at Kansai Medical University in Osaka, and his team found that the BM-MNC cell treatment showed improvement in several major parameters.[20] Patients treated with the bone marrow-derived mononuclear cells performed better on tests designed to determine blood pressure, reported less pain, and were able to walk pain-free for farther distances.[20] (See figure at left.) Tateishi-Yuyama and his colleagues followed up with a randomized controlled study, which found similar results.[20] Tateishi-Yuyama hypothesized that the population of EPCs within the BMC population was responsible for much of the repair, in conjunction with pro-angiogenic factors released by the bone marrow-derived cells.[20] Those who reviewed the study also noted that the bone-marrow cell population contained approximately 500 times the number of hematopoietic stem cells as the cell population received by the control group.[19]

Since Tateishi-Yuyama et al.'s study, eighteen other clinical studies have been conducted which used a similar composition of bone marrow-derived cells. Taken together, these studies comprise hundreds of patients. Sixteen of the eighteen studies showed clinical improvement in one or more areas, whereas two of the eighteen studies showed equivocal results.[19] In many instances, the percentages of amputations decreased, while patients reported feeling less pain.[19]

These results are encouraging, and indicate that stem cell-based therapies may play a role in treating peripheral artery disease and its symptoms, including limb ischemia. Such a therapy would reduce the number of amputations performed in the United States and abroad, and increase overall vascular health for hundreds of thousands of at-risk patients.

But few of these clinical trials have been randomized controlled studies, and each trial has involved a small number of participants. To translate these results into a therapeutic treatment, larger trials are needed.

Meanwhile, large trials are already underway to bring a stem cell-based cardiac treatment to market. In fact, though it may seem cutting edge, clinical trials using stem cells for treating heart failure have been going on in the United States for over a decade.

Angiographic analysis of collateral vessel formation after bone marrow-derived mononuclear cell transplantation.

Collateral branches were strikingly increased at (A) knee and upper-tibia and (B) lower-tibia, ankle, and foot before and 24 weeks after marrow implantation. Contrast densities in suprafemoral, posterior-tibial, and dorsal pedal arteries (arrows) are similar before and after implantation.[20]

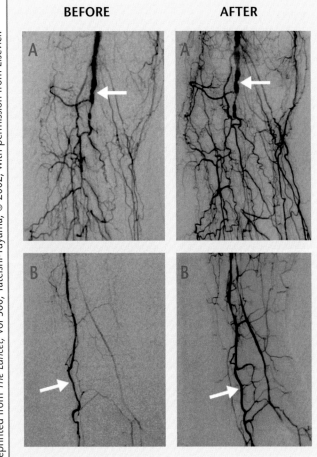

BEFORE   AFTER

A   A

B   B

The History of Clinical Trials for Heart Failure

"We had our first patients in the United States in 2000," Dib remembers, "and we weren't even the first ones. The first patients who received stem cells for heart failure were in France, under Dr. Philippe Menasche, (MD), then of the Bichat Hospital, in Paris. The United States started immediately after."

Menasche and his team took stem cells from the thigh muscles of seven patients and placed them within the patients' hearts during a bypass operation. The results suggested that these muscle cells were differentiating into viable cardiomyocyte-like cells. At around the same time, Dr. Patrick Serruys (MD, PhD), increased a patient's ejection fraction by 6 percent with a stem cell treatment in a research trial in the Netherlands.[21]

In the first United States-based clinical trial, Dib took a similar approach to Menasche's:

At that time the cells we took were from the muscle. They are called skeletal muscle-derived stem cells, or myoblasts. We transplanted these myoblasts into the hearts of patients who were undergoing bypass surgery. The trial was, firstly, proof of feasibility and safety. These cells survived in the heart, made new muscles, and expressed proteins that make them fatigue resistant, just like heart muscles.

Fatigue resistance is not an important attribute for skeletal muscles, but cardiac muscles can never rest. For the stem cell-derived muscles to develop fatigue resistance was a major accomplishment. "It's important," Dib affirms. "It means that the environment is interacting with these cells, and that the cells are responding to appropriate cues and signals."

Those earlier trials demonstrated that stem cells, in this case cells taken from skeletal muscle, can offer improved clinical outcome for patients. The stem cells that were used—myoblasts—differentiated into cells that helped the heart regain function. Today's clinical trials have built upon these original proof-of-principle tests, bringing us inexorably closer to a mainstream treatment, and expanding our knowledge of how various stem cells can treat different aspects of the same disease. A decade ago, clinicians investigated using myoblasts as a tool to repair the heart. Today, we are exploring several different cells, building a veritable stem cell toolbox for cardiac repair.

Researchers around the world have begun the process of passing stem cell-based treatments through these tripartite trials. In Germany and Switzerland, Phase II of a clinical trial, the Repair AMI trial, was recently completed. This trial used bone marrow-derived progenitor cells to treat patients with acute myocardial infarction. Presenting the conclusions of the trial back in 2005, Dr. Volker Schachinger (MD), professor at Johann Wolfgang Goethe University in Frankfurt, Germany, declared that the result "shows for the first time that it is possible to regenerate damaged heart tissue."[22] A larger trial, he explained, would allow his team "to see whether these effects translate into reductions in clinical end points. If these are successful, this would open up a whole new way of treating heart disease."[22]

Schachinger's team is currently looking into conducting a Phase III clinical trial.[22] Dr. Dib affirms the importance of a larger clinical trial. "The results demonstrated improvement in heart function and showed a better clinical outcome. Based on that, the research team in Germany is planning to move forward with a Phase III clinical trial." And once that trial is completed, if the results are in keeping with the previous two trial phases, this stem cell treatment can become available to the world at large.

Moving Toward Allogeneic Trials

The Repair AMI trial used a cross-section of bone marrow-derived progenitor cells, comprising a mixture of different stem cell types as well as more differentiated cells, as its cell source. This is similar to the methodology of the trials aiming to repair limb ischemia and treat peripheral artery disease. While the use of bone marrow-derived mononuclear cells has shown some benefit, a new generation of clinical trials has turned towards allogeneic stem cells with the goal of effecting even greater repair.

"In the United States, we are now in a Phase II, large clinical trial, with over 200 patients," Dib explains, "We are applying bone marrow-derived stem cells to patients within seven days of a myocardial infarction." The difference is that while the Repair AMI trial used autologous stem cells, the American study uses allogeneic stem cells. "The ability to use allogeneic stem cells," continues Dib, "represents a major advancement in this field, for acute myocardial infarction and for stem cell therapy in general. With allogeneic stem cells, one donor can provide enough stem cells for between 10,000 and 20,000 treatments." With more advanced technology, it is now possible to expand that number twenty-fold, so that several healthy donors could be the cell source for millions of heart failure patients.

The first clinical study using allogeneic mesenchymal stem cells, a Phase I clinical trial led by Dr. Joshua Hare (MD) of the University of Miami, was concluded in 2009. The results of the randomized controlled study demonstrated that "in 4 specific areas of pre-specified safety monitoring—cardiac arrhythmias, pulmonary function, cardiac performance, and patient global symptomatic status—the treated patients exhibited significantly improved outcomes relative to the placebo group, consistent with a therapeutic benefit." The treated patients also experienced an average 6.7% improvement in LVEF after six months.[23]

In a paper published in the *Journal of the American College of Cardiology*, Hare and his team explain why these cells are advantageous compared to other cell sources, most notably autologous bone marrow mononuclear cells:

> *The use of allogeneic hMSCs (human mesenchymal stem cells) has a number of important advantages. They likely represent an enriched population of cells with therapeutic capacity. They are readily prepared from healthy donors and may be used as an allogeneic, and thus 'off-the-shelf' agent. They are easy to administer, as evidenced by the intravenous approach used in this study. Finally, and most compelling, there are a wealth of pre-clinical data in rodent and larger animal models supporting their efficacy in cardiac repair.[23]*

The Future

Dib is the principal investigator of a study utilizing mesenchymal precursor cells to treat heart failure patients. In this capacity, he oversees clinical trials at six different medical sites in the United States, including the Texas Heart Institute, the Minneapolis Heart Institute, and a site at the University of Pittsburgh. His current study is just one of the 21 clinical trials, in different phases, currently being conducted at 43 different research institutions around the country.[2]

Recent research that Dib finds exciting, uses a myocardial matrix to deliver stem cells directly to the infarcted area of an AMI-affected heart. "The limitation right now for stem cells is that their retention rate is low in the area of transplantation. Even with direct injection, retention rate does not exceed 15%." A low retention rate means that not all the cells are staying in place; rather, many migrate away from the center of the damage. While stem cell treatments offer promise for cardiac conditions, they may be vastly more effective if more stem cells stayed within the targeted area. "If we mix the stem cells with the matrix, we have a much higher likelihood of having a much higher retention rate," he says.

Other studies have caught Dib's attention, including a clinical trial on using CD34+ stem cells, a type of hematopoietic stem cell, to treat patients with coronary artery disease. The results from the 164 patients enrolled in the trial, Dib remarks, "show some hope and promise" and hint at the possibility of using stem cells to enhance bloodflow in the heart, easing chest pain and increasing longevity for patients who grapple with coronary artery disease.

With several studies nearing their post-Phase III finish line, it seems likely that stem cell therapy will soon find its way routinely into the cardiology units of hospitals around the world. These treatments have the potential to save limbs by affecting peripheral blood flow, and similarly may save lives by treating heart failure and related cardiac conditions.

Hare, director of the University of Miami's Interdisciplinary Stem Cell Institute and one of the pioneers of allogeneic stem cell therapy for heart conditions, believes that these studies will begin a major medical transition in the cardiac arena. "Stem cell therapy shifts the whole paradigm for treating heart disease, whether it's caused by heart attack, arrhythmia, or cardiomyopathy," he said in a 2010 interview. "My prediction is that in 10 to 15 years, thanks to this new ability to repair damage, heart disease will no longer be the number one killer in the country."[2]

Fighting back against the number one killer of Americans is a laudable goal, and one that deserves widespread support. As a number of stem cell-based clinical trials near completion, there may be good reason to believe that all of society will soon benefit from stem cell solutions to this serious problem.

Chapter 11
Ophthalmic Conditions

It was MA's sight that left him first. The vision in his left eye deteriorated, while the vision in his right eye became dark and blurry. MA, an engineer, was constantly using his computer for work-related activities, but the words on the screen became more and more difficult to read. "The words started doubling," he explained. "Not just a little, but significantly. I could hardly work. After 40 minutes, it became difficult to work on the computer." Straining his eyesight in order to continue working, MA soon developed a series of unbearable headaches.[A]

MA knew that his vision loss was due to an enemy he had been fighting all his life: diabetes. He had developed the systemic disease in childhood and had learned how to manage it, just as millions of other patients do, with regular insulin shots to regulate his blood sugar. But MA was now in his late fifties, and he could feel the disease taking its toll on his body. He felt his arms and legs growing weaker and he began having trouble moving, eventually coming to the point where he could not walk without assistance.

Retina

Cornea

Pupil

Lens

Cross-section of a normal eye.

But it was his vision loss that eventually forced MA to take time off from his job. MA knew that he was in danger of losing his livelihood and his sight to diabetes. With this in mind, he began looking into whether stem cells could give him the upper hand against the disease. MA is one of the few people who have received stem cell transplantation to restore their sight.

There are many warning signs that indicate someone is at risk for losing their sight: a loss in the ability to see at night, dark spots that float across the field of vision, or trouble identifying details. These are all early symptoms for three common ophthalmic diseases: retinitis pigmentosa, diabetic retinopathy, and macular degeneration. All three conditions are degenerative, leading to worsened vision and even blindness over time. None of these conditions currently has a cure.

For MA, the condition that threatened his sight was diabetic retinopathy, one of the leading causes of blindness in the United States today.[1] The vast majority of diabetics are at risk of developing diabetic retinopathy (DR); there are over 23 million diabetics in the United States alone.[2, 3] Diabetes affects the entire body, which means that those afflicted by DR are already struggling to manage the other complications of diabetes. Diabetic retinopathy adds a significant financial burden for these people; medical costs incurred from diabetic retinopathy in the United States are estimated at over $500 million a year.[4]

Diabetic Retinopathy: The Pathology

Diabetic retinopathy (DR) is a condition caused by diabetes mellitus, commonly known as diabetes. Diabetes, a systemic disease, occurs when the body is unable to adequately process glucose due to insulin deficiency or a malfunction in the receptors that would normally respond to insulin triggers. Since a diabetic is unable to process excess glucose, high levels build up in the blood. The hyperglycemic blood begins degrading vascular cells, like those supporting the small blood vessels within the eye. These small blood vessels are thus deprived of a support structure. Meanwhile, in the blood vessels themselves, the glucose-altered blood slows the flow and may cause ischemia. A vessel that is clogged with thick and viscous blood, similar to one that is blocked by a blood clot, will lead to the death of nearby cells that are deprived of important nutritional support. Furthermore, the hyperglycemic blood of a diabetic will also cause small vessels to hemorrhage. The extravagated blood gets into other parts of the eye and unbalances sensitive retinal cells. Beyond pooling into unwanted areas, these blood cells contain iron, which is an important component of hemoglobin but can also create a toxic microenvironment if not controlled. In proximity to a collection of damaged cells, the iron will promote a stronger inflammatory response, causing even more damage.

Diabetic retinopathy occurs when the vascular cells in the retina of the eye begin to die due to these diabetes-induced irregularities with the eye's blood flow. A DR-afflicted eye will often have a series of abnormal new blood vessels, which form as a result of the body's attempt to bring more blood to the back of the eye.[5]

"When the original small blood vessels deteriorate, they can't bring oxygen to the retinal tissue," explains Dr. Paul Tornambe (MD), an ophthalmologist who serves as a clinical researcher and director of the Retina Research Foundation of San Diego. Tornambe, former president of the American Society of Retina Specialists, elaborates on the retinal tissue's response: "The tissue either dies, or screams for more oxygen and nutrition, and the body responds to that by bringing abnormal blood vessels into the retina, which then hemorrhage."[B] These abnormal blood vessels are fragile and permeable, and their hemorrhaging causes further damage to the eye.

Retinal cells are a type of brain-derived neural cell and are responsible for converting light into electrical signals that the brain can interpret as vision. When they die, the brain no longer receives these signals, and a diabetic's vision becomes more and more blurred,

Fundus photos show a normal eye on the left and proliferative retinopathy on the right. This occurs when abnormal new blood vessels and scar tissue form on the surface of the retina.

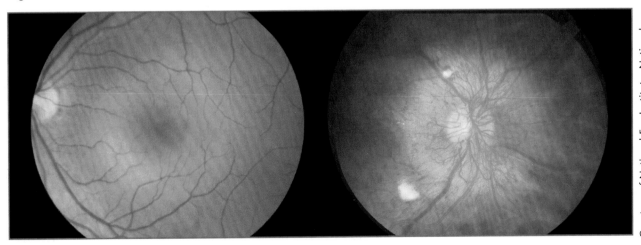

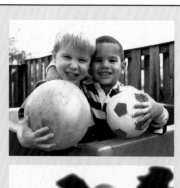

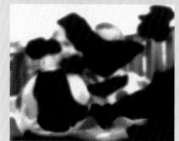

The top photo represents what a person with normal vision would see, the bottom is vision impaired by diabetic retinopathy.

often leading to complete blindness. The first set of symptoms includes specks of debris such as blood or vitreous opacities in the visual field, often referred to as floaters. Eventually, these floaters may become larger, and more permanent, as the vessels of the eye continue to leak blood.

Fortunately, the pathophysiology for diabetic retinopathy is well understood, and thus a possible solution to the problem of DR presents itself: improve the circulation of the eye by repairing and strengthening the pre-existing small blood vessels. While this does not address the systemic disease, it may provide improvements in the retinal damage.

Using Stem Cells to Treat Diabetic Retinopathy

To determine the potential impact that stem cell treatments may have on DR, Tornambe reviewed the data from a clinical study using mesenchymal stem cells to treat seven people with diabetic retinopathy. "What the study showed," Tornambe says, "is that the eyes that were treated with stem cells saw improved blood flow to the retina. This was demonstrated very objectively with Doppler flow velocity studies," which use ultrasonic bursts to measure the velocity of blood flow in a certain area—in this case, the ophthalmic artery. Tornambe continues, "When the circulation is improved to the retina, the retina gets oxygen and nutrition, and it does not die. It does not make abnormal blood vessels that bleed. And, hopefully, it will preserve vision."

The study that Tornambe referred to used MSCs, which have well-established vasculotrophic properties. MSCs produce the growth factors that modulate the development of new blood vessels, such as the protein endostatin. Recent research has shown that endostatin's effects extend to the arena of the eye, inhibiting abnormal neovascularization in the tissue area responsible for supplying nutrients to the retina.[6] There is interesting research supporting the inverse correlation between endostatin and diabetic retinopathy.[8] Down's Syndrome, a condition associated with a decreased risk of diabetic retinopathy, is known to increase endostatin levels.[7] The current hypothesis is that the up-regulation of endostatin caused by Down's Syndrome is the reason diabetic retinopathy is less likely in these individuals.[9] The MSCs may have the ability to up-regulate endostatin and other angiogenic inhibitors, and therefore reduce the formation of abnormal blood vessels. MSCs also produce trophic factors, such as angiopoietin-1, which strengthen pre-existing blood vessels, bolstering them against the degrading effects of hypergly-cemic blood.[10] MSCs also release additional trophic factors such as **ciliary neurotrophic factor (CNTF)**, which "modulates survival of retinal neuronal cells," ensuring the survival of threatened neuronal cells.[10] Recently, an Oregon-based research group examined how MSCs were able to address retinal degeneration through the use of these growth factors. The team concluded, "MSCs may prove to be the ideal cell source for auto-cell therapy for retinal degeneration and other ocular vascular diseases."[10]

Stem Cells as "Little Doctors"

Previously, we have explained that MSCs promote angiogenesis. In this case, however, they work to inhibit neovascularization. These results seem contradictory, but in reality illustrate the versatility of stem cells. Stem cells work to restore homeostasis to an area of the body that is in disequilibrium. If the area needs more blood vessels, stem cells can up-regulate pro-angiogenic factors. If the area has aberrant vascularity, the stem cells can induce the opposite effect. This is one advantage that stem cell-based medicine has over pharmacologic solutions to disease: a cell can change its behavior to better treat the underlying pathophysiology. A drug cannot. It is this versatility that Dr. Yanai of Jerusalem's Hebrew University-Hadassah Medical School was referring to when he described stem cells as "little doctors."[11]

MSCs are not the only "little doctors" that can treat ophthalmic conditions. Retinal cells are derived from neural stem cells, so NSCs and their derivates may also prove to be a potent treatment option. NSCs would be able to differentiate into new retinal cells, to replace dead ones. As well, their Chaperone Effect could rescue cells in danger of dying. Some research has indicated that allogeneic neural stem cells are immuno-privileged, meaning "the immune system will not attack them," and thus have excellent implications for the treatment of CNS disorders as well as retinal disorders such as diabetic retinopathy.[12]

Dr. Michael Young (PhD) of Harvard Medical School explained that our growing understanding of the immuno-privileged status of NSC cells "could have an enormous effect on how we perform brain or retinal transplantations in the future."[13]

Just as the MSC-NSC combination has offered improvement in case study patients for stroke and spinal cord injury, similarly it may offer a powerful treatment option for diabetic retinopathy and other degenerative eye diseases.

Ciliary neurotrophic factor (CNTF): is a protein that in humans is encoded by the CNTF gene. The protein encoded by this gene is a polypeptide hormone and nerve growth factor whose actions appear to be restricted to the nervous system where it promotes neurotransmitter synthesis and neurite outgrowth in certain neuronal populations including astrocytes. The protein is a potent survival factor for neurons and oligodendrocytes and may be relevant in reducing tissue destruction during inflammatory attacks.

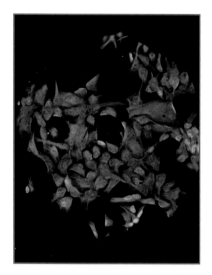

In vitro expanded fetal neural progenitor cells.

MA noticed the difference; he had fewer headaches and reported that his vision had improved approximately 80%.

Restoring Sight

Tornambe had studied the results of seven patients, several of whom had received NSCs in addition to MSCs. MA, whose story was presented at the beginning of the chapter, was one such patient.

He enrolled in a clinical study in June 2006, receiving three stem cell treatments over a period of two years. During the first treatment, he received an injection of neural progenitor cells in each eye, as well as an infusion of mesenchymal stem cells. For the subsequent two treatments, he received just neural cells, again in each eye.

MA started noting improvements within a few weeks after his first treatment. In post-treatment follow-ups, conducted in August and September 2006, doctors noticed improvement as well. Clinicians observed that the electric response threshold of the retina in both of MA's eyes had decreased. The electric response threshold is a measure of how much stimulation is needed before any type of excitable cell transmits an electrical impulse. For retinal cells, this measurement refers to the amount of light that is needed before the retina sees that a light is shining. For MA, his lowered response threshold meant that he was able to see in dimmer light, resulting in clearer vision. MA's response threshold decrease was shown at 3 months to be approximately "25% below pretreatment level in the right eye; 50% below pretreatment level in the left eye."[14] The thickness of his retinal nerve fiber layer had also increased significantly, indicating greater numbers of healthy retinal cells.[15] Further tests, conducted in April 2007, confirmed that his eyes were improving.[15]

The graph to the right illustrates MA's improvements after stem cell therapy.

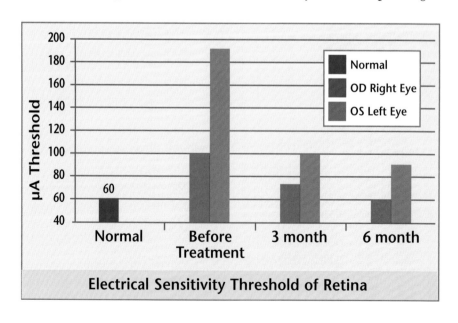

Electrical Sensitivity Threshold of Retina

MA noticed the difference; he had fewer headaches and reported that his vision had improved approximately 80%. "The double vision is greatly reduced, and I can see much better," he said in a follow-up session.[16] He was eventually able to read up to five hours without taking a break. MA's improvements eventually enabled him to return to work.

MA was engaged in a clinical study to address his diabetic retinopathy, but a treatment that would reduce the manifestations of diabetes in the eye could possibly reduce the problems diabetes caused in other parts of the body, as well. It appears that the MSCs were able to do more for MA than just treat his diabetic retinopathy; they may also have reduced the severity of his diabetes. After his first treatment, MA started reporting better mobility, but he also was able to reduce his insulin intake by 50 percent.

The results of the patients in this study, Tornambe noted, seemed to show that "this treatment could be used to treat a large spectrum of the diabetic population, regardless of duration of disease or

Retarding Diabetic Retinopathy

The following chart summarizes the three year follow up results of four patients with diabetic retinopathy. The patients had a single treatment with neural and mesenchymal stem cells and were serially evaluated at the Federov Eye Institute in Moscow. These preliminary results indicate that stem cell treatment may help stabilize or improve eye function above baseline for extended periods of time.

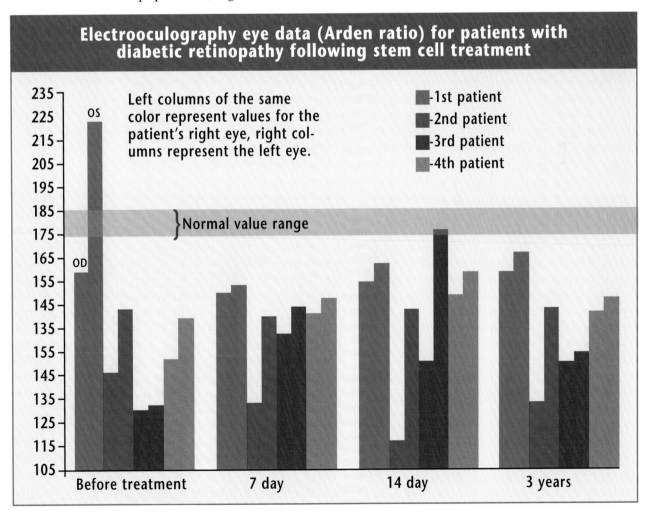

Electrooculography eye data (Arden ratio) for patients with diabetic retinopathy following stem cell treatment

Left columns of the same color represent values for the patient's right eye, right columns represent the left eye.

- 1st patient
- 2nd patient
- 3rd patient
- 4th patient

Normal value range

Before treatment 7 day 14 day 3 years

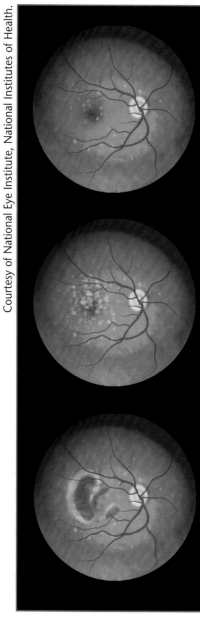

Macular degeneration: top early intermediate (dry), middle intermediate (dry) and lower neovascular (wet).

disease severity."[17] MA's result also illustrates that stem cell treatments may improve function in other areas affected by diabetes.

As scientists further develop cell matrices and other methods to influence stem cells' homing abilities, the future for diabetic retinopathy patients may become even brighter.

Macular Degeneration

Age-related macular degeneration, or AMD, is the foremost cause of blindness among the elderly. Dr. Robert Klein (MD), a professor at the University of Wisconsin, Department of Ophthamology and Visual Sciences, recently completed a study on the prevalence of macular degeneration in the United States. One in fifteen Americans aged 40-years and older have signs of AMD, approximately 7.2 million people.[18] However, this is a 9% decrease in the prevalence since a prior study was done in 1994; this may be attributable to improvements in diet, exercise and blood pressure.[18] While the exact cause of AMD is still debated, it generally occurs when the macula, a section of the retina, becomes damaged.

There are two forms of macular degeneration:

1. *Central Geographic Atrophy, or "Dry" Macular Degeneration:* For reasons that are not yet fully explained, the cells of the macula begin to break down. The problem may originate with the retinal photoreceptor cells themselves, or with the retinal pigment epithelium (RPE) cells, which supply the retina with oxygen and nutrients and which also remove waste products from the eye. Whatever the cause, the result is a build-up of cellular debris called "drusen" and the gradual failing of key retinal cells. As Tornambe describes it, "the retina basically wears out."

2. *Neovascular or Exudative ("Wet") Macular Degeneration:* As a consequence of "dry" AMD, the body will often try to supply the affected area with more blood. Thus, factors like VEGF are up-regulated while other inhibiting factors go through abnormal changes, an occurrence that may result in aberrant blood vessel growth. These weak blood vessels begin leaking blood onto the macula, destroying retinal cells and creating scar tissue within the retina. Although not all cases of dry AMD will lead to a wet form of the disease, the presence of central geographic atrophy is a pre-requisite for neovascular macular degeneration.

Both forms of macular degeneration cause the loss of central vision, in many situations making it impossible to recognize faces.

The dry form of the disease is far more prevalent, with approximately 90% of all macular degeneration cases being dry. However, wet macular degeneration is far more likely to result in blindness.

Both forms of macular degeneration are mainly linked to age, so much so that many physicians often refer to macular degeneration as age-related macular degeneration. In the United States, the National Eye Institute cautions that almost a third of all people above the age of 75 are at risk for AMD.[19] Both the wet and dry forms of AMD are progressively degenerative, and they both lack effective treatment options. There is currently no cure for AMD.

In the United Kingdom, where over 500,000 people are affected by macular degeneration, a research group known as The London Project to Cure Blindness has been working diligently to advance stem cell treatments for AMD. The group began with animal trials, restoring sight to a group of rats that suffered from an AMD-like condition. The results were encouraging, but rat models of AMD have long been acknowledged to be imperfect indicators of AMD in humans. The researchers realized they needed to move forward with human trials, in order to have a good indication as to whether the stem cell treatments would work.

The Project advanced their work by using autologous cells to treat a small group of AMD patients. The results were encouraging. "In some cases, the transplants were so successful that the patients were able to read, cycle and use a computer," reported a journalist who spoke with scientists from the Project.[20] Currently, the Project is preparing to investigate the use of embryonic stem cells to treat AMD in a clinical setting. The Project's clinical trial, expected to start at the beginning of 2011, is only the second clinical trial with embryonic stem cells for any clinical condition ever attempted (as of the date of this publication).[21, 22] The London Project acknowledges that, "considering that these will be the first human embryonic stem cell trials in man in the UK, the project really will be breaking new ground."[23]

The Project is attempting to use stem cells to produce new retinal pigment epithelial cells, which are among the hardest affected by macular degeneration. It is the failure of the RPE cells, in AMD and in other retinal diseases, which cause other cell types to subsequently die off. Replace the atrophying RPE cells with healthy ones, the researchers of the Project maintain, and an efficacious treatment for AMD will have been created. Pharmaceutical research

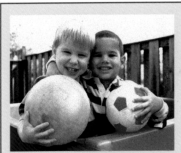
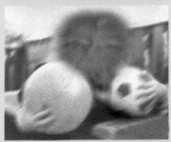

The top photo represents what a person with normal vision would see, the bottom is vision impaired by age related macular degeneration.

Courtesy of National Eye Institute, National Institutes of Health.

"This could have a tremendous effect on a huge population who have no current therapy."

giant, Pfizer, seems to agree; they announced their financial backing of the Project in April of 2009.[21]

The researchers have discovered how to place the stem cells on an artificial membrane, which is then inserted in the back of the retina, negating the need for the cells to home to the site of the degeneration. Dr. Pete Coffey (PhD), Director of the London Project and Professor of Cellular Therapy and Visual Sciences at the University College London, believes that the treatment, which has already shown effective proof-of-principle with the previous adult autologous trials, could quickly transition to mainstream medicine, saying, "This could have a tremendous effect on a huge population who have no current therapy."[20] And although 14 million people have been rendered legally blind due to AMD in Europe alone, Coffey envisions this potential treatment as not limited to one continent, but "as a global therapy."[23]

Other Stem Cells and Macular Degeneration

Other research has found additional possibilities for stem cell therapy. Dr. Martin Friedlander (MD, PhD), of the Scripps Research Institute, in San Diego, California, has delivered hematopoietic stem cells (HSCs) to mice with abnormal vasculature in the eye, a model resembling diabetic retinopathy and wet AMD. The cells subsequently "stabilized and prevented deterioration of the eye. In addition to rescuing blood vessels, the cells had a 'neurotrophic rescue effect' in which neurons of the eye were saved," not unlike the neurotrophic effect manifested by stem cells in other clinical treatment situations.[5] Furthermore, these cells appeared able to differentiate into microglial cells, promoting vascular repair.[5]

The reparative role of microglia has been disputed, but a study from a Japanese research group based in Kyoto University provided further evidence that transplanted microglial cells, such as those differentiated from transplanted HSCs, actually "play a protective role in retinitis pigmentosa" and similar retinal diseases.[24] The more microglial cells in the retina, then, the better, and HSCs appear to be able to differentiate into these supportive cells. A study published in the *American Journal of Pathology* also demonstrated that HSCs may be able to transdifferentiate into RPE and other cells that could assist in retinal repair, providing further support for the hypothesis that "HSCs could serve as a therapeutic source for long-term regeneration of injured retina and choroid in diseases such as age-related macular degeneration and retinitis pigmentosa."[25]

"HSCs could serve as a therapeutic source for long-term regeneration of injured retina and choroid in diseases such as age-related macular degeneration and retinitis pigmentosa."

Writing in *The Journal of Clinical Investigation*, Friedlander's team declared that the "profound vasculotrophic and neuro-trophic effects" of the stem cells used in their investigation may offer hope not just to those who are going blind, but to those who have just started experiencing symptoms of retinal degeneration.[26] They argued, "since nearly all of the human inherited retinal degenerations are of early, but slow, onset, it may be possible to identify an individual with retinal degeneration, treat them intravitreally with an autologous bone marrow stem cell graft, and delay retinal degeneration with concomitant loss of vision."[26]

In other words, some type of stem cell preventive regimen could postpone blindness indefinitely for patients suffering from retinal degenerative diseases. While Friedlander's team used autologous stem cells, allogeneic cells may offer the advantage of being less senescent than the cells taken from AMD patients. The average AMD patient is of a more advanced age, a fact reflected in the acronym AMD (age-related macular degeneration.) Immune-privileged allogeneic stem cells from a younger donor may be more potent than the patient's own stem cells.

Friedlander has more recently begun looking at the possibility of induced pluripotent stem cells, and how they might be used to treat AMD. His research is being funded by grants from the California Institute for Regenerative Medicine and the National Eye Institute, reflecting the degree of confidence state and federal authorities have in the potential of stem cell therapy to achieve clinical results. For Friedlander, who also works as a clinician, treating AMD is not just a scientific endeavor. "The clinical reality," he explained in a 2009 interview, "is that 6 to 8 percent of people over the age of 75 are legally blind from this disease."

And, by all accounts, AMD is likely to become a more serious problem in North America. "We are the age of the Baby Boomers," Tornambe exclaimed. "You ain't seen nothing yet."

"We are the age of the Baby Boomers," Dr. Tornambe exclaimed, "You ain't seen nothing yet."

Retinitis Pigmentosa

Compared to diabetic retinopathy and macular degeneration, retinitis pigmentosa (RP) is relatively less common. A genetic disorder, it affects approximately 1 in 4,000 people in the U.S. In retinitis pigmentosa, genetic mutations cause the malfunction of cells around the retinal pigment epithelium. Retinitis pigmentosa

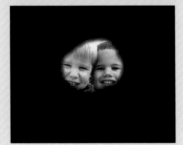

The top photo represents what a person with normal vision would see, the bottom is vision impaired by retinitis pigmentosa.

affects rod photoreceptor cells near the epithelium; as the photoreceptor cells die off, vision loss occurs.

A person with an RP-expressed phenotype will usually lose the ability to see in the dark, a condition known as nyctalopia or night blindness. As more photoreceptors or epithelial cells die off, peripheral vision worsens, until an RP patient is only able to see through a "tunnel" of vision at the center of the visual field.

There are many different genes that, through mutation, can cause RP. This mutation leads to visual degeneration, as unhealthy retinal cells begin dying off. A successful stem cell treatment must accomplish the task of replacing these dead photoreceptor cells with new ones. Professor of ophthalmology at the University of Oxford, Dr. Robert MacLaren (MD, PhD) explains that, because retinitis pigmentosa only affects certain cell types, the resulting degeneration "initially leaves the inner neural circuitry intact and new photoreceptors need only make single, short synaptic connections to contribute to the retinotopic map."[27] However, maximum effect will be achieved only if the new cells are not deficient. This fact argues against the use of autologous stem cells to treat RP, as an autologous treatment would simply inject cells containing the same defect which resulted in the death of the original photoreceptor cells.

The most promising stem cell treatment might be an allogeneic transfer of cells that have already been primed to produce photoreceptors. As an illustration of this possibility, MacLaren and his team conducted an animal study in which they transplanted retinal progenitor cells from non-RP mice into mice with retinal degeneration. The transplanted cells were found to "differentiate, form functional synaptic connections with downstream targets in the recipient retina and contribute to vital function."[27]

It is important to remember that retinal cells are actually neural cells; they are essentially the mediator between the rest of the eye and the brain. As such, retinal progenitor cells are derived from neural stem cells. Studies have also suggested that neural progenitor cells employ trophic effects to rescue endogenous retinal cells. For example, an animal study, led by Dr. Mark Kirk (PhD) of the University of Missouri, placed neural cells derived from embryonic stem cells within the eyes of retina-damaged adult mice. Kirk's team found that the transplanted cells "enhanced survival of host retinal neurons, particularly photoreceptors."[28] Neural stem cells, through their neurotrophic effects, may also be able to enhance the survival of endogenous retinal cells.

Slowing the Progression of Retinitis Pigmentosa

Recently, Tornambe studied the results of a Stemedica-sponsored animal study that employed undifferentiated neural stem cells, along with retinal pigment epithelial progenitor cells and ciliary body progenitor cells. "The study that we recently reviewed was with rats with retinal dystrophies. These rats were doomed to be blind at 36 weeks, but the stem cells were able to tremendously modify and slow the progression of the deterioration to the point that many of the cells looked normal."

The ciliary body progenitor cells, which come from the triangular ciliary muscles that can be seen in the corner of the eye, were generally ineffective; in short, they were the wrong cell type to use for a retinal condition. But the RPE progenitor cells and neural stem cells were apparently able to effect repair.

The RPE/NSC combination seems uniquely suited to offer an effective multi-cell solution to retinitis pigmentosa. The RPE progenitor cells work to strengthen the cell population that supports the retinal cells, and thus restore balance to the retinal microenvironment. Epithelial cells play a primary role in regulating retinal homeostasis. They are the gatekeepers of the retina, determining which small molecules enter and exit. Their health is vital to the health of the retinal photoreceptors. As Tornambe summarized, the animal trial demonstrated that "RPE stem cells injected into the suprachoroidal space prevented the animal's RPE cell's degeneration as well as preventing degeneration of the overlying photoreceptors." Meanwhile, the NSCs are apparently able to differentiate into functioning photoreceptor cells, and through the Chaperone Effect they can rescue photoreceptor cells that otherwise would die off, treating the primary cause of the vision loss.

The rats in the animal study had a retinal dystrophy that was similar to retinitis pigmentosa. "In the animals that had the stem cells inserted, the retinal dystrophy progressed much more slowly," explains Tornambe. "At the conclusion of the study, the histology of the retina was almost normal in the cases of those eyes that had the stem cells, compared to the controls, and the electro-physiologic studies showed responses in those eyes that had the stem cells inserted, as compared with the control eyes."

Electrophysiologic studies are a common tool to determine response in animal studies. "With an animal, you can't just ask them to look at an E chart and tell you what they see," Tornambe jokes.

"The study that we recently reviewed was with rats with retinal dystrophies. These rats were doomed to be blind at 36 weeks, but the stem cells were able to tremendously modify and slow the progression of the deterioration to the point that many of the cells looked normal."

"What's even more exciting, and this is a real mystery to me, is that we would treat only one eye, and yet the untreated eye in these rats would also improve. There's some crossover effect, and I'm still trying to figure out why that is."

"But you can use techniques such as electrical stimulation, and then measure the subsequent impulse. And in places where the control rats had completely extinguished impulses, the stem cell-treated animals showed impulses as a result of the stimulation. So something was clearly happening."

Tornambe was surprised by how effective the stem cells appeared to be in promoting the rats' vision. "What's even more exciting," he explains, "and this is a real mystery to me, is that we would treat only one eye, and yet the untreated eye in these rats would also improve. There's some crossover effect, and I'm still trying to figure out why that is." One hypothesis is that the positive outcome of the untreated eye was achieved through the stem cells' systematic release of cytokines and other growth factors, inducing the endogenous stem cells of the untreated eye to mobilize.

This study represents one contribution to the field of stem cell research regarding ophthalmic disease. Other contributions include a recently-concluded study at the Columbia University Medical Center, where researchers used mouse embryonic stem cells to replace diseased retinal cells in a mouse model of RP. The lead author of the resulting paper, Dr. Stephen Tsang (MD, PhD) declared, "This research is promising because we successfully turned stem cells into retinal cells, and these retinal cells restored vision in a mouse model of retinitis pigmentosa."[29]

In the Columbia study, sight was restored in a quarter of the mice that received the ESCs. However, complications were found in some of the mice, including benign tumors.[29] This is one of the concerns with using embryonic stem cells, and one of the reasons that adult stem cells may be a better choice for human use.

"This research is promising because we successfully turned stem cells into retinal cells, and these retinal cells restored vision in a mouse model of retinitis pigmentosa."

Tornambe sees stem cells as the future of RP treatments. "In some diseases where we can intervene in a slowly progressive disease, for example, like retinitis pigmentosa, instead of having to make completely new tissue, we might be able to re-model or re-engineer affected tissue with stem cells, so that it becomes healthy tissue. At this time," he continues, "I don't know of any other way to regenerate tissue. We've tried retinal tissue transplants, for example. That doesn't work. With the exception of corneal transplants, we have had very limited success with transplanted eye tissue. Maybe in the future we will overcome the hurdles of retinal transplants, but I think that the answer is more likely to come from stem cells."

Chapter 12
Wound Care

There is hope for the nearly 35 million patients worldwide who suffer annually from chronic wounds, as well as the estimated 6.5 million with burns severe enough to require professional treatment.[1] Significant treatment advancements have occurred through the use of anti-infectives, skin ulcer management, moist dressings, pressure relief (including negative pressure) and biological dressings. These technologies are helping to drive double digit growth in a wound care market set to hit $12.5 billion by 2012.[2]

Many factors are fueling this growth, the key drivers being an aging population, an ever-rising epidemic of diabetes, and the prevalence of vascular disease. Chronic skin wounds are classically divided into three categories of ulceration: diabetic, pressure and venous. Each of these will be discussed in this chapter. First, however, it is helpful to take a closer look at the skin to understand both normal function as well as the pathology of a chronic wound.

The skin is the largest organ in the body, comprising about two square meters (21.5 square feet) and 16% of the average person's

Wound Type	Worldwide Prevalence	CAGR* 2007-2016
Burns	6.5 million	1.3%
Pressure Ulcers	8.5 million	6.9%
Venous Ulcers	12.5 million	6.7%
Diabetic Ulcers	13.5 million	9.3%
*CAGR: Compound annual growth rate. Data is from MedMarket Diligence, LLC.[1]		

body weight. It serves a variety of functions, the most critical of which is barrier protection. It keeps harmful agents, such as bacteria, out. The skin regulates temperature through blood vessel dilation—to dissipate heat, or contraction—to conserve heat. Sweat and sebum provide lubrication to the skin. Ultraviolet light stimulates the skin to synthesize Vitamin D that affects calcium and bone metabolism.

There are two layers to the skin. The epidermis is the outermost layer. It is a very thin layer varying in depth anywhere from 150 to 300 microns. To put this in perspective, the diameter of a typical hair averages 80 microns. The epidermis contains the skin cells, or keratinocytes. They grow from the basal layer and shed between 14 and 28 days.

The dermis is 2-3 millimeters in depth. This layer is comprised of connective tissue in the form of collagen and elastin fibers. These substances are secreted by the fibroblasts in the extracellular matrix. The dermis contains nerves, blood vessels, glands and hair fibers. The macrophage cells that respond to inflammation are housed here.

Stem and progenitor cells are found in four regions of the skin: the junction of the epidermis and dermis, the bottom of the sebaceous gland, the bulge of the hair follicle, and the dermal papilla. These cells play a vital role in regenerating and repairing wounds.

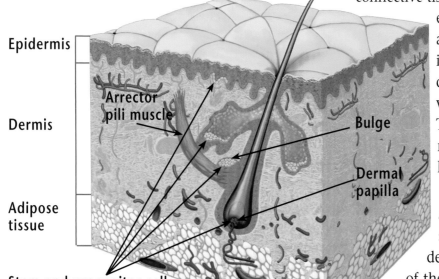

Epidermis

Dermis

Arrector pili muscle

Bulge

Dermal papilla

Adipose tissue

Stem and progenitor cells are found at the junction of the epidermis and dermis, the bottom of the sebaceous gland, the bulge of the hair follicle, and the dermal papilla.

The Stages of Wound Healing

We are all familiar with the heat, redness, tenderness and swelling that accompany a skin wound and the progression to healing. Wound healing takes place in a series of steps, the first of which is the inflammatory response that occurs within minutes of an injury. Once the skin is injured, a type of soluble signaling protein known as **cytokines** are secreted by the body's white blood cells. Just as adrenaline prompts the central nervous system to immediately respond to a threat, the cytokines jump-start the wound healing process. They initiate a cascade of biological reactions that begins with homeostasis. Vessels constrict to control bleeding and platelets in the blood begin forming fibrin clots. Histamine, released from the body's mast cells, enables serum to enter the wound, accompanied by white cells (the primary type being neutrophils.)

The neutrophils begin a cleaning process, engulfing bacteria and other cellular debris. They then give way to another type of white blood cell known as a monocyte. These white blood cells are transformed into macrophages. The macrophages are the vultures of the wound healing process. They secrete nitrous oxide that kills pathogens; they also secrete proteases, one class of which is known as matrix metalloproteinases (MMP) that break down the damaged tissue which they then ingest.

Once the inflammatory process ceases, the stage of early wound repair begins. This is marked by three simultaneous events governed by a category of signaling proteins known as growth factors. The three events are epithelialization, neoangiogenesis and provisional matrix formation.[A, 3]

- *Epithelialization:* This is the process whereby the body attempts to cover the denuded surface with skin. This process is directed by the fibroblasts in the dermis that influence the keratinocytes to proliferate and move to close the surface of the wound. The fibroblasts secrete the growth factor KGF-2 (keratinocyte growth factor) and the cytokine IL-6 (interleukin-6) working in conjunction with nitrous oxide.

- *Neoangiogenesis:* This involves the creation of the endothelial cells and the capillaries necessary to supply the healing wound with blood flow. This process is started by the macrophages releasing cytokines, however in the early wound healing phase it is primarily the keratinocyte expression of VEGF (see Chapter

Cytokines: small cell-signaling protein molecules that are secreted by numerous cells of the immune system and are a category of signaling molecules used extensively in intercellular communication. Cytokines can be classified as proteins, peptides, or glycoproteins; the term "cytokine" encompasses a large and diverse family of regulators produced throughout the body by cells of diverse embryological origin.

Cytokines and Factors in Early Inflammation

The following cytokines and factors are released by the inflammatory neutrophils, and later, macrophages in the earliest stage of wound healing. The cytokines also serve to stimulate the fibroblasts, endothelial cells and the macrophages to secrete more cytokines.

- PDGF: Platelet-derived growth factor
- IL-1: Interleukin-1
- TNF-α: Tumor necrosis factor-a (assay)
- G-CSF: Granulocyte colony-stimulating factor
- GM-CSF: Granulocyte-macrophage stimulating factor

Growth Factor Signaling

Growth factors influence healing through three different signaling methods:

1. Autocrine: the cell signals itself.

2. Paracrine: the cell signals its immediate neighbors.

3. Endocrine: one or more cells signal remote cells via the blood stream.

Dr. Robert Goldman (MD), Assistant Professor in the Department of Rehabilitation Medicine, University of Pennsylvania, notes that autocrine and paracrine communication are important in coordinating the wound healing process and are effective at extremely low concentrations.[3] These low concentrations are effective because of the avid and precise binding of growth factor proteins to cell surface receptors.[4]

10) that is responsible for this neoangiogenesis. Fibroblasts also express VEGF.

• *Provisional Matrix Formation:* The matrix provides the structural support for the wound to contract. The macrophages initiate this formation through the secretion of cytokines TNF-α and PDGF. Fibroblasts then take over the process. In response to stimulation by PDGF they begin synthesizing the glycosamino-glycans and fibronectin that are important components of the matrix. Over a 7-14 week period, TGF-ß induces the fibroblasts to form Type I collagen, allowing contraction of the wound to take place. This early contraction, along with the epidermal covering, closes the wound.

Late wound repair may continue for as long as a year. The collagen meshwork becomes thicker and remodeled so as to gain additional strength. Fibroblasts do this work, stimulated by TGF-ß, which also inhibits some of the activity of the MMPs that were active in the early inflammatory phase.

When the wound is large and unable to easily close, rather than become neatly organized and smooth, the collagen fibers proliferate and form a mass of tangled fibers that contain few pigmented cells. In short, the wound is healed with a scar. When this tightened tissue occurs near a joint, it may result in a contracture, which restricts range of motion. Another type of disordered wound healing is known as a keloid, which is marked by an overproduction of disorganized collagen in response to a wound. Keloid-prone patients have alterations to their TGF growth factors.

Understanding Chronic Wounds

Chronic wounds are those that exhibit delayed healing. There are many reasons for this—among them diabetes, infection, advanced age, friction, anemia, inadequate blood supply and nutritional deficiencies. As we have noted, the major types of chronic wounds are diabetic, venous and pressure.

• *Diabetic Ulcers:* Diabetes hardens blood vessels, impairs circulation, and reduces peripheral nerve sensation. For these reasons, an ulcer that would normally heal quickly may result in a chronic wound in a diabetic. This can become life-threatening, especially when the wound is on the lower extremity, an extremely common occurrence. One study of diabetics found that 15% of the 150 million diabetics worldwide suffer from foot ulcerations.[5] "Approximately 15 to 20 percent of the esti-mated 16 million persons in the United States with diabetes mellitus will be hospitalized with a foot complication at some time during the course of their disease."[6] The wound, refusing to heal, becomes an entry point for infections that can spread to the rest of the body. Partially formed blood clots at the inju-ry site may break apart and clog nearby blood vessels, causing ischemia. This helps explain why over 60% of all lower-limb amputations (excepting those that are necessary due to trauma, such as a car crash) occur in diabetics.[7]

- *Pressure Ulcers:* Pressure ulcers are also known as decubitus ulcers. They are a major problem for bedridden patients, par-ticularly the elderly who are prone to having thin skin and longer wound healing time. The pressure sore forms as the result of tissue damage at the point where a bony prominence comes into contact with an object such as a bed or a chair. The most commonly involved areas are the pelvic bones, sacrum, hips, ankles, and heels. Pressure ulcers have been categorized by the National Pressure Ulcer Advisory Panel (NPUAP) into four stages, reflecting the amount of anatomical tissue lost (see chart). Preventing and effectively managing pressure ulcers is an important measure of quality for US healthcare facilities.

- *Venous Ulcers:* These skin ulcers are the most common type of leg ulcer. A venous stasis ulcer occurs when the valves in the veins of the leg malfunction, stretching the veins and allow-ing blood to pool in a certain area. The epidermis over this area tends to thin and take on a discolored brown appearance as melanin and hemosiderin (iron containing pigment) get deposited in the tissue. The skin appears leathery and edema-tous. The resultant ulcer often forms on the lower leg in an area where the neighboring blood vessels have already broken down, making the venous stasis ulcer particularly resistant to treatment. One of the most common areas is the inner ankle. As with the ulcers mentioned earlier, infection is likely. In addi-tion to biological wound dressings, these wounds are treated by extrinsic compression that helps to reduce the swelling and extravagated blood.

Chronic wounds (wounds that will not heal within a normal time period) pose enormous problems for affected individuals, their caregivers, and society at large. These wounds affect more than

PRESSURE ULCER FOUR STAGES

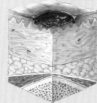

Stage 1: Intact skin with non-blanchable redness of a localized area usually over a bony prominence. Darkly pigmented skin may not have visible blanching; its color may differ from the surrounding area.

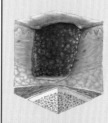

Stage 2: Partial thickness loss of dermis presenting as a shallow open ulcer with a red pink wound bed, without slough. May also present as an intact or open/ruptured serum-filled blister.

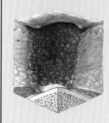

Stage 3: Full thickness tissue loss. Subcutaneous fat may be visible but bone, tendon or muscle are not exposed. Slough may be present but does not obscure the depth of tissue loss. May include undermining and tunneling.

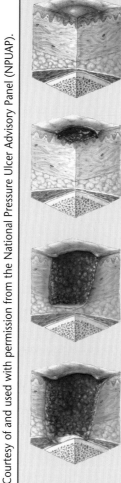

Stage 4: Full thickness tissue loss with exposed bone, tendon or muscle. Slough or eschar may be present on some parts of the wound bed. Often include undermining and tunneling.

Courtesy of and used with permission from the National Pressure Ulcer Advisory Panel (NPUAP).

five million Americans, and cost an estimated $20 billion a year.[8] Modern medicine has been unable to provide satisfactory answers to many of these five million Americans. "The best available treatment for chronic wounds achieves only a 50% healing rate that is often temporary."[9]

The Emergence of Biological Dressings

Biological dressings, comprising cells from an assortment of sources, are now routinely used in the management of skin wounds. These cell-based therapies assist in repairing and/or replacing the wounded tissue. Some cellular products can also help restore normal functionality to the skin such as sweating, sebum production, or hair replacement.

As more biological dressings come to market, scientific attention is increasingly being drawn to the type of cells used, as well as the sources of these cells. Improvements in wound healing outcomes will be driven by the choice of biological material used, as well as the wound healing factors they secrete. An additional important factor will be the delivery system used. Among the common allogeneic sources in commercially available products are:

- Acellular cadaver dermis,
- Porcine skin or small intestine mucosa,
- Foreskin fibroblasts and keratinocytes, and
- Donor keratinocytes.

These cells are layered or seeded onto a variety of matrixes that, depending upon the product, may include nylon mesh, silicone, bovine or horse collagen, polyglycolic acid, or hyaluronic acid.

In addition to allogeneic sources, autologous skin fibroblasts and substitutes have been used in the treatment of leg ulcers. As with many types of autologous treatment, different levels of efficiency are achieved.[10] This is due, in large part, to the long time needed to cultivate the patient's own tissue. With these limitations in mind, the selection of allogeneic cell type becomes paramount.

Fetal Cells: Enhanced Efficiency and Effectiveness for Wound Healing

It is no surprise that the search for an ideal allogeneic cell has focused on the study of fetal skin cells. Scientists have long known that an in-utero wound to a fetus heals without scarring, and with little concomitant inflammation. Could this benefit extend to the treatment of adult wounds with fetal skin cells? According to Dr. Lee Ann Laurent-Applegate (PhD), University Hospital CHUV, Department of Musculoskeletal Medicine, Cellular Therapy Unit, in Lausanne, Switzerland, fetal skin cells offer multiple advantages over other sources. Applegate has studied the application of fetal skin cells on a collagen matrix for chronic wounds and burns.

In her studies with this technology, she has noted that the new wound collagen is deposited in a very organized pattern that is indistinguishable from uninjured tissue. Using fetal skin cells, it is possible to regenerate all layers of skin as well as normal appendages such as hair follicles, sebaceous and sweat glands.[10] There are significant manufacturing advantages that fetal cells, taken at 14

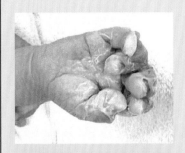
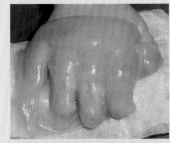
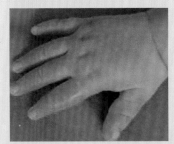
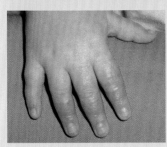

The photos above are of a 14 month old female who suffered second and third degree burns from scalding coffee. She was treated with fetal cell constructs. *Top:* Before treatment; *Second:* Fetal cell construct after application; *Third:* 2 weeks post treatment; *Bottom:* Follow-up 15 months post treatment.[11, 12]

Top and Bottom images: Reprinted from Applegate, L. A., *Skin Pharmacol Physiol*, 22:63-73, © 2009, with permission from S. Karger AG, Basel. Second and Third images: Reprinted from Applegate, L. A., *The Lancet*, 366:840-842, © 2005, wiht permission from Elsevier.

The Difference Between Scarring and Scarless Collagen[12]

Why does an adult wound result in a scar, while an in-utero fetal wound does not? The answer may be found in the type of collagen produced. In the fetus, the fibroblasts produce more type III collagen with the wound made up of 30-60% type III. Adult wounds comprised only 10-20% type III, with a greater percentage of type I collagen. In comparison to type I collagen, type III fibers are smaller and finer, allowing for a more organized deposition. The growth factor TGF-ß has also been shown to play an important role in this process.

weeks of gestation, have, including:

- Rapid growth in culture,

- Resistance to oxidative stress,

- No expression of HLA (thus they are immune privileged and do not incur rejection),

- Expandability without potency loss: 900 million biological bandages can be fabricated from one master bank, and

- Minimal initial tissue requirement: a master bank can be built from one skin organ donation (no need for multiple donors).

Applegate reported on the use of the fetal skin constructs to treat 13 skin ulcers in 9 patients over 3 to 31 weeks. Of these 13 ulcers, eight closed completely, four were significantly ameliorated in size but not completely closed. One patient who noted substantial progress was lost to follow-up.[10] In other studies, allogeneic skin substitutes that used fetal foreskin have shown decreased healing times for diabetic foot ulcers and non-bearing wounds.[13, 14]

Applegate noted similar success using fetal skin constructs in a study of deep second and third degree burns in pediatric patients.[11] Complete closure of the burn occurred at just over two weeks with no hypertrophic granulation tissue. Furthermore, no retraction or secondary skin breakdown occurred. When the constructs were applied over extremities, the joints healed with full range of motion.

Growth Factors: The Search for a Silver Bullet

We have seen how cell choice makes a difference in efficiency of wound healing. Because so much of the wound healing effect is mediated by growth factors, researchers have spent considerable time and attention in this arena. Similar to the drug discovery process, the earliest research has centered around attempts to identify a singular growth factor, one that ultimately can be manufactured synthetically through a recombinant process.

One of the first to be considered has been VEGF. In a study led by Dr. Robert Galiano (MD) of Northwestern Memorial Hospital in Chicago, topically applied VEGF was introduced to the wounds of diabetic mice. The VEGF-treated mice healed more than twice as fast as untreated mice, with the VEGF wounds showing "increased epithelialization, increased matrix deposition, and enhanced cellular proliferation" compared to the control group.[15] The researchers noted that the VEGF also induced a significant up-regulation of platelet-derived growth factor-B and fibroblast growth factor-2. These two growth factors influence both platelet and fibroblast activity.

Although the results of the animal study were uniformly positive, there was one small proviso: VEGF treatment originally induced some leakage in the newly formed vasculature near the wounds.[15] It is possible that the concomitant application of other regulatory factors, such as angiopoietin, might have reduced this vascular reaction, but the study had only used one growth factor.

VEGF is not the only singular growth factor that has been tested on wound healing. A study with the Sonic Hedgehog (SHH) protein, which regulates the interaction between the outer and inner linings of blood vessels, showed that the use of this peptide enhanced wound healing in a mouse model by promoting increased wound vascularity.[B, 16] Other studies have focused on colony-stimulating factors and keratinocyte growth factors for venous stasis ulcers. The colony-stimulating factors aid wound healing by stimulating the macrophages and monocytes, leading to an increase in granulation volume.[17] Keratinocyte growth factor (KGF-2) studies of rats showed that this growth factor aids epithelialization, but does little for wound contraction.[18]

Of all the singular growth factor treatments, only one is approved for treatment by the FDA in the United States. Platelet-derived growth factor-BB (PDGF-BB) has been approved for the treatment of neuropathic diabetic ulcers; it is used off-label for other wound types. Known as becaplermin (REGRANEX® gel), it is produced from genetically engineered yeast cells in which the gene for the Beta chain of PDGF has been inserted. In a multicenter, randomized, prospective double-blind placebo-controlled trial, PDGF-BB demonstrated 20% improvement in wound closure of lower extremity diabetic ulcers after 20 weeks of treatment.[19] The best results appeared to be obtained in wounds that had been aggressively debrided.[20]

The Power of More than One Growth Factor

But why use just one isolated growth factor, when stem cells are able to up-regulate and secrete so many different factors? After all, "optimum healing of a cutaneous wound requires a well-orchestrated integration of the complex biological and molecular events of cell migration and proliferation and extracellular matrix deposition, angiogenesis, and remodeling."[9] That is to say, there are a lot of

Why is Fetal Skin More Biologically Potent than Neonatal Foreskin?[21]
Differences in gene expression for cytokines and growth factors helps to explain the difference in biological effect of these two skin sources. Two of note: regulation for some of the TGF-ß genes were increased as much as six fold. Down-regulation of the growth factor GDF-10 (important for wound healing) was 11.8 times greater.

"Optimum healing of a cutaneous wound requires a well-orchestrated integration of the complex biological and molecular events of cell migration and proliferation and extracellular matrix deposition, angiogenesis, and remodeling."

different variables that need to be understood, or rather optimized, for better clinical results. A stem cell, through its production of multiple types of growth factors with multiple mechanisms of action, may be far better suited to heal a complex wound than a single recombinant created protein. With this broader efficacy in mind, researchers turned their attention to a well-profiled stem cell: the mesenchymal stem cell.

Mesenchymal stem cells, the cells that differentiate into connective tissue, have been used in conjunction with many other types of stem cells, partly to optimize the other cells' results. In a wound-healing situation, however, the connective tissue comprises much of the tissue in urgent need of repair. For this reason, MSCs are on the forefront of researchers' efforts for wound treatment.

MSCs, HSCs and Wound Care

MSCs had already gained a well-established history in treating acute radiation syndrome, with mechanisms of action that promised additional benefits if applied to wound healing. But starting in 2003, several studies began piquing academic interest in the possibility of using MSCs, and other stem cell types, to repair dermal wounds.

A pilot study in 2003, followed by a single-patient study in 2005 and another small-number patient study in 2007, used bone marrow aspirate to treat chronic wounds.[22, 23, 24] The results were encouraging, but it was hard to draw conclusions about which specific cells were inducing healing.

An animal study conducted at the University of Washington Medical Center helped explain the results. The Washington researchers, led by Dr. Carrie Fathke (MD), used bone-marrow cells in mice to measure collagen deposition and wound repair. The bone marrow cells included three stem cell types: EPCs, HSCs, and MSCs. The researchers sought to understand how these and other cells could work in concert to heal wounds, but they also attempted to examine each cell's effects in isolation by separating the hematopoietic and mesenchymal cells and then treating mice with each cell type. Their results "suggest[ed] a potential divergence in the role of the two bone marrow components."[25] The hematopoietic cells produced more cells during the beginning of the wound healing process, but the mesenchymal cells worked to "maintain a stable population in the skin throughout the wound repair process."[25]

The study demonstrated that "there is a unique contribution from both hematopoietic and MC lineages during the early phase of wound healing and later remodeling phase."[25] The findings regarding mesenchymal cells, however, were arguably more exciting, for three reasons. First, mesenchymal stem cells are far easier to obtain than most other cell types, making them a more compelling option for stem cell-based treatments.[26] Second, HSCs have more immuno-compatability issues than MSCs, again giving MSCs the advantage in translating scientific data to clinical results. And finally, the evidence that MSCs were more useful for later stages of repair seemed applicable to a chronic wound situation where the original inflammatory response had not manifested effective healing.

The University of Washington study, like the small-number clinical studies, aroused scientific interest, but it also raised unresolved questions. Fathke et al. admitted that "because our MC [mesencyhmal cell] selection method enriches for MC without eliminating contaminating HC [hematopoietic cells], additional experiments are necessary to confirm these findings."[25] Similarly, additional experiments were needed to resolve which cellular elements of the bone marrow aspirate, in the clinical studies, were most responsible for effecting repair.

Though other stem cell types can replace injured cells, HSCs can differentiate into different blood cells to fight infection (white blood cells), nourish the wounded area (red blood cells), and begin the process of repair (platelets). The administration of HSCs may be especially useful during the early phases of wound healing, when the body needs white blood cells to fight off invading bacteria and cleanse cellular debris as part of the inflammatory response. A 2009 review article points out that "the obvious source for the leukocytes that migrate to the wound site during the early, inflammatory phase are bone marrow-derived hematopoietic stem cells, which have long been recognized to give rise to all blood cell lineages."[27] Because HSCs express HLA that might cause an immunorejection or even graft-versus-host disease, however, HSCs may be one of the few stem cell types for which an autologous source is preferred.

The scientific establishment is focusing much of its attention on the mesenchymal stem cell, conducting a variety of animal studies and clinical trials. In fact, animal trials using mesenchymal stem cells were already underway before Fathke et al. published their own findings on how MSCs compared to other cell types.

MSCs were used to treat mini-pigs with skin wounds.[28] "The cells differentiated into vascular endothelial tissue," explains a 2010

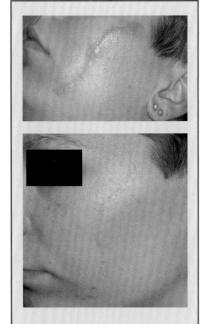

Combination Treatment of Hypertrophic Scars

This case study, presented at the 2008 meeting of the American Society for Laser Medicine and Surgery (ASLMS) by Dr. Nikolai I. Tankovich (MD, PhD) and colleagues shows before and after treatment of one-year old hypertrophic scar. The patient received two identical treatments two months apart. The after photo on the bottom (slightly enlarged) shows results at four months. The patient was treated, at the same session, with a 1540nm fractional non-ablative laser along with an injection of fibroblast progenitor cells primed to produce collagenase. Collagenase is an enzyme that helps to break down the disordered scar tissue.

review, "forming new blood vessels and thus improving wound healing."[29] A contemporary study treated burn-wounded rats with autologous and allogeneic MSCs, resulting in "a rapid decrease in the burn area."[29, 30] In one study, researchers used human-derived MSCs to treat mice with injuries to the skin and spinal cord.[31] Improved healing was observed in the spinal cord (see Chapter 6) and the skin. Another study has shown that mesenchymal stem cells can form several different types of skin cells, including keratinocytes.[32] As scientific knowledge of MSCs use in wounds grew, researchers began wondering how MSCs might be used to treat burns.

The First Clinical Use of Stem Cells for Burn Victims

In 2005, a paper published in the Russian scientific journal *Kletochnye Tecknologii v Biologii I Meditisine (Cell Technologies in Biology and Medicine)* told the story of S., a 45-year old female patient who had suffered devastating burns two years earlier.

Dr. Masrur F. Rasulov (MD) and his team of scientists, from the Institute of Transplantology and Artificial Organs in Moscow, explain that S.'s clothes "inflamed during fire and stuck to the skin," burning her at the "neck, left half of the face, left upper limb, left half of the chest, lower third of the left thigh, and anterior surface of both shins, total area up to 40% body surface."[33] Many of those burns were third degree burns.

"Despite the 20-day treatment," Rasulov et al. wrote, "respiratory, cardiovascular, and hepatic [liver] insufficiency progressed."[33] S. required repeated blood cell infusions in order to remain stable. In addition to traditional wound care, the hospital team performed multiple and extensive debridements (removal of dead tissue). However, necrosed tissue would re-form in different wound sites "because of poor blood supply and wound infection."[33] S.'s wounds were manifesting "weak epithelial growth at some sites (at the wound edges)," but the wound-healing process was moving at a frustratingly slow pace.

After approximately one month of limited improvement with traditional treatment, S. received an application of fibroblast-like mesenchymal stem cells (FMSC). These cells were allogeneic MSCs that had been primed to "pre-differentiate" into fibroblasts, the connective tissue cells that stimulate collagen production and produce the extracellular matrix.[33] Fibroblasts are integral to the wound healing process, and Rasulov et al. hypothesized that they would effect significant wound repair. They were right. In their own words detailing S.'s condition, the researchers explained that, three days after the first FMSC transplant:

> *The greater part of granulating surface of burn wounds was covered with granulations, patient's status improved; she easier contacted with other people, pain in the burn wounds was relieved. Visually, numerous small bright red vessels appeared; these new capillaries were plethoric [filled with too much blood] and profusely bled even after careful dressing removal.[33]*

With improved underlying tissue, S. was then able to undergo autodermoblasty, a painful but necessary process that remains an important part of wound repair for serious burn patients. It consists of removing strips of the patient's own skin, cultivated from unwounded areas of the body, and laying them on top of the wounded area. The intention is that the body will reincorporate the skin into the wounded site, but the process is far from foolproof.

The wounded area must develop working vasculature and an extracellular matrix to supply the grafted skin with oxygen and nutrients, and quickly, before the skin cells die off. New tissue must form to connect the skin to the wounded area. Meanwhile, debris in the wound will obstruct the healing process, even with regular debridement. Connecting a skin graft to a wound becomes much more difficult if there is a layer of dead tissue in the way.

Rasulov et al. hoped that the FMSCs would lay the groundwork for the skin grafts to successfully integrate themselves, or "take." In November 2003, S. had skin removed from her thighs and placed onto the area of her burns, covering approximately 60% of the wound surface. At the same time, S. received additional transplants of FMSC on the wounds, and around the skin grafts. The first benefit of the FMSC transplantation was seen a mere 30 minutes after the first autodermoplasty. "Due to formation of a protective film by transplanted FMSC covering the entire burn surface, plasmarrhea drastically decreased as early as during the first 30 min."[33] The study authors use the term "plasmarrhea" to refer to the weeping of plasma, the colorless fluid that forms part of the blood. The FMSC helped stop the plasma from leaking out of S.'s open wounds.[33]

Days later, the medical team observed the beginning of the granulation processes followed by new blood vessels and skin formation

Earliest Tissue Replacement for Burns in the United States

In 1981, a burn patient was treated in Boston by first removing a small piece of skin. The cells were expanded outside the body, put on gauze and placed back on the wound.

According to Dr. Anthony Atala (MD), Director of the Wake Forest Institute for Regenerative Medicine, this is the earliest report for this treatment.[38]

"Transplantation of allogeneic FMSC appreciably accelerated recovery of homeostasis and promoted healing of thermal burn, thus accelerating convalescence of a patient with burns."

around the grafted areas, "due to high capacity of allogenic FMSC to stimulate epithelial and endothelial growth." Ten days after the autodermoplasty, the researchers observed that 99% of the transplanted skin grafts had successfully reconnected to the subdermal tissue.[33]

Thirteen days after her first autodermoplasty, S. received a second set of skin grafts. Approximately two weeks after that, she was discharged from the hospital. The researchers concluded that "transplantation of allogeneic FMSC appreciably accelerated recovery of homeostasis and promoted healing of thermal burn, thus accelerating convalescence of a patient with burns." Furthermore, they proposed that autodermoplasty "can be performed sooner with more rapid take of SG" when fibroblast-like mesenchymal stem cells were used to stimulate wound healing in conjunction with the skin graft procedures.[33]

No treatment could restore S.'s skin to how it was before the fire, but allogeneic adult stem cells were able to contribute to her recovery, helping her integrate more healthy skin into the wound, accelerating healing, and assisting in getting her out of the hospital and back to reclaiming her life.

Chronic Wounds and Burns

The clinical studies continued to progress; in 2006, a diabetic with a foot ulcer received a combination of MSCs and fibroblasts.[34] "The outcome," explains a 2010 review, "was a steady decrease in wound size and increase in vascularity."[29] In 2007, a young Chilean victim of radiation burns was treated with locally applied autologous MSCs, and rapid wound healing was observed.[35] The same year, skin cancer patients' acute wounds were treated with autologous MSCs, and demonstrated a "major decrease in wound size."[29, 36] The following year, twenty patients with chronic wounds received MSCs from a collagen sponge graft. Eighteen of the twenty patients experienced complete wound healing, a 90% success rate.[37] More recently, research teams have begun cultivating mesenchymal stem cells from adipose tissue, comparing them to bone marrow-derived MSCs to see if different lineages of mesenchymal stem cells might produce different results.

With this growing body of research, clinicians have gained a better understanding of how these stem cells are able to effect repair of chronic wounds. A scientific team at the University of Wisconsin notably summarized the role of mesenchymal stem cells:

Ten days after the autodermoplasty, the researchers observed that 99% of the transplanted skin grafts had "taken," successfully reconnecting to the subdermal tissue.

Functional characteristics of mesenchymal stem cells that may benefit wound healing include their ability to migrate to the site of injury or inflammation, participate in regeneration of damaged tissues, stimulate proliferation and differentiation of resident progenitor cells, promote recovery of injured cells through growth factor secretion and matrix remodeling, and exert unique immunomodulatory and anti-inflammatory effects. Thus, in contrast to most pharmacologic agents targeting single pathophysiologic pathways, mesenchymal stem cells could affect tissue healing and regeneration through many different routes.[39]

The Wisconsin researchers also point out that mesencyhmal stem cells can address tissue hypoxia, inflammation, repetitive ischemic injuries, and cellular aging; all elements that can contribute to chronic wounds.[39]

Mesenchymal stem cells are remarkable for their ease of cultivation, immunocompatibility, and their ability to catalyze or advance healing pathways. They have shown promise in a variety of clinical indications, but in wound healing, their ability to create connective tissue and "provide the microenvironmental support for hematopoietic cells" allows them to make an especially pronounced contribution.[39] As previous chapters have demonstrated, however, no single type of cell has a monopoly on repair. Other types of adult stem cells that have shown promise include **keratinocyte** progenitor cells, abreviated as KSCs, endothelial progenitor cells, and hematopoietic stem cells.

Keratinocyte Progenitor Cells and Wound Healing

It has been well established that different species have different rates of healing when it comes to dermal wounds. For example, "full thickness skin wounds heal more rapidly in rabbits than human beings, with greater contraction, and less scar formation," noted a paper in British medical journal, *The Lancet*.[39] Part of the reason seems to be that rabbits simply have more hair than humans. It was first noticed in 1976 that hair follicles could produce skin cells that would re-establish missing skin tissue, and more recent stem cell research has uncovered an explanation: hair follicles have their own source of progenitor cells.[42] These keratinocyte progenitor cells reside in the part of the skin that sheaths the bulge of the follicle itself. From there, they rally to the epidermis "during times

> ### MSCs and Wound Healing
> MSCs exert their wound healing effects through the production of diverse growth factors that activate dermal fibroblasts causing them to increase proliferation and migration, as well as secrete collagen. The antioxidant effects of MSCs also protect fibroblasts from oxidative stress. Among the factors released by MSCs are vascular endothelial growth factor, hepatocyte growth factor, insulin-like growth factor, platelet-derived growth factor, and transforming growth factor ß.[41]

Keratinocytes: make up 95% of epidermal cells, and are responsible for the creation of keratin. Going from epidermis to dermis, keratinocytes are also known as prickle cells, granular cells, and basal cells.

of need," such as a skin wound, where they can differentiate into needed skin cells.[42] A 2005 study at the University of Pennsylvania School of Medicine found that "about one-third of the coverage of the wound came from the progenitor cells in the hair follicle."[43] Dr. George Cotsarelis (MD), the senior author of the resulting paper, who identified this source of stem cells back in 1990, expressed hope that "in the future, we think that we will be able to design treatments that enhance the flow of cells from the hair follicle to the epidermis in the hope of enhancing wound healing and treating patients with wounds."[43, 44]

Epithelial, or keratinocyte, cells in the skin are located within the bulge of the hair follicle, around and below the arrector pili muscle. Cotsarelis has found these follicular stem cells to be an excellent tool for wound repair. Another main population of stem cells in the skin come from the basal layer of the epidermis and are often referred to as interfollicular epidermal stem cells. These skin stem cells were noticed in animal populations in the early 1980s, but a subsequent explosion of scientific studies into these interfollicular epidermal stem cells began in the next decade.[44]

Scientists have noted that the "two KSC [keratinocyte stem cell] populations are endowed with considerable plasticity and could be interchangeable to a certain extent," implying that both stem cell types could offer similar clinical results for wound healing and other dermatologic issues.[45] However, Dr. Pritinder Kaur (PhD), of the Epithelial Stem Cell Biology Laboratory at the Peter MacCallum Cancer Centre in Melbourne, Australia, cautions:

An important factor often overlooked in KSC biology is that only a minute proportion of primary epidermal cells isolated from the skin actually adhere to tissue culture plastic and subsequently form a measurable colony... The limitations of current culture techniques then have profound implications for both basic stem cell research and clinical applications.[44]

Kaur continues by pointing out that scientific advancement is necessary to move keratinocyte cells further along the transition from science to medicine. "Clearly, a lot remains to be done to improve culture conditions for ex *vivo* expansion of patient keratinocytes so that more of the precious harvested cells are employed for therapy."[44]

Other types of skin stem cells have been uncovered, as well. In 2009, researchers at the Howard Hughes Medical Institute (HHMI) in Maryland confirmed the discovery of a new type of skin stem cell.[47]

Skin Stem Cell Plasticity

Dr. Robert Hoffman, Professor of Surgery at the University of California, San Diego Medical Center, and his team were able to show that stem cells isolated from the hair-follicle bulge were able to differentiate into neurons, glia, keratinocytes, smooth muscle cells, and melanocytes *in vitro*.

Furthermore, these cells were able to differentiate into neurons after being transplanted into mice.

These cells also express the neural stem cell marker, nestin.[46]

These cells, which researcher Dr. Freda Miller (PhD) dubbed skin-derived precursors (SKP), reside in the dermis, below the epithelial region in which previous populations of stem cells have been located.

This is not the first time that the Howard Hughes Medical Institute has induced a breakthrough in our understanding of skin stem cells. HHMI researcher Dr. Elaine Fuchs (PhD) is a well-known stem cell pioneer, having discovered an epidermal stem cell population approximately a decade ago. Fuchs's scientific explorations were first hailed as a possible cure for baldness; now, her insights are recognized as having paved the way for current research into wound care.[48]

As Miller sees it, her dermal stem cells could be used in a complementary way to epithelial cells. The two cell types, dermal and epidermal, would be able to repair both levels of the skin in a wound care situation. "Stem cell researchers like to talk about building organs in a dish," explained Miller in an interview last year. "If you have all the right players—dermal stem cells and epidermal stem cells—working together, you could do that with skin in a very real way."[47]

Endothelial Progenitor Cells (EPC) and Beyond

Research into endothelial progenitor cells has revealed that, by secreting growth factors and cytokines, and through their promotion of angiogenesis, EPCs "may be regarded as an attractive therapeutic option for the treatment of chronic wounds, which remain a major clinical problem, especially in diabetic patients."[49] An animal study conducted by a team of scientists at the Sungkyunkwan University School of Medicine in Seoul, Korea, demonstrated how EPCs induce wound healing. Their findings included:

- EPCs released significant levels of growth factors, including VEGF and platelet-derived growth factor BB (PDGF-BB). PDGF-BB is known to stimulate fibroblasts to produce the extra-cellular matrix, effecting significant wound repair. In fact, PDGF-BB is sometimes administered to chronic wounds alone.

- EPCs "produced in abundance several chemoattractants of monocytes and macrophages that are known to play a pivotal role in the early phase of wound healing."[49]

- EPCs promote angiogenesis, being "directly involved in the formation of new capillaries in the granulation tissue."[49] The researchers noted that transplanted EPCs were not just up-regulating angiogenic factors, but also differentiating into the endothelial cells needed to grow new vascular tissue.

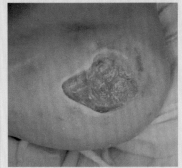

Limb salvage after marrow implantation. The top image shows a non-healing ulcer on the patient's heel. Improvement can be seen in the bottom image 8 weeks after implantation.

EPCs, the researchers concluded, had the potential to effect meaningful repair to chronic wounds.

Though other stem cell types can replace injured cells, HSCs can differentiate into different blood cells to fight infection (white blood cells), nourish the wounded area (red blood cells), and begin the process of repair (platelets). The administration of HSCs may be especially useful during the early phases of wound healing, when the body needs white blood cells to fight off invading bacteria and cleanse cellular debris as part of the inflammatory response. A 2009 review article points out, "the obvious source for the leukocytes that migrate to the wound site during the early, inflammatory phase are bone marrow-derived hematopoietic stem cells, which have long been recognized to give rise to all blood cell lineages."[27]

Progenitor cells from other tissue sources are also being used in wound healing. Dr. Minori Ueda (DDS, PhD), from the Department of Oral and Maxillofacial Surgery, Nagoya University School of Medicine, has been conducting research on skin applications involving two different stem cell populations: deciduous teeth and gingival mucousal cells.[41, 50, 51] In addition to being a rich source of growth factors, he has shown that these stem cells increase collagen synthesis and activate the proliferation and migration of the fibroblasts.[50]

Delivery Systems

One of the remaining limitations of stem cell therapy is that there may not be enough cultured cells to effect a clinical result. With KSCs, in Dr. Kaur's words, "What goes into a culture dish is not necessarily equivalent to what we read out."[44] Other stem cell types have similar problems with expansion, such as cardiac stem cells. And even if large numbers of stem cells are introduced to the body, not all of them home into the appropriate area.

In order to mitigate or erase all of these problems, the clinician tries to ensure that the stem cells home into the exact area of injury, and stay there. Promising advances in this area include cell matrices, genetically altered cells or cells that have been primed in a cell culture to act a certain way, and even imbuing cells with magnetic properties.

With dermal wounds, clinicians have different options for how to deliver the cells to the body, allowing for experimentation to discover which delivery mechanisms ensure that the stem cells will stay in place. Some of the stem cell delivery mechanisms that have been used to great effect with dermal wounds include:

- *Fibrin Spray:* Dr. Vincent Falanga (MD) of the Departments of Dermatology and Biochemistry at Boston University School of Medicine, is credited with developing a fibrin spray used to deliver mesenchymal stem cells to cutaneous wounds. Fibrin is a protein which, in conjunction with platelets, forms the clot of a wound. Sprayed on a wound, the fibrin forms a mesh into which the stem cells are embedded. Falanga and a colleague, Dr. Jisun Cha (MD) of Roger Williams Medical Center, declared that the spray "may represent a rather ideal way of introducing cells, and not just stem cells (perhaps even soluble mediators), into injury sites."[26]

- *Mucosal epithelial cell spray:* Taking advantage of the high proliferative ability and long biological activity of mucosal epidermal cells, Ueda has created a sprayed application of cultured mucosal epithelial autografts. Ten patients with deep dermal burns were included in a prospective study. The average total-body-surface burn was 17.7%; the average Abbreviated Burn Severity Index (ABSI) was 6.3 points. Patients had excellent results with the average period of epithelialization for the wound surface occurring at 12.5 days. The Vancouver Scar Scale at follow up was 1.5 points, which indicated an excellent cosmetic outcome.[51]

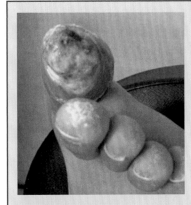
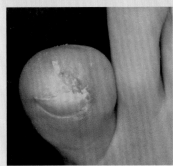

Limb salvage after marrow implantation. Top image shows ischemic necrosis on the patient's big toe. The bottom shows improvement 8 weeks after implantation.

Reprinted from Tateishi-Yuyama, *The Lancet*, 360:427-435, © 2002, with permission from Elsevier.

- *Matrices:* A patient presenting a chronic ulcer received a collagen matrix seeded with bone marrow cells in 2005, before a skin graft. "Although, we recognize that a single clinical case is not the basis for solid conclusion," the study's authors admit, "the treatment successfully induced healthy granulation tissue without any side effect and eventual closure of a nonhealing chronic wound that had not responded to a year of conventional therapy."[23] In a previously mentioned 2008 clinical study, twenty patients with chronic wounds received their MSCs through a collagen sponge applied to the injured area; the wounds healed in 90% of the patients.[37] Today, intelligent matrices are being designed to generate specific signals that will optimize cell homing, mobilization, and adhesion mechanisms.[29]

These delivery systems "may serve as a scaffold for mesenchymal stem cell attachment and native cell recruitment, with the potential to further improve tissue regeneration," explain the doctors at the

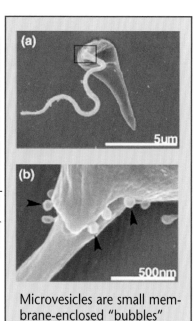

Microvesicles are small membrane-enclosed "bubbles" which can transport key genes and proteins to neighboring cells.

Division of Plastic and Reconstructive Surgery at the University of Wisconsin-Madison.[39]

Addressing the Challenge of Scalability

For a stem cell or growth factor treatment to ultimately prove successful as a commercial product, it must be scalable. The treatment should be easily deliverable to large populations in diverse settings. This presents a challenge for the delivery of allogeneic-live stem cell products. To maintain viability, these products must be kept frozen before being thawed out. Once thawed, the products must have the equivalent or near equivalent viability and potency of the fresh product. Years of developing proprietary technology has made this possible, representing the leadership position that several companies in the private sector now hold within the stem cell field.

However, even with the best freezing techniques, there still exist limitations to delivery. The ideal cell-based product would have the following specifications:

• Biologically active at room temperature,

• Containing all necessary growth factors for wound healing,

• Deliverable in a variety of formats,

• Scalable—able to be quickly reproduced in large amounts, and

• Produced under current Good Manufacturing Practices (cGMP) conditions.

Stemedica Cell Technologies has recently advanced the field of wound healing through the use of a proprietary patented stabalization technology. In this process, the cell is preserved, no longer living, and reduced to a dried powder that contains the full complement of cytokines and growth factors of the original stem cell. A unique advantage of this method is preservation of the cell's microvesicles, small membrane-enclosed "bubbles" that can transport key genes and proteins to neighboring cells.

Treatment options are numerous for a dried, biologically active product with all the necessary factors for wound healing. The product could be directly applied to a wound, integrated into a gel, or seeded onto a matrix of either a new or existing product. Rather than attempt wound healing with a single growth factor, the rationale is strong for applying a growth factor cocktail to the wound. One wound care study noted that:

Although many attempts have been made to improve chronic wounds by administering angiogenic growth factors such as VEGF, clinical results have been discouraging, with only modest improvements in the length of time to closure, in breaking strength, and in neuropathy.[49]

Similarly, the release of a few growth factors with limited viability is no comparison to a stem cell treatment that would utilize an optimal balance of over a hundred growth factors and cytokines. If stem cells are our "little doctors," then their unique protein secretions may be the best therapeutic regimen.

Preserving stem cell wound care factors through this proprietary technology has ramifications beyond the world of wound care, but for millions of people who deal with chronic wounds, this scalable and effective stem cell-based solution may offer significant healing.

Toward a New Future

Wound care is a field in which new solutions are urgently needed, but more than that, it is a field which would benefit from "a new paradigm of treatment."[29] Today, a variety of stem cell types have entered different phases of scientific exploration and clinical development. Simultaneously, clinicians are experimenting with new ways to apply stem cells. This has resulted in advancements in the number of stem cells that remain viable and that operate within the treatment area, or take, better optimizing clinical outcomes. Similarly, stem cell-based wound healing factor treatment may soon become another clinical breakthrough, one that could offer relief to millions.

With this new paradigm, stem cell treatments could become the standard of care for burn victims, diabetics, and the elderly. As these treatments become increasingly scalable due to innovation in the private sector, stem cells may even find application on the battlefield healing the wounds of soldiers with combat-related injuries. No matter the patient, stem cells may offer a meaningful treatment option, especially for wounds that will not heal through conventional therapies.

Chapter 13
The Future

"You talk about the potential for cures with cell-based therapies. If you look at the big picture, about three-quarters of healthcare expenditures are driven by chronic and degenerative diseases for which stem cells are potentially relevant. That includes diseases like diabetes, like heart failure, etc," explained Brock Reeve, Executive Director of the Harvard Stem Cell Institute, at a forum held at Harvard Business School on April 15, 2010. Reeve, who is also the half-brother of the late actor and stem cell research advocate Christopher Reeve, continued by saying:

> If stem cells ultimately are successful, there's a big 'whack' out of healthcare costs that we can take with this sort of approach. And I would suggest that so far, a lot of the pharmaceutical treatments have only been able to deal with symptoms, as opposed to fundamental cures. So the promise of stem cells, an exciting part, is the promise for the cure. [A, 1]

The group that Director Reeve was addressing included representatives from the worlds of venture capital, medicine, pharmaceuticals, healthcare and even insurance. Reeve's co-presenters also comprised a diverse group; he was followed by Dr. George Daley (MD, PhD) the decorated hematologist and past-President of the International Society for Stem Cell Research, but he was also preceded by Dr. Devyn Smith (PhD), Senior Director of one of Pfizer's Strategic Management Groups.

The assorted collection of both speakers and attendees at this event helps to reflect that the possibilities of stem cell medicine have wide ramifications for the worlds of science and healthcare, but also for various other disciplines. Investor interest in the stem cell field is exploding, while "Big Pharma" wonders whether the next stem cell "cure" will help them develop a new product or perhaps make some of their current drugs more effective.

"Historically in this space, both the venture capital industry has under-invested, and the pharmaceutical industry has under-invested." Reeve said. This is because "biotech companies are becoming product companies; they are not as oriented on R&D as they used to be." But as the technology and knowledge base expands, so does investor interest in partnering with stem cell companies and research initiatives around the world.

Within the next few years, adult cellular therapies are expected to transition from an industry worth tens of millions of dollars, to an industry whose revenues are measured in the billions.[2] Pharmaceutical companies have begun paying attention. For example, Pfizer pledged in November 2009 to invest up to $100 million in regenerative research, a category which includes both adult and embryonic stem cells.[2] If biotech companies are product-oriented companies, as Reeve says, then their increasing investment in stem cells reflects their belief that there will soon be a cell-based product entering the market.

Financially, the impact of a commercial stem cell product "would be staggering," write University of Minnesota Medical School professors Dr. Leo Furcht (MD) and William Hoffman. "To put this in perspective," they elaborate,

> *Consider that the global market for just one drug that makes more red blood cells from blood-forming stem cells—erythropoietin—is approximately $4 billion annually. Imagine the*

value of a drug that could regenerate heart muscle for people who have had heart attacks or who have heart failure for other reasons.[3]

But biotech companies are doing more than simply imagining these drugs; they are working hard to bring them to the market today. Robin Young, a financial analyst who observes the stem cell market and who has been named one of the best analysts "on the street" by *The Wall Street Journal*, has predicted that sales for stem cell-based treatments will reach $8.5 billion by 2016.[3] Kalorama Information, a market research company, predicts that stem cell technology will most likely reach more than $11 billion by the end of 2020.[4]

Hurdles to Progress

There are three major "gating factors" that can slow down the progress of a company as it attempts to get a stem cell-based therapy (SCBT) to market: technology, regulation, and investment. The development of safe and efficacious cell technology is a process that takes place within the company. Regulation, on the other hand, is a process with an extra set of variables, as companies work to meet the standards of regulatory agencies. Investment involves yet another set of variables, as private and public investors judge the likely success of a stem cell-based product.

For an allogeneic stem cell company, it is not enough to appropriately manufacture stem cells. There must also be a system in place to disseminate live cells on a global scale. Previously, a stem cell product made in California but sent to Europe or Asia would not survive the trip. Today, a new generation of proprietary cryogenic technology exists that allows for the cells to be frozen, shipped, and thawed, with a negligible difference in viability. It is due to this advance in technology that stem cell companies are able to realize the goal of global growth.

Furthermore, cutting-edge stem cell research has recently begun exploring the idea of using stem cells stabilized at room temperature. This proprietary process allows for the delivery of important stem cell factors without the need for freezing. Because freezing is not used, different application methods can be utilized to introduce the stem cell factors to the area of need.

There are still some areas where stem cell companies can continue improvement. For example, more information is needed

In the FDA's defense, the task of regulating prospective SCBTs is made even more challenging when one considers how rapidly the stem cell field is advancing. It seems like new stem cell discoveries occur every week, and regulators must keep abreast of new developments that may offer insight into the safety or efficacy of a proposed treatment.

to determine methods of delivery and dosimetry (the number of stem cells a patient should receive). Dozens of clinical studies have tried to answer this question, but more large-scale clinical trials are needed in order to further confirm and refine protocols.

While stem cell companies wrestle with these questions, they are beholding to national regulatory agencies. In the United States, this agency is the Food and Drug Administration (FDA), which is responsible for granting or withholding clearance to all new drugs or therapies in the United States market. Every stem cell company must embark upon the process of proving their cells' safety and efficacy to the FDA.

Stem cell-based treatments fall under several categories of regulated products: biologic products, drugs, devices, xenotransplantation products, and human cells, tissues, and cellular and tissue-based products.[5] Additionally, since the advent of embryonic stem cells, the FDA has crafted a set of guidelines that apply more specifically to embryonic stem cells. All of these regulations are in place to ensure safety for the patient population, but unfortunately they also ensure that the regulatory road is a long one. A more streamlined process would be beneficial to getting stem cell based therapies into the market at a faster pace.

A recent *Time* magazine article repeated some of the more common criticisms of the FDA, among which are the allegations that "the FDA is just plugging along. It's a small agency with a fine old tradition dwarfed in both budget and political power by the pharmaceutical giants it is being asked to police."[6] These issues may manifest themselves during a review of SCBTs, when the "small agency" must make sure that it understands all of the issues regarding a proposed new therapy, which is a difficult task given the complexity of stem cell biology. The result can be an unnecessarily elongated regulatory timeline.

In the FDA's defense, the task of regulating prospective SCBTs is made even more challenging when one considers how rapidly the stem cell field is advancing. It seems like new stem cell discoveries occur every week, and regulators must keep abreast of new developments that may offer insight into the safety or efficacy of a proposed treatment.

The FDA's current approach is limited in its accommodation of a multi-cell treatment paradigm. Given current regulatory procedures, only one stem cell-based therapy is tested at a time. This precludes effective measurement of a therapy that uses two or more stem cell types until each of the stem cells types have been individually approved for a certain indication. Yet years of clinical results have already shown that multi-cell treatment regimens can achieve better results than single-cell treatments.

But as the pace of research accelerates, so eventually will the transition through the regulatory path. Institutions are integrating stem cell medicine in a growing body of basic science, providing regulatory bodies with an enhanced understanding of how stem cells work within the body.

Similarly, the investment community's confidence in stem cell treatments has grown as basic research has advanced. The biggest issue that has restrained the investment community from entering the stem cell space has been misunderstandings over the therapeutic and financial capability of a stem cell-based treatment. More simply put, investors want to know, does it work? Can it be made into a major product? What is the timeline?

A review of the scientific literature, and a look at patient populations struck by an epidemic of degenerative and trauma-induced conditions, makes clear the fact that SCBTs offer the capability to provide measurable benefit to millions, if not billions of people. Increasingly, investors have come to this realization. Like most of the general public, investors see SCBT as a long-term proposition, an investment which would take decades to pay off. However, the many clinical studies around the world have demonstrated that stem cell treatments are already here. As the general public becomes better versed in the possibilities of stem cells, so too will investors realize that investment in SCBTs represents an exciting opportunity for financial growth.

Stem cell companies can tackle "orphan diseases" that major pharmaceutical companies have avoided, a fact that makes investment in SCBTs even more appealing than investment in traditional biotechnology ventures. An example is epidermolysis bullosa, a rare disease that can cause a patient's skin to literally fall off when touched.[7] Private companies and public institutions, noting that a certain disease has a very small patient population, are unwilling to invest millions in researching a treatment. For traditional biopharmaceuticals, orphan diseases represent a losing investment. But, stem cell companies are able to approach the problem in a different way, because they are looking for a cell-based, not a

Orphan Diseases

Most orphan diseases are "orphaned" because they are rare, affecting perhaps a few thousand people. But the term "rare disease" is quite misleading. There are thousands of rare diseases that affect the global population. EURORDIS, an organization dedicated to improving the lives of Europeans with rare diseases, has concluded that 6-8% of the European population suffer from a rare disease, a number encompassing some 30 million people.[10] In the United States, the number is slightly smaller. The Office of Rare Diseases, part of the National Institutes of Health, estimates that approximately 25 million Americans suffer from a rare disease.[11]

pharmacological, solution. As such, they are uniquely suited to offer realistic treatment solutions for orphan diseases, reaching out to a patient population that other biotechnology companies traditionally avoid.

The FDA appears to recognize this. Since 1983, the regulatory administration has been able to confer "Orphan Drug Status" on a company's efforts to tackle an orphan disease. The privileged status conveys a series of government incentives. Today, the FDA has granted several companies in the stem cell space Orphan Drug Status, showing faith in SCBT's ability to take on these small-scale diseases.[8, 9] From orphan diseases to conditions that strike down the elderly, the pace of stem cell research into clinical translation is accelerating.

As we come even closer to having stem cells enter the realm of mainstream medicine, we get a tantalizing glimpse of the future: new ways to apply stem cells, new treatment protocols for potential stem cell therapy, new uses of stem cells for drug discovery, and new players in the stem cell field. This final chapter explores these myriad possibilities, taking a comprehensive look at emerging trends and discussing the future of stem cells as medicine.

It's a Stem Cell World

As we have pointed out, the patients that stand to benefit from these potential treatments are not limited to one country, nor is the scientific research. Stem cell research is quickly becoming the next Space Race, with various countries pouring money and resources into their research institutions. As Furcht and Hoffman wrote,

In no field have governments and research universities prepared to seize the emerging field for their own competitive advantage as much as in stem cell research. Some countries are well out of the starting gate; others are trying to find the racetrack.[3]

Many of the leading countries are situated in Asia. A *Nature* article explains that "many of the world's leading stem cell biologists and cloning specialists hail from countries such as South Korea and Japan," and that "these pioneers are willing to share knowledge and techniques with scientists from less developed neighbours in the region, who are keen to enter the game."[12]

Whether developed or not, many of these countries see stem cell research as a way to firmly establish themselves as scientific leaders, bringing in massive foreign investment and bolstering national prestige. Robert Higgins, a venture capitalist who moderated the aforementioned Harvard Business School event, recalled when Dr. Shinya Yamanaka (MD, PhD), of the Institute for Frontier Medical Sciences at Kyoto University, discovered induced pluripotent (iPS) stem cells. Immediately after this major scientific breakthrough he said, "The Japanese government showed up the next day, committed tens of millions of dollars, and built an entire institute around him. We're talking about an enormous commitment, at the highest levels of government."[B, 1] Higgins, also a Senior Lecturer at Harvard Business School, continued: "The Japanese write about this in passionate, nationalistic terms. They see the stem cell area as the biggest opportunity for them in science and technology, and they are pouring money into it."

On the discussion panel, Dr. Daley explained that the Japanese are not the only ones who associate stem cells with national prestige and success: "The other day, the former head of the Economic Development Board of Singapore, Philip Yo, called me and asked, 'What are you not able to do [with stem cells] in the United States? We want to invest in that!'"[C, 1]

Singapore, Japan, China, India, and South Korea are all well-developed Asian countries which seem to possess the strong government support and technical prowess that allow for such rapid advancement in the stem cell field, and they are utilizing these advantages accordingly.[12] China's expenditure on scientific research has reached $44 billion, with stem cell research receiving priority funding.[13] With more money comes more research; China now ranks fifth in the world in number of published stem cell studies.[14] Similarly, India's stem cell sector, including research and stem cell therapies, is expected to surpass $500 million by the end of 2010.[15] Even less developed Asian countries are rapidly following in their footsteps. In 2006, for example, the Thailand Research Fund started a $50 million grant program for stem cell research.[12]

Asia is just one region in which national governments have begun exploring what stem cells could mean for their economies. The Middle East and Eastern Europe, even Latin America and the Caribbean, have become players in the stem cell field. Countries within the former Soviet Union, as well, continue to conduct research with the goal of clinical translation. While "we are still a major player" in the field of stem cell research, Dr. Daley explained, "we'd certainly do a lot better if we had an equal amount of capital"

"The Japanese write about this in passionate, nationalistic terms. They see the stem cell area as the biggest opportunity for them in science and technology, and they are pouring money into it."

China's expenditure on scientific research has reached $44 billion, with stem cell research receiving priority funding.[13] With more money comes more research; China now ranks fifth in the world in number of published stem cell studies.

American hospitals have been losing their lead in medical tourism, as highly-trained doctors and new technology increasingly make their way overseas.

as researchers from other countries. "I'm envious of the freedom that some of my international colleagues have had."

Part of this freedom comes from regulatory committees that are less restrictive of stem cell research, allowing scientists and clinicians from different countries to move at a faster pace. Some of this difference manifests itself in countries' various attitudes towards using stem cells to treat patients. In the United States, stem cell-based treatments are not yet available, with the exception of clinical trials. Meanwhile, other countries may offer these same treatments. This regulatory mismatch has meant that two different countries may be worlds away from each other in terms of their approach to stem cell treatment, while remaining within traveling distance of one another. This fact has had profound ramifications for the stem cell world.

Medical Tourism

With the advancement of stem cell science and the proliferation of clinical studies all over the world, there has been a rise in "medical tourism" for stem cell treatments. Medical tourism refers to when patients travel abroad to receive medical procedures. Medical tourism is motivated by many rationales, and takes many forms. The patient who travels to Mexico to undergo a less expensive dental procedure is engaging in medical tourism, as is the patient who flies to Europe to receive a surgical procedure not covered by their insurance. Medical tourism is a fairly frequent phenomenon; up to 500,000 Americans receive a medical procedure abroad every year.[16] Traditionally, medical tourism has been a two-way street; American hospitals treat tens of thousands of foreign patients, with annual revenue for American medical tourism totaling more than $1 billion.[17] Recently, however, American hospitals have been losing their lead in medical tourism, as highly trained doctors and new technology increasingly make their way overseas.

Stem cell treatments have recently become a growing subset of medical tourism. Because stem cells for use in a therapeutic procedure have not yet been approved by the FDA, many Americans who believe their condition can be helped by stem cells have gone abroad for treatment. An entire industry has grown around this phenomenon, with companies arranging stem cell treatments at facilities around the world.

But with the sudden and rapid growth of interest in stem cell treatments, there have emerged many "hucksters" who seek to profit from the hope of the sick. These individuals may promise more than they deliver, bypass critical safety studies, and take chances with the lives of patients. The infamous PLoS Case, described in Chapter 2, demonstrates the terrible effects that can occur if the cell cultivation or treatment protocol is inappropriate.

Any medical procedure has a risk of side effects, and these risks increase when the procedure is still developing. Stem cells are crossing the bridge from science to mainstream medicine, but they are no panacea. Over the course of this book, we have presented you with a few examples of individuals whose lives have been positively affected by clinical treatment that has utilized stem cells as medicine. It is important to remember that all of these patients were enrolled in clinical studies, that these patients were observed and treated by highly-qualified clinicians at respected and accredited institutions, and that many of the patients also participated in more traditional modes of therapy (such as physical therapy) during their stem cell regimen. Even more importantly, these patients received stem cells that were properly manufactured and were held to stringent safety standards.

Even with the most impressive results, none of the patients we have mentioned were cured of their condition; instead, they achieved functional improvements which allowed them to regain a measure of independence and dignity, and which raised their quality of life. There are some medical tourism companies that promise a stem cell cure for conditions such as Alzheimer's and spinal cord injury. Others have promised cures for diseases, such as AIDS, for which little to no stem cell research has been done.[18] To promise a cure to desperate patients is to prey on peoples' sense of hope. Similarly, no doctor or scientist can be sure that a stem cell treatment will help any one individual, so companies or doctors who guarantee results from a stem cell treatment are acting unethically. The patient testimonials presented within the pages of this book are meant to illustrate the potential of stem cell therapy, but they reflect individual results, and any doctor will reinforce the fact that peoples' bodies will respond differently to the same medicine.

Crossing the Great Divide

Many scientific and medical experts believe that no stem cell treatments should be performed anywhere, under any conditions. Until the science has been fully explored, they argue, it is unethical to treat people. A similar, albeit less extreme, position is that stem cell treatments should be relegated to the province of clinical trials.

No doctor or scientist can be sure that a stem cell treatment will help any one individual, so companies or doctors who "guarantee" results from a stem cell treatment are acting unethically.

Other members of the stem cell field view the problem differently. Rather than determining that all non-clinical treatment is wrong, they instead see a space for ethical and responsible application of stem cells for the seriously ill. Drs. Olle Lindvall (MD, PhD), Professor at the Wallenburg Neuroscience Center in Sweden, and Dr. Insoo Hyun (PhD), Associate Professor of Bioethics at Case Western Reserve University, laid out this position in a 2009 paper in the journal *Science*.[19] The authors point out that seriously ill patients may be unable or unwilling to enroll in clinical trials, and thus, require other treatment options:

From many patients' point of view, consenting to medically innovative care may be preferable to enrolling in a clinical trial, especially where patient care is decidedly not the purpose of the trial—expanding knowledge is. Patients with precious little time might not care much about expanding knowledge; what they care about is getting better and surviving. Demonizing stem cell tourism will never squelch this vital instinct. Acceptable channels must be made available to seriously ill patients.[19]

"The difficulty," the authors explain, "lies in being able to distinguish clearly between objectionable stem cell tourism and legitimate attempts at medically innovative stem cell-based interventions."[19] Objectionable stem cell tourism, of course, should be unacceptable under all circumstances, but responsible stem cell-based interventions could be acceptable if held to appropriate standards.

Responsible stem cell treatments could even perform a service for the medical community, Lindvall and Hyun argue:

In the last 40 years, only 10 to 20% of all surgical techniques were developed through a clinical trial process. Some specialties, such as cardiac transplant and laparoscopic surgery, developed entirely without clinical trials. Responsible medical innovation could be an important avenue for the development of stem cell-based therapies that follow a surgical paradigm or otherwise do not fit neatly into the square peg of the clinical trial process.[19]

If there is a space for legitimate non-clinical trial stem cell therapy, the authors stress, it is only in the presence of "rigorous oversight and scientific integrity," as well as standards that protect patients.[19] The authors point out several requirements that must be in place for a stem cell therapy to be viewed as responsible. These requirements echo those put forth by the International Society for Stem Cell Research (ISSCR), a nonprofit stem cell research organization that published a list of guidelines for the clinical translation of stem cells, in December 2008.

The ISSCR, acknowledging the "distinction between the commercial purveyance of unproven stem cell interventions and legitimate attempts at medical innovation outside the context of a formal clinical trial," created a list of guidelines to steer responsible physician application of non-clinical trial treatments.

The ISSCR also prepared an accompanying document, the *Patient Handbook on Stem Cell Therapies*, which helps inform prospective patients of what to look for to determine the legitimacy of an offered stem cell therapy. In the handbook, they include this advice:

To begin, ask for evidence that:

- *Preclinical studies have been published, and reviewed and repeated by other experts in the field.*

- *The providers have approval from an independent committee such as an Institutional Review Board or Ethics Review Board to make sure the risks are as low as possible and are worth any potential benefits, and that your rights are being protected.*

- *The providers have approval from a national or regional regulatory agency, such as the Food and Drug Administration or the European Medicines Agency for the safe conduct of clinical trials or medical use of a product for this disease.[21]*

Drawing from our own experience in visiting dozens of stem cell manufacturing facilities, hospitals that have begun experimental stem cell treatments, and clinics from around the world, we must emphasize that any safe and efficacious stem cell treatment use stem cells that have been properly manufactured. This includes a battery of safety studies, as well as tests to ensure that the cell population is actually stem cells, as opposed to cells that have already been differentiated. Previous clinical and pre-clinical trials which reported lackluster results may have used regular cells for their treatment, as opposed to multipotent stem cells. For both the health of the stem cell industry and that of prospective patients, hospitals must be able to guarantee that they are using true stem cells from a trusted and accredited manufacturer. Any institution that intends to offer stem cell therapy must meet all of these criteria, in order to be considered responsible and ethical.

Excerpt from *Patient Handbook on Stem Cell Therapies.*

For further recommendations from the ISSCR, including questions that every patient should ask, you are encouraged to read the Patient Handbook online at: http://www.isscr.org/clinical_trans/pdfs/ISSCRPatientHandbook.pdf

Below are the recommendations from the ISSCR's *Guidelines for Clinical Translation of Stem Cells*:[20]

Recommendation 34: Clinician-scientists may provide unproven stem cell-based interventions to at most a very small number of patients outside the extent of a formal clinical trial, provided that:

(a) there is a written plan for the procedure that includes:
  i. scientific rationale and justification explaining why the procedure has a reasonable chance of success, including any preclinical evidence of proof-of-principle for efficacy and safety;
  ii. explanation of why the proposed stem cell-based intervention should be attempted compared to existing treatments;
  iii. full characterization of the types of cells being transplanted and their characteristics as discussed in Section 4, Cell Processing and Manufacture;
  iv. description of how the cells will be administered, including adjuvant drugs, agents, and surgical procedures; and
  v. plan for clinical follow-up and data collection to assess the effectiveness and adverse effects of the cell therapy;

(b) the written plan is approved through a peer review process by appropriate experts who have no vested interest in the proposed procedure;

(c) the clinical and administrative leadership supports the decision to attempt the medical innovation and the institution is held accountable for the innovative procedure;

(d) all personnel have appropriate qualifications and the institution where the procedure will be carried out has appropriate facilities and processes of peer review and clinical quality control monitoring;

(e) voluntary informed consent is provided by patients who appreciate the intervention is unproven and who demonstrate their understanding of the risks and benefits of the procedure;

(f) there is an action plan for adverse events that includes timely and adequate medical care and if necessary psychological support services;

(g) insurance coverage or other appropriate financial or medical resources are available to patients to cover any complications arising from the procedure; and

(h) there is a commitment by clinician-scientists to use their experience with individual patients to contribute to generalizable knowledge. This includes:
  i. ascertaining outcomes in a systematic and objective manner;
  ii. a plan for communication outcomes, including negative outcomes and adverse events, to the scientific community to enable critical review (for example, as abstracts to professional meetings or publications in peer-reviewed journals); and
  iii. moving to a formal clinical trial in a timely manner after experience with at most a few patients.

A stem cell treatment represents a serious medical procedure, and no person should even consider undergoing a treatment without asking critical questions from the treatment provider, as well as independent specialists, and receiving clear answers. Whether considering a clinical trial or an innovative clinical study, prospective patients should always receive a medical opinion from their own doctor, as well as the opinion of medical specialists within the field. While stem cells represent an exciting advance in medical science, no one should let enthusiasm or hype unduly influence them to make an ill-informed decision regarding their health, or the health of their loved ones.

Cells and Drug Discovery

Stem cells have been much lauded for their ability to effect repair directly. But some scientists are equally or more excited by the stem cell's ability to recreate perfect testing conditions for new drugs. Induced pluripotent cells (iPS), in particular, could be taken from diseased patients and grown into the offending cell type. For example, cells from Parkinson's patients could be differentiated into motor neurons. The stem cell differentiation process, explains a *Harvard Magazine* article, would "allow researchers to watch a given disease unfold... The iPS cells will allow researchers to watch, over and over, how diseases progress, so they can test ways to intervene."[22] Scientists could also introduce experimental drugs to the diseased cells, testing to see how they react. More elaborate drug testing models could even use the same stem cells to differentiate into cell types that might be adversely affected by the drugs, like liver or heart cells.

Using stem cells as a vehicle for drug testing would have several benefits. First, it would be safer than current drug testing models, which jump directly from animal studies to testing on humans. With stem cells, scientists could see the effects of a drug on a human cell before undergoing costly pre-clinical or clinical trials. Stem cells could also be used to screen for side effects of drugs that are already on the market. For example, if a heart failure patient is allergic to warfarin, the active ingredient in many blood thinners, testing a blood-thinning drug on that patient's stem cells would reveal whether the drug would trigger an allergic reaction.

Second, stem cells could spur new medical research investment from pharmaceutical and venture capital companies, by dramatically lowering the barriers to entry for introducing a new drug to the

Stem Cell Clinical Trials

To see the list of ongoing and completed clinical trials in the United States, including trials that are accepting volunteers for stem cell procedures, visit www. clinicaltrials.gov, a database maintained by the National Institutes of Health.

market. Research and biopharmaceutical companies often spend hundreds of millions of dollars attempting to get a new drug to market. These drugs must go through the gauntlet of FDA-mandated clinical trials, and many progress to Phase III trials, only to fail. One recent report conducted by Windhover Information, Inc., studied 656 Phase III trials. Out of these trials, 278 failed, marking a failure rate of over 40%.[23] For the companies financing these trials, this represents major financial losses. These dismal results help explain why even large companies are reticent to fund testing for new drugs that could help prospective patients, especially those suffering from orphan diseases. With a stem cell testing program, however, these companies would be able to know whether their drugs will work, at a fraction of the normal cost. With reduced barriers to entry, the pace of private research can be expected to dramatically accelerate.

And thirdly, stem cells would also be responsible for reducing the timeframe for new drug development. Arranging and conducting clinical trials for a new drug is often a drawn-out and elaborate process. In contrast, *in vitro* tests of new drugs on stem cell-derived cells would give researchers more immediate and more easily reproducible results, hastening the process by which a new drug either fails to demonstrate efficacy or successfully enters the market.

Besides being directly applied as medicine, then, stem cells can also be seen as tools to further advance our knowledge of disease, and to create medical solutions to pressing health problems.

New Ways to Apply Stem Cells

Despite the incredible advances that have been made in stem cell science over the past decade, there are still areas where improvement could bring an enhanced clinical result. For example, administration of stem cells to the central nervous system (CNS) requires injections to the spine.

In order to be effective, transfused neural stem cells must cross the blood brain barrier (BBB), a protective barrier that keeps the sensitive CNS cells from being affected by the rest of the body. In the same way that a military base has its own checkpoints to prevent undesirables from entering, so does the BBB prevent "civilian" cells from entering the CNS. If clinicians wish to introduce stem cells to the brain or spinal cord, they must either introduce cells outside the CNS and hope that some cells get through the "checkpoints", or they must break through the BBB and introduce the cells directly to the treatment area.

But what if the transfused stem cells were given a special "pass" to enter the BBB, using an avenue that connects the CNS to the rest of the body? In that case, clinicians would be able to deliver stem cells more directly to the treated area.

Researchers from Tuebingen, Germany and St. Paul, Minnesota seemed to have discovered one such "pass" in 2009, by developing a novel stem cell delivery system. The researchers suspended stem cells in fluid, then used a nasal spray to deliver the cells to lab mice. In an article published that year, the researchers explained that "cells applied intranasally can migrate to the intact brain through the cribiform plate along the olfactory neural pathway and possibly along other routes of migration."[24] The olfactory neural pathway is a set of neurons that connects the nose to the brain; it is the pathway that allows our brain to process smells. In this situation, the olfactory neural pathway acted as a special "VIP checkpoint" giving permission for the stem cells to enter.

The researchers postulated that they could achieve even more potential clinical benefit by increasing the number of stem cells that successfully reached the brain through the olfactory neural pathway. They tried applying the nasal spray after pre-treating their lab animals with hyaluronidase. Hyaluronidase is known to increase tissue permeability by breaking down hyaluronic acid. For this reason, hyaluronidase has been used for years in order to remove cosmetic fillers made from hyaluronic acid in the instance of an over-injection. In this study, the researchers found that pre-treating the lab animals with hyaluronidase before applying the stem cell nasal spray nearly tripled the number of stem cells which reached the olfactory bulb of the brain.[25]

The success of the study "opens new avenues for the use of this method as a non-invasive alternative to the current traumatic surgical procedure of transplantation," explain the authors of the study in their paper.[24] "The IN [intranasal] delivery method provides the option of chronic treatments which may enhance the number of delivered cells in order to achieve therapeutic benefit."[24] And a nasal spray is just one conceivable way to deliver future stem cell treatments. Eyedrops, given the right formulation, could someday be used to deliver stem cells directly to the eye, a process which might be more useful for accelerating healing after eye surgery than for retinal degenerative diseases. Or stem cells might conceivably be delivered through sublingual absorption, quickly entering the bloodstream without the need for an injection.

Cells applied intranasally can migrate to the intact brain through the cribiform plate along the olfactory neural pathway and possibly along other routes of migration.

New topical applications are increasingly becoming a reality as well, as stem cell treatments appear to be poised for conjunctive use with dermatologic procedures. As we saw in the previous chapter, stem cells can be applied topically to injured skin, which has already been compromised. But in healthy skin, the stem cells cannot penetrate the stratum corneum and enter the body. If another device were to temporarily open up passageways in the skin, however, the stem cells could enter the body and affect repair in a certain area without the need for injection.

Thankfully, the field of dermatology has developed an entire subset of devices designed to do just that. Chemical peels and microdermabrasion devices are designed to scrub away the top layer of the skin so that healthier skin can regrow in its place, while fractional laser devices have been developed to create tiny holes in the skin so that it can optimally regenerate new, healthier tissue with minimal downtime. The advances in dermatology have allowed for more effective treatment of scars and disfiguring skin conditions, such as port wine stains.

But the effects of these laser devices could be multiplied, if they were used in conjunction with stem cells. The lasers would initiate skin remodeling by stimulating the wound response, while topically-applied stem cells and stem cell factors would bring their various mechanisms of action to bear, dramatically improving the result.

In envisioning a future where stem cell therapy plays a part within mainstream medicine, the possibilities of combination therapy are nearly limitless. Many pharmaceutical drugs, for example, aim to up-regulate certain molecular factors. Paired with stem cells, these effects could be multiplied, making the drugs far more effective. Or, as stem cells modulate the regulation of many different molecular factors, they could be used to mitigate side effects from a certain drug. For example, if stem cells were used as the delivery device for certain pharmaceutical compounds, they could modulate the compound's toxicity, making the drug safer for long-term use. And through their ability to clean up the cellular microenvironment, stem cells could provide more fertile ground for the drug's mechanism of action to take effect.

Stem cells have always been "team players," initiating a Chaperone Effect that rescues and activates endogenous cells.[26] Much of the repair they effect in the body is through their encouragement of other cells, and through their ability to lay the ground-

The effects of these laser devices could be multiplied, if they were used in conjunction with stem cells. The lasers would initiate skin remodeling by stimulating the wound response.

work for a healthier cellular environment to emerge. So it is no surprise that they are well poised to serve as an adjunctive treatment to other modalities.

A Bold Vision

As stem cells continue along this pathway to clinical translation, they offer to radically change the way we approach managed care. Diseases that previously were death sentences may soon meet their match, in the form of powerful cell-based medicine. Stem cell treatments could change the healthcare, insurance, and pharmaceutical industries. Old drugs that were aimed at delaying the onset of a disease would become relics, in favor of stem cells that could turn back the tide of pathogenesis. Patients with neurodegenerative diseases could schedule appointments for their neurologist several times a year, for an examination and a stem cell treatment in the same way that they schedule appointments for their dentist or dermatologist. For some conditions, patients will be able to take doses of stem cells in the same way that we now take daily pills, as scientists invent and perfect new methods of application. As our understanding of the human genome progresses, we may be able to detect genetic predispositions for disease in newborns. Knowing this, doctors could embark on a preventive stem cell treatment regimen for patients who are more likely to develop degenerative diseases.

This is our vision for the future, and it is a profoundly ambitious one. We still have much work to do before we approach a world without any "no-option" patients. We are making strides toward this future, every day. Researchers around the world are exploring the stem cell's mechanism of action, uncovering new pieces of this grand scientific puzzle. As our understanding of the cells themselves grows, so does our appreciation of their multitude of effects on the body. As more clinical trials and medical innovations take place, we begin to see how patients around the world can benefit from this potential therapy. There are still a multitude of questions that must be answered before stem cells are ready to be offered as medicine, but an entire community of scientists and doctors around the world are hard at work to provide answers.

Convergence

The phrase "clinical translation" refers to a long road connecting scientific discovery to mainstream medicine. That road began

As stem cells continue along this pathway to clinical translation, they offer to radically change the way we approach managed care. Diseases that previously were death sentences may soon meet their match, in the form of powerful cell-based medicine.

Creating New Organs

In a keynote speech to the 25th Army Science Conference, Dr. Anthony Atala discussed how his team has overcome three challenges to the creation of replacement organs: an inability to expand cells *in vitro*, inadequate biomaterials, and inadequate vascularity. Wake Forest researchers began by targeting the cells that lead to regeneration during normal injury and expand these cells *in vitro* by using specific growth factors. They select the committed progenitor cells that are specific to each organ. The tissue is integrated with specific 3D scaffolds comprised of compatible biomaterials. This allows for the creation of artificial organs such as bladders or tracheas. The researchers have solved one of the greatest challenges, providing adequate vascularity. Tissue larger than an eraser pencil will not grow unless it is provided with blood supply. Branching allows for this tissue to obtain the necessary vascularity. To date, Wake Forest has created more than a dozen different tissues; the majority come from autologous sources; exceptions being nerves, livers and pancreas.[27]

over 100 years ago, with Maximov's discovery of hematopoietic stem cells. And as generations of scientists across the globe learned more about the potential therapeutic properties of these amazing cells, a destination emerged. With each clinical trial, stem cells take another step down the road to clinical translation, and the fields of stem cell science and stem cell medicine draw closer together.

As the clinical translation road becomes increasingly well traveled, so too have lines of communication and collaboration opened between different sectors of the stem cell field. Cross-discipline institutes are forming at major universities, whose research becomes the starting point for clinical trials at world-renowned hospitals, whose efforts may be funded by the government but whose cell lines may come from the private sector. State-based stem cell policies become national stem cell policies, while researchers from different nations join together to form international cooperatives like the International Society for Stem Cell Research. As Furcht and Hoffman put it:

> It's too soon to know which country will win the stem cell race. What is certain is that the power of biomedical imagination and information technology spills over international boundaries more freely than ever… The global exchange of stem cell research information is growing in tandem.[3]

Meanwhile, the political debate over embryonic/adult cells gives way to an ethic of intellectual curiosity in the scientific world. As previous generations of stem cell researchers remained united by their profession during the Cold War, so do today's scientists refuse to be pulled in by political conflict over which stem cells are best. While embryonic stem cells fuel further breakthroughs at the lab bench, adult stem cells increasingly venture out into the arena of clinical trials and human treatment.

And in an increasingly interconnected world, a global community of researchers and clinicians has emerged to tackle the challenge of moving stem cells from bench to bedside. Convergence is the new paradigm. It is this spirit of convergence, of cooperation and shared hope for the future, which will further propel stem cells down the road of clinical translation. A century ago, stem cells emerged as a new scientific endeavor. Today, we are on the cusp of another endeavor, one that will revolutionize healthcare by establishing stem cells as medicine.

About Stemedica Cell Technologies, Inc.

Stemedica is a world leader in developing, manufacturing and distributing allogeneic adult stem cell products for human use in clinical trials. These products address the debilitating nature of complex diseases and physical trauma. The Company was formed in 2005 by a management team with experience in building successful organizations. Stemedica's products and services are provided to decision makers in government regulatory agencies, hospitals (where there is regulatory approval), academic, research institutions, pharmaceutical and healthcare companies.

Our explicit goal is to set the international standard for excellence in safety and quality. Stemedica's developmental efforts stand on the shoulders of the rich history of stem cell discovery and clinical experience of scientists and physicians from around the world. To this end, we are indebted to our colleagues from Russia, Europe, Canada, Japan, Korea, China and other countries whose research and clinical experience have proven to be invaluable.

STEMEDICA™

Multiple Cell Technology

Stemedica's proprietary processes and procedures provide the company with the capability to isolate, extract, expand, manufacture and master bank multiple unique lines of immune-privileged adult stem cells. These proprietary lines provide Stemedica with the ability to customize specialized formulations that are required to address complex diseases and other debilitating conditions.

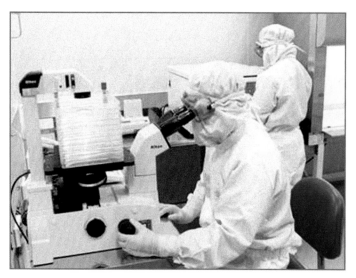

Company Mission

Stemedica's core mission is to develop, manufacture and distribute adult stem cells that have the potential to save, restore and improve lives by reversing the debilitating nature of complex diseases and physical trauma. Stemedica's management and employees are dedicated to executing this mission with great passion and with business and scientific discipline.

Stemedica has a deep appreciation for the impact its scientific and medical technologies have on the lives of patients, their families, and friends. To this end, the company will continue to strive for excellence in science, medicine, technology and in its business practices.

Research and Product Development Focus

The company's research, product development and manufacturing are focused on four primary medical areas:

- *Neurological Diseases:* Diseases and conditions such as: Alzheimer's, Parkinson's, ischemic stroke, traumatic brain injury, and spinal cord injury.

- *Sight Restoration:* Diseases of the eye such as: diabetic retinopathy, retinitis pigmentosa, and age-related macular degeneration.

- *Cardiovascular:* Functional improvement related to acute myocardial infarction, cardiomyopathy and heart failure.

- *Bone and Soft Tissue:* Repair of bone and soft tissue conditions including: scars, burn scars, and acute and chronic skin wounds.

Demand for Stemedica's products is increasing as the world's population continues to grow, traditional medical remedies fail to provide adequate results and people desire to experience a higher quality of life as they live longer.

Technology Advantage

Stemedica has developed unique stem cell lines and related stem cell factors that allow researchers and clinicians to employ multiple formulations. The company uses proprietary processes and procedures for manufacturing and banking its adult stem cell products. Technology advantages include:

- Diverse and multiple product offerings derived from numerous tissue source origins;

- Stem cells that are immune privileged—stem cell transplantation does not require immunosuppressant agents or HLA matching;

- Stem cells with proven viability, potency and migratory properties;

- Proprietary master banking processes that insure cell preservation;

- Protocols, templates, training and educational programs related to stem cell transplantation;

- Extensive bio-safety testing at certified laboratories. Tests include tumorigenicity, acute and chronic toxicity and others (see Chapter 1 for detailed list of tests);

- Comprehensive portfolio of intellectual property;

- Superior scalability source donations and proprietary preservation processes and procedures; and

- Ability to safely ship cells worldwide.

The Stemedica scientific team has developed technologies that enable our manufacturing and quality personnel to create master banks of multi-stem cell products. For example, extracting bone marrow from one 19-year-old donor enables Stemedica to create enough stem cells for physicians to treat over 300,000 patients.

Manufacturing

Stemedica has been licensed by the State of California's Food and Drug Branch to manufacture stem cells for human use under FDA cGMP standards of compliance as well as Swissmedic and European Union and Korean FDA guidelines. The company is currently manufacturing and shipping stem cells to countries around the world that are conducting clinical trials. Patients suffering from medical conditions such as those previously indicated are being treated in these trials.

The company has an unparalleled capacity to manufacture quality stem cell products. Through its facilities in San Diego, California, its partnership in Switzerland with DFB BioScience, and with its joint venture in South Korea, these facilities allow Stemedica to manufacture its multiple allogeneic stem cell products to meet international safety and quality standards.

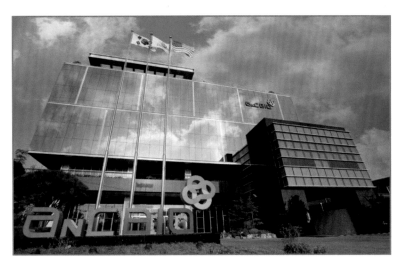

Stemedica-AnCBio headquarters in Seoul, Korea.

Commitment to Quality

Stemedica employs rigorous and highly advanced controls, processes and procedures that follow all the safety testing outlined in Chapter 1. All safety tests are audited and certified by independent laboratories.

In addition to exceeding the safety testing requirements of the FDA, Stemedica's stem cells are tested for viability, potency and migration properties. Tests conducted by independent research institutions have repeatedly demonstrated that Stemedica's stem cells meet the highest standards of performance available.

Management, Advisors, and Board of Directors

Stemedica has built an experienced team of international and domestic scientists and medical professionals who have been involved for the past six years in extensive research and stem cell product development. These efforts include:

1. Confirming the safety, reliability and efficacy of the company's science and technology;

2. Advancing the company's protocols for isolating, expanding, processing, manufacturing and master banking of stem cells; and,

3. Refining Stemedica's methodologies and standard operating procedures used in clinical application.

The team has expertise in stem cell research and clinical trials, medically-based technology transfer from foreign countries, applying for and receiving FDA clearances, commercialization of new products and technologies, and the utilization of cutting-edge marketing strategies.

A prominent Board of Directors and a Board of Scientific and Business Advisors support the company's management by providing a professional forum to review the company's management practices, business development tactics, product and service offerings and long-term strategic objectives.

Stemedica's Worldwide Reach

Stemedica's management has established strategic relationships with regulatory agencies, ministers of health, leading hospital officials, scientists and physicians throughout the world, including China, South Korea, Mexico, Russia, India, and countries in Central and Eastern Europe, the Middle East, Central America, and South America. These alliances will help support our ongoing research and product development efforts.

These relationships have resulted in joint venture manufacturing, distribution agreements and clinical trials using Stemedica cells and protocols. Many countries have granted regulatory approval to import Stemedica's stem cells as the product of choice to conduct clinical trials for varying debilitating injuries and diseases.

We have an opportunity to provide a better life for our fellow citizens around the world, our children, our grandchildren and ourselves. Diseases and medical conditions for which there are no effective treatment options may not be eradicated, but it is our sincerest belief that stem cells are the future of medicine, and the future is already here.

About the Authors

Roger J. Howe, PhD, Founder and Executive Chairman & Maynard A. Howe, PhD, Founder, Vice Chairman & CEO

Drs. Roger and Maynard Howe bring a diverse background to Stemedica. Over the past 30 years, they have launched several successful ventures in adult stem cell technology, medical device, information systems, and behavioral sciences including marketing, customer and quality survey research. They have experience in: a) recruiting and leading exceptional teams of nationally and internationally recognized scientists, physicians, technicians, executive teams and board members; b) managing intellectual property, regulatory and FDA processes and procedures; and, c) setting up distribution and managing sales channels throughout North America, Europe, South America and parts of Asia. They have also led fund raising initiatives to secure private, institutional and venture capital investments as well as coordinated and negotiated the exit strategies and plans for each company.

Prior to serving as founders of Stemedica Cell Technologies, Inc., they were instrumental in launching Reliant Technologies (now Solta, Nasdaq: SLTM) and Cardiovascular Systems, Inc. (Nasdaq: CSII).

Reliant Technologies (now Solta) is comprised of a team of scientists, engineers and physicians that developed, tested and launched the revolutionary medical laser for skin rejuvination known as Fraxel®. This device created a new category of aesthetic science known as fractional photothermolysis. Reliant Technologies has achieved a strong intellectual property position with several issued and pending patents. In addition, prior to its sale, Reliant secured multiple FDA clearances for its technology and established global distribution.

Cardiovascular Systems, Inc. (CSI) develops and commercializes interventional technologies for the treatment of cardiovascular disease. CSI is a leader in providing clinically proven, safe and effective vascular solutions, with its mission of saving limbs and restoring patients' ability to walk pain-free, remain productive and live independently. CSI has FDA approval for peripheral artery disease and is currently in clinical trials for the treatment of the coronary artery. The company has a portfolio of over 83 international and US patents issued and 74 pending.

In addition to Reliant Technologies and Cardiovascular Systems, the Howes also co-founded NIS, a leading customer, quality and market research company specializing in conducting branding campaigns, marketing assessments, and trend research in both business-to-business and business-to-customer environments for major Fortune 500 corporations. NIS was selected by the U.S. Federal Government to execute its proprietary algorithm technology on behalf of the Equal Access Mandate (Judge Greene) for allocating telephone users to long distance carriers following the breakup of AT&T. This resulted in the surveying, processing, analysis and allocation of over 100 million personal and business long distance users in North America. NIS was sold to National Computer Systems and later to Person, plc (NYSE: PSO).

The Howes are co-authors of numerous articles and top selling business books. They are nationally and internationally recognized speakers and lecturers. Their benchmark book *Quality on Trial: Bringing Customer Relationships into Focus*, is in its second edition and has been published in several languages. Other books include a five part implementation manual series, *Business to Business Marketing Management System*, McGraw-Hill; *Team Dynamics in Developing Organizations*, Kendall-Hunt; *Preventing Workplace Violence*, Alliant Press; *Building Profits Through Organizational Change*, American Management Association.

Nikolai I. Tankovich, MD, PhD, Founder, President & Chief Medical Officer

Dr. Nikolai Tankovich was born in Siberia after his grandparents' family had been deported there from the capital of Russia by the Bolshevik government. Graduating high school with honors, he was accepted to Moscow University where he received a Masters degree in Physics and a Doctorate (PhD) in Biophysics for his thesis, "Hydrodynamics and Mass Transfer of Magnetic Drug Carriers in Blood Flow." After finishing his dissertation, Dr. Tankovich continued his education and graduated with honors from Moscow's Medical Semashko University, specializing in general surgery. He completed residency training in oncology and became a surgical oncologist.

Dr. Tankovich became Director of the Medical Biophysics Lab at the Kurchatov Atomic Energy Center (in 1982) where he conducted research on the use of laser and electromagnetic radiation in biology and medicine. Working as a physician at the Cancer Research Center, he specialized in the diagnosis and laser treatment of malignant tumors and bone marrow disease.

Following his publication on the use of magnetron's electromagnetic radiation for the resonance release of stromal and hematopoietic stem cells from bone marrow into the blood flow, he was invited by the University of California, Irvine (UCI) to conduct research on stromal bone marrow release by millimeter electromagnetic wave radiation. This research was performed at the University of California, Santa Barbara using the free electron laser and presented at the International Center for Research on Cancer (Lyon, France). Dr. Tankovich was invited by Dr. Arnold Beckman and the Bechtel Corporation to further his work at the Beckman Laser Research Institute and Clinic as a visiting Professor of the Department of Surgery.

Dr. Tankovich has pursued many diverse applications for the use of lasers in medicine and surgery. Building upon his earlier discoveries in Russia, he pioneered laser hair removal. He was issued the first patent on hair removal by the U.S. Patent and Trademark Office in 1993 which he licensed to the Thermolase Corporation. Serving as vice-president of Thermolase, the company in 1996 reached a market capitalization of $1.6 Billion. As other companies moved into the hair removal space, Thermolase sold its hair removal technologies and diversified into the biotech sector.

Pursuing a long-term interest in stem cells, in 1997 Dr. Tankovich completed a series of *in vivo* experiments employing stem cells to grow hair. He filed his first application on this technology that year and was granted a patent in 2000 for harvesting, expansion and implantation of stem cells to grow hair. He has also patented technology on laser use to remodel skin by attracting cell progenitors to the micro injured papillary dermis and epidermis. He licensed this technology to Reliant Technology, Inc. in 2004 (acquired by Solta Medical, Inc.)

Dr. Tankovich continues to explore the multiple applications of stem cells in medicine and is a frequent lecturer at universities around the world including Oxford University (United Kingdom), Kitasato University (Japan), University of New South Wales (Australia),

Calude Bernard University (France), the University of Moscow (Russia), the University of Lausanne (Switzerland) and others.

He has over 50 scientific publications, is author of more than 100 international and U. S. Patents and has presented his research at more than 100 conferences and meetings. Dr. Tankovich has been awarded the Kurchatov's Medal from the Atomic Energy Commission for his input into atomic science for medicine.

David A. Howe, MD, MBA, DC, CCN, Senior Vice President & Medical Director

Dr. Howe brings over 35 years of experience as a medical practitioner to his role at Stemedica as Senior Vice President and Medical Director. Over the past five years, Dr. Howe has been involved in stem cell studies with internationally recognized stem cell scientists and physicians in several countries. In addition, he has developed treatment methodologies for patients suffering from diseases and conditions for which there are no cures. He has documented successful outcomes and has assisted in the development of clinical protocols for the treatment of patients with Alzheimer's, Parkinson's, spinal cord injury, stroke, retinal eye conditions, multiple sclerosis, as well as several orphan diseases. In addition, he has trained physicians in several countries in stem cell transplantation methodologies using multiple cell lines to treat the diseases and conditions indicated above.

In his capacity as Medical Director at Stemedica, he has worked with international medical ethics committees, independent review boards and government regulatory agencies that approve treatment protocols and monitor the safety and efficacy of stem cell treatment. He is a frequent speaker, guest lecturer and panelist at national and international conferences on stem cell research, multiple cell technology and transplantation methodologies.

Dr. Howe is the founder and former owner of the San Diego Clinic of Preventive Medicine, a private medical clinic specializing in current treatments in alternative, as well as mainstream medicine. Dr. Howe is a member of the American College for Advancement in Medicine, a member of the American College of Osteopathic Pain Management, and a member of the Board of Directors for the World Trade Center.

James R. Tager

James Tager has been writing professionally for six years. He serves as a contributing editor of *The Aesthetic Guide*, and moderates THE Aesthetic Show, an annual conference on innovative cosmetic technologies. He specializes in the creation of online training programs for a variety of surgical and medical procedures. He also assists physicians with their online marketing efforts.

James has attended London School of Economics, the Universidad de San Pablo (Madrid, Spain), and Duke University where he received his BA in Political Science, *cum laude* in 2009. At Duke, he was the Recipient of the William J. Griffith University Service Award for "Outstanding Contributions to the Global Community" and the Robert S. Rankin American Government Award for "Leadership and Academic Achievement." He has served as president of the Duke Human Rights Coalition and as a columnist and staff writer for various academic publications. He is currently enrolled at Harvard Law School (JD '13) where he is pursuing his passion for safeguarding international human rights.

About Stemedica's Scientific & Medical Team

Alex Kharazi, MD, PhD, Chief Technology Officer

Dr. Alex Kharazi completed his Medical degree in Internal Medicine and Pathology in 1978 in Kiev at the Medical Institute in the Ukraine. From 1978 to 1981 he was a postdoctoral fellow at the Kiev Institute of Gerontology. Dr. Kharazi received extensive training in cell biology and immunology, including tissue culture and subsequently earned his PhD in Immunology. His research interests were focused on restoring immunity in aged mice using stem cells from young adult mice. While studying the role of the thymus in the development of the mouse immune system, he collaborated with Friedenstein's lab in Moscow on the physiological contribution of chemical factors produced by thymic stromal cells (microenvironment).

In 1989, he was invited to work as a research fellow in the Department of Pathology at the Tokyo Metropolitan Institute of Gerontology in Japan. There he studied early progenitors for adult thymic epithelial cells and successfully established adult thymic epithelial cell lines. He received extensive training in immuno-cytology and flow cytometry.

In 1991, Dr. Kharazi was invited to the University of California, Los Angeles to serve as chief pathologist of a United States Environmental Protection Agency controlled study on the effects of magnetic fields on the incidence of lymphoma in mice. While at UCLA he deepened his understanding of Good Laboratory Practices (GLP) and regulatory affairs. The results of the study were reported to the United States Congress. From 1998 through 2005, Dr. Kharazi served as chief scientist of the Immunotherapy laboratory at St. Vincent Medical Center in Los Angeles, California. There, his research interests focused on cancer treatment using tumor vaccines, which were designed and manufactured to activate a patient's own immune system. He successfully designed and prepared a breast cancer vaccine using genetic engineering; the vaccine is currently in the patent application process. He also conducted scientific work on the role that dendritic cells play in the generation of anti-tumor immune response. Dr. Kharazi has extensive experience in conducting FDA approved clinical trials.

His peer-reviewed publications appear in over 20 scientific journals. In addition, his published abstracts are reported in 31 publications and he has contributed to several chapters in scholarly textbooks. Dr. Kharazi has presented his research at numerous national and international scientific conferences. He is an active member of many distinguished societies such as The American Association for Cancer Research. In addition, he served as a consultant to several research companies and he has also been a faculty member at the University of Southern California in Los Angeles, as well as other University of California institutions.

Lev Verkh, PhD, Chief Regulatory & Clinical Development Officer

Dr. Lev Verkh holds a PhD degree in Biophysics and a Master of Science in Physics from the State University of New York at Buffalo, and Bachelor of Science degree in Theoretical Physics from Odessa State University. He is author or co-author of over 40 peer-reviewed publications.

His clinical and regulatory experience includes 23 years working for Pfizer, Baxter BioScience, Alliance Pharmaceutical Corporation and Alpha Therapeutic Corporation. He has directed national and multi-national Phase I, II, III and IV clinical trials in cardiology, oncology, peripheral vascular diseases, hematology, blood disorders and imaging methods. Through his efforts and the efforts of his teams, he has received FDA approval for several products that are currently on the market.

Under his direction and leadership, Stemedica successfully worked with the FDA and received an Investigational New Drug approval for the first clinical trial in ischemic stroke patients using Stemedica adult allogeneic bone marrow stem cells.

In addition to directing Stemedica's clinical trials within the United States, Dr. Verkh assists foreign regulatory agencies in establishing guidelines for stem cell technologies in medicine. He is also responsible for assisting in the organization and supervision of clinical trials outside the United States that utilize Stemedica technology.

Eugene Baranov, PhD, Vice President of Global Research

Dr. Baranov is recognized for his experience as a researcher, innovator and educator for application of physical chemistry, biophysical methods and imaging technology in cancer research and biotech related disciplines. He has published more than 60 articles (including publications in such highly-ranked scientific journals as *Cell, Cancer Cell,* and *Proceedings of the National Academy of Sciences of the U.S.A.*) He has presented the results of his research at over 30 conferences and seminars worldwide.

Dr. Baranov has been an educator at several international universities and an inventor of three U. S. patents. He was also a consultant for several U. S. companies specializing in nutrition, cosmetics and cancer research. Dr. Baranov's research has been significant in many areas. These include: anthracycline drugs' cell membrane transport kinetics and their interaction with DNA; the development of vital fluorescent dye and laser based technology for early cancer diagnosis and clinical usage; the implementation of a double derivative method for data image analysis of collagen structure in normal and pathological tissues (breast cancer and diabetes); the application of fluorescent, polarized and nanosecond time-resolved spectroscopy for studies of drug interactions and their molecular complexes with their targets.

Ludmilla Kharazi, MD, PhD, Senior Scientist

Dr. Ludmilla Kharazi received her Medical degree from Kiev Medical Institute, Ukraine and her PhD from the Institute of Gerontology, Academy of Medical Sciences of Ukraine. Her research focused on age-related changes of brain neuromediators, such as dopamine and serotonin. During her postdoctoral work she researched Parkinson's disease using animal models. Dr. Kharazi continued to concentrate on the aging of the adult animal central nervous system and has produced over ten publications in the areas related to mechanisms of aging and longevity and the effects of stress.

At the National Genetics Institute she focused her efforts on developmental tasks related to testing blood samples for various viruses using PCR technology. At AmCyte Corporation, she was involved in research of gene expression by progenitors for insulin producing cells. She is one of the leading cell culture specialists and has developed proprietary processes, standard operating procedures and technologies for various stem cell cultures, as well as methods for their isolation, expansion, purification and characterization.

Alexei Lukashev, PhD, Director, Laser Stem Cell Division

Dr. Alexei Lukashev has over 20 years of experience in advanced research and development in solid state and eximer lasers, nonlinear optics and interaction of laser radiation with matter. Dr. Lukashev currently works with a laser for hydrogen bond modification that was invented while he was working at Moscow's General Physics Institute with Nobel Prize winner and academician A. Prokhorov.

Dr. Lukashev has a track record of new product development for the medical and semiconductor industries including lasers for hair removal, vascular treatment and skin resurfacing. He has also participated in the development of optical methods of non-invasive cancer diagnostics and was the managing director of development and manufacturing of DermaChiller 4, an FDA-approved hand-held device for cooling the skin during laser and medical procedures. Dr. Lukashev currently holds 7 United States patents and has been published in 36 peer review journals and conference proceedings. He presents his works at international conferences such as SPIE Biomedical Optics, the Association of Research in Vision and Opthalmology (ARVO), and the American Society of Laser Medicine Surgery (ASLMS).

He is currently developing methods of using laser radiation with stem cell therapy to treat posterior eye dysfunctions such as retinitis pigmentosa, age-related macular degeneration, and retinal vessels occlusion. Dr. Lukashev studies photothermal and photomechanical mechanisms of releasing signaling proteins, cytokines and endogenous stem cells in the retina with specially designed laser pulses.

Tim Brown, MS, JD, Director, Intellectual Property

As Stemedica's Director of Intellectual Property, Tim Brown's role is to achieve patent protection for the company's intellectual property and technology. He has extensive experience in drafting and managing patent applications and dockets concerning stem cell and related technology through all stages of prosecution including: researching and drafting opinions relating to patentability and freedom to operate, providing strategic guidance for patent portfolio development, assessing and negotiating in-licensing opportunities, preparation of discovery documents, preparation of infringement complaints, drafting office actions, and managing outside intellectual consultants and advisors.

Mr. Brown is an attorney licensed to the state of California and before the United States Patent and Trademark Office. He has a Master of Science in Biotechnology from Johns Hopkins University, an MBA from California Polytechnic State University, and a JD from California

Western School of Law. Before joining Stemedica, Mr. Brown worked as a Patent Examiner for the United States Patent and Trademark Office (Alexandria, Virginia) analyzing the patentability of medical diagnostics, antiviral therapies and commercial software.

Yuri Kudinov, MD, PhD, Research Scientist

Dr. Yuri Kudinov received his Medical degree in Internal Medicine from the National Medical University Kyiv, Ukraine and his PhD from the Institute of Gerontology, Academy of Medical Sciences of Ukraine specializing in Immunology and Allergy. As a research scholar at the University of Southern California, Saint Vincent Medical Center Immunotherapy Laboratory, he specialized in the development and preparation for administration of cancer vaccines in FDA approved clinical trials. His research and publication focused on resistant tumor cell lines of different histological origins related to mesothelioma, colon and hepatocellular carcinoma cells.

Dr. Kudinov has a high level of proficiency in flow cytometry, general immunophenotyping, cytokine flow cytometry, cell analysis, apoptosis assays, immunohistochemistry, *in vitro* cytotoxic assays, chromogenic endpoint limulus amoebocyte lysate testing and statistical analysis.

He has extensive experience in rejuvenation of the aging immune system, stimulation of immunogenicity of whole-cell cancer vaccines, and quality control testing of multipotent stem cells including large scale expansion of mesenchymal stromal cells and neural progenitor cells in perfusion bioreactors. He is known for his ability to optimize cell culture conditions to enhance production of therapeutic stem cell growth factors, as well as his expertise in the preservation and stabilization of isolated therapeutic stem cells and growth factors.

Grigory K. Vertelov, PhD, Research Scientist

Dr. Grigory Vertelov received his PhD in Organic Chemistry, and his Masters degree in Chemistry and Medicinal Chemistry from Moscow State University, Russia. His postdoctoral work as a research scholar in the Department of Chemistry, Princeton University (New Jersey), focused on the synthesis of phosphonic acids, oligothiophenes, surface modification—monolayer deposition on the oxide surfaces and organic semiconductors and transistors.

In addition to his research efforts, he has taught courses at the graduate level and participated in managing research projects in the departments of chemistry, biology, physics and materials engineering at

Auburn University, the University of Alabama, Moscow University, Russia, and University of Nice Sophia Antipolis, France.

The focus of Dr. Vertelov's research efforts is on developing new chemical compounds to enhance transfection efficiency of mesenchymal stem cells. He is capitalizing on his experience and expertise in working with nanoparticles to conjugate them with plasmid DNA and create complexes that will be introduced into mesenchymal stem cells. Following DNA translation, the cells are expected to secrete the cytokines of interest to promote the healing process at the site of injury. He has over a dozen publications and abstracts.

M. G. Muraldihar, PhD, Research Scientist

Dr. M. G. Muraldihar received his PhD in Molecular Genetics from The Ohio State University and his Master of Science degree in Biochemistry from M. S. University of Baroda, India. He has over 20 years of experience in molecular biology with an emphasis on DNA/RNA analysis, cloning, genomic and cDNA library construction/screening, in-situ hybridization, PCR/aPCR sequencing, *in vitro* transcription, recombinant protein expression/production, drosophila genetics, and RFLP mapping and transgenics. In the field of cell biology he has extensive experience in tissue culture, transfection (stable and transient) transduction, protein expression, SDS-PAGE, FACS, viral propagation/titre and enzyme-kinetics. His work in bioinformatics has included genomic/proteomic analysis tools, microarray analysis, software development/testing and PCR primer/probe design.

Dr. Muraldihar has served as a senior research scientist and principal scientist at several organizations including Polyclone Bioservices in the United States, India and Europe where he designed and developed projects in bioinformatics. At the La Jolla Institute of Molecular Medicine, California, his focus was on adenoviral-based vaccines against HIV. Research projects at the Children's Hospital of Los Angeles focused on the development of lentivectors for gene-therapy of pancreatic disease and the transdifferentiation of hematopoietic stem cells to islet cells. At the Salk Institute, California his research focused on neuronal development in drosophila and at the University of California, San Francisco studies were conducted in therapeutic targets of scistosoma mansoni, the parasite responsible for human schistosomiasis. He has several peer review publications.

Chang-Hun Huh, MD, PhD, Clinical Research Scientist

Dr. Huh is an Assistant Professor in the Department of Dermatology, Seoul National University Bundang Hospital. He received both his MD and PhD degrees from Seoul National University College of Medicine. His PhD thesis was "The Influence of Adipose-Derived Adult Stem Cells on Epidermis of Living Skin Equivalent." He holds active leadership positions in the Korean Dermatologic Laser Association, the Korean Society for Aesthetic and Dermatologic Surgery, the Korean Society of Cosmetic Dermatology, and the Korean Hair Research Society. He serves as a reviewer of many established international journals including *International Journal of Dermatology, Archives of Dermatological Research, Journal of Dermatological Treatment, Journal of Dermatology*, and *Annals of Dermatology*.

His research interests include stem cell biology, hair and scalp disease, photo-medicine, skin cancer and wound healing. Dr. Huh is the recipient of numerous international awards. Since 2001, he has authored over 80 articles in domestic and SCI ranked international journals.

Riccardo Emilio Nisato, PhD, E-MBA, Director, Clinical Development

Dr. Riccardo Nisato holds a Masters in Pharmacology (University Paris V & Hospital Xavier Bichât), a Masters in Medical Biology (University of Geneva), a PhD in Biology (University of Geneva), a postdoctorate (École Polytechnique Fédérale de Lausanne, EPFL, Switzerland) and an Executive MBA-Management of Technology (joint MBA, EPFL-HEC Lausanne, Switzerland and McCombs School of Business, Austin, Texas).

He is a respected biologist and has worked and taught at several universities and hospitals in Europe, the United States and South Africa. Dr. Nisato has published a number of peer reviewed scientific articles and book chapters, presented at numerous international conferences, and received several awards for his research. He also initiated and managed collaborations with major pharmaceutical corporations, med-tech companies and start-ups.

Dr. Nisato has over ten years experience in molecular and cell biology (he engineered the first human lymphatic endothelial cell line used by research laboratories worldwide), bioengineering, small and large animal experimentation, and current Good Manufacturing Practice (cGMP) cell manufacturing. He also collaborated extensively with key opinion leaders, researchers and surgeons involved in cell-based clinical trials and approved therapies for skin burn treatments for children and adults. His strategic consultancy, requested by the Board of the Hospital, established the basis for project development of the cGMP platform for cell therapy at the University Hospital of Lausanne, Switzerland.

In addition to his biology-related expertise, Dr. Nisato has in dept knowledge of technology and regulatory management as he evaluated and participated in fundamental and clinical projects (up to marketing authorization). He frequently interacts with Swiss Health Authorities such as the Swiss Veterinary Office, Federal office of Public Health (FOPH), and Swiss Agency for Therapeutic Products (Swissmedic).

Ike Whan Lee, PhD, President, Stemedica-AnCBio

Dr. Ike Lee received his PhD in Molecular and Cellular Biology from the University of Georgia and his Master of Science degree in Microbiology from Yonsei University Graduate School in Seoul, Korea. He also received postdoctoral training at the Harvard Medical School and Beth Israel Medical Center in cardiology and cell biology. Dr. Lee is President and CTO of AnC Bio, the joint venture partner of Stemedica-AnCBio. AnC Bio is a leader in stem cell technologies, cell therapy and cell culture manufacturing in Korea. Under Dr. Lee's leadership, the company is actively establishing global operations of providing cell therapy products as well as cell culture-based vaccines.

With his expertise in the development and commercialization of biomedical technologies, Dr. Lee has been actively working in the establishment and operation of biotech start-up companies in the United States, Belgium and Korea, as well as consulting with the Korean government in developing biomedical complexes through the collaboration of universities, hospitals, biotechs and financial organizations. In his capacity as an executive of the biotech companies, Dr. Lee has led research and development activities, as well as managed technologies and intellectual properties for clinically relevant technologies in stem cell therapy and tissue regeneration. Dr. Lee has accumulated extensive experience in establishing research and development projects based on the in-licensed technologies and organizing multi-institutional collaboration/alliance to maximally utilize the resources and to facilitate the best development of the technologies.

References

Chapter 1 Understanding the Promise of Stem Cells

1. Ramalho-Santos, M., & Willenbring, H. (2007). On the origin of the term 'stem cell.' *Cell Stem Cell, 1*(1), 35-38.

2. Kempen, J. H., O'Colmain, B. J., Leske, M. C., Haffner, S. M., Klein, R., Moss, S. E., . . . Eye Diseases Prevalence Research Group. (2004). The prevalence of diabetic retinopathy among adults in the United States. *Archives of Ophthamology, 122*(4), 552-563.

3. Faul, M., Xu, L., Wald, M. M., & Coronado, V. G. (2010). *Traumatic Brain Injury in the United States: Emergency Department Visits, Hospitalizations and Deaths 2002 - 2006* (pp. 25). Atlanta, GA: Centers for Disease Control and Prevention, National Center for Injury Prevention and Control.

4. American Heart Association. (2010). *Heart Disease and Stroke Statistics—2010 Update*. Dallas, Texas: American Heart Association.

5. U.S. National Institutes of Health. (2010). Search stem cells: found 3172 studies. Retrieved from http://www.clinicaltrials.gov/ct2/results?term=stem+cells.

6. Mason, C., & Manzotti, E. (2010). 2010: The pace of RegenMed 2.0 Gathers Momentum. In B. F. Siegel, R. E. Margolin, & R. M. Isasi (Eds.), *World Stem Cell Report - 2010* (pp. 10-11).

7. Elliott, D. (Host), & Krulwich, R. (Reporter). (2006, July 1). Bacteria outnumber cells in human body. *Weekend All Things Considered*. Retrieved from http://www.npr.org/templates/story/story.php?storyId=5527426.

8. Smith, A. (2006). A glossary for stem-cell biology. *Nature, 441*, 1060.

9. Parkinson's stem cell advance. (2002, January 8). *BBC News*. Retrieved from http://news.bbc.co.uk/2/hi/health/1748928.stm.

10. Kattan, A. (2009, June 16). Adult stem cells are a promising market. *Fortune Magazine: Fortune Tech Daily*. Retrieved from http://money.cnn.com/2009/06/16/technology/adult_stem_cell_therapy.fortune/index.htm.

11. Flynn, C. M., & Kaufman, D. S. (2007). Donor cell leukemia: Insight into cancer stem cells and the stem cell niche. *Blood, 109*(7), 2688-2692.

12. Greaves, M. F. (2006). Cord blood donor cell leukemia in recipients [Letter to the editor]. *Leukemia, 20*(4), 744-745.

13. Cooper, M. D. (2003). In Memoriam: Robert A. Good May 21, 1922 - June 13, 2003. *The Journal of Immunology, 171*, 6318-6319. Retrieved from http://www.jimmunol.org/cgi/content/full/171/12/6318.

14. Zhang, Z. Y., Teoh, S. H., Chong, M. S., Schantz, J. T., Fisk, N. M., Choolani, M. A., & Chan, J. (2009). Superior osteogenic capacity for bone tissue engineering of fetal compared with perinatal and adult mesenchymal stem cells. *Stem Cells, 27*(1), 126-137.

15. Goldstein, L., & Schneider, M. (2010). *Stem Cells for Dummies* (pp. 63). Indianapolis, IN: Wiley Publishing, Inc.

16. Koustas, W. T. (2011, January 19). Regenerative Sciences—FDA Struggle Continues [Web log message]. Retrieved from http://www.fdalawblog.net/fda_law_blog_hyman_phelps/2011/01/regenerative-sciences-fda-struggle-continues.html.

17. Amariglio, N., Hirschberg, A., Scheithauer, B. W., Cohen, Y., Loewenthal, R., Trakhtenbrot, L., . . . Rechavi, G. (2009). Donor-derived brain tumor following neural stem cell transplantation in an ataxia telangiectasia patient. *Public Library of Science: Medicine, 6*(2), e1000029.

Chapter 2 A Russian Story

1. Maximov, A. (1917, December 19). [Letter to Samuel Huntington]. University of Chicago Library, Special Collections, Chicago, IL.

2. Konstantinov, I. E. (2000). In search of Alexander A. Maximow: the man behind the Unitarian theory of hematopoiesis. *Perspectives in Biology and Medicine, 43*(2), 269-276.

3. DiDio, L. J. (1986). Remembering Alexander Alexandrowitsch Maximow. *Tokai Journal of Experimental and Clinical Medicine, 11*(3), 151-153.

4. Furcht, L., & Hoffman, W. (2008). *The Stem Cell Dilemma: Beacons of Hope or Harbingers of Doom?* New York, NY: Arcade Publishing, Inc.

5. Ramalho-Santos, M., & Willenbring, H. (2007). On the origin of the term "stem cell." *Cell Stem Cell*, *1*(1), 35-38.

6. Maximow, A. A. (2009). The lymphocyte as a stem cell, common to different blood elements in embryonic development and during the post-fetal life of mammals. *Cellular Therapy and Transplantation*, *1*(3).

7. Friedenstein, A. J. (2009). On stromal-hematopoietic interrelationships: Maximov's ideas and modern models. *Cellular Therapy and Transplantation*, *1*(3). (Reprinted from Modern Trends in Human Leukemia VIII, 1989, Ed. R. Neth).

8. Horne, C. F. (2009). *Source Records of the Great War*, Volume 1: Causes. Whitefish, MT: Kessinger Publishing, LLC.

9. Konstantinov, I. E., Mejevoi, N., & Anichkov, N. M. (2006). Nikolai N. Anichkov and his theory of atherosclerosis. *Texas Heart Institute Journal*, *33*(4), 417-423.

10. Urlanis, B. (1971). *Wars and Population*. New York, NY: Beekman Publishers.

11. Mikhaîlovna Ivanova, G., Flath, C. A., & Raleigh, D. J. (2000). *Labor Camp Socialism: The Gulag in the Soviet Totalitarian System*. Armonk, NY: M.E. Sharpe

12. Novik, A. A., Ionova, T. I., Gorodokin, G., Smolyaninov, A., & Afanasyev, B. V. (2009). The Maximow 1909 centenary: A reappraisal. *Cellular Therapy and Transplantation*, *1*(3). doi: 10.3205/ctt2009-en-000034.01

13. Konstantinov, I. E. (1998). Nikolai S. Korotkov: a story of an unknown surgeon with an immortal name. *Surgery*, *123*(4), 371-381.

14. Maximov, A. (1919, March 30). [Letter to Professor Bensley, Petrograd]. University of Chicago Library, Special Collections, Chicago, IL.

15. Foot, C. (1927, June 18). [Letter to Alexander Maximov]. University of Chicago Library, Special Collections, Chicago, IL.

16. Maximov, A. (1927, June 22). [Letter to Chandler Foot]. University of Chicago Library, Special Collections, Chicago, IL.

17. Downey, H. (1928, December 12). [Letter from Hal Downey to William Bloom]. University of Chicago Library Special Collections, Chicago, IL.

Footnotes

A. The name can also be spelled "Maximow," a reflection of German pronunciation at a time when German was considered the language of science.

B. Kalyuzhny, V. (2010, January). Personal e-mail correspondence.

C. The unnamed "Professor" in the letter is almost certainly a reference to Professor Huntington.

D. Konstantinov. "Nikolai N. Anichkov." Although Maximov had died the year before, Aschoff's letter makes it unclear whether he was aware of his colleague's passing. If not, this ignorance can be attributed to the slow rate of transferring news between America and Europe at the time.

Chapter 3 From Disaster to Recovery

1. Afanasyev, B., Elstner, E., & Zander, A. R. (2009). A.J. Friedenstein, founder of the mesenchymal stem cell concept. *Cellular Therapy and Transplantation*, *1*(3), 35-38. doi: 10.3205/ctt-2009-en-000029.01

2. Gardner, M. (1957) *Fads and Fallacies in the Name of Science*. New York, NY: Dover Books.

3. Burnham, D. (1977, November 26). C.I.A. papers, released to Nader, tell of two Soviet nuclear accidents. *The New York Times*. Retrieved from Medvedev, Z. (1979). *A Nuclear Disaster in the Urals*. New York, NY: W.W. Norton and Company, Inc.

4. Medvedev, Z. (1979). *A Nuclear Disaster in the Urals*. New York, NY: W.W. Norton and Company, Inc.

5. Carlson, B. M. (1968). Regeneration research in the Soviet Union. *The Anatomical Record*, *160*(4), 665-674.

6. Afanasyev, B., Elstner, E., & Zander, A. R. (2009). Editorial – The Maximow 1909 centenary: A reappraisal. *Cellular Therapy and Transplantation*, *1*(3), 31-34. doi: 10.3205/ctt-2009-en-000034.01

7. Friedenstein, A. J. (2009). On stromal-hematopoietic interrelationships: Maximov's ideas and modern models. *Cellular Therapy and Transplantation*, *1*(3). (Reprinted from *Modern Trends in Human Leukemia VIII*, 1989, Ed. R. Neth).

8. Kuznetsov, S., & Robey, P. G. (2000). A look at the history of bone marrow stromal cells. *Graft Review, 3*(6), 278-283.

9. Drize, N., & Ornatsky, O. (2009). Obituary: Joseph Lvovich Chertkov, M.D., Ph.D. 1927-2009. *Experimental Hematology, 37*, 876-877. doi: 10.1016/j.exphem.2009.04.007

10. Mitchell, G. (Presenter), & Coukell, A. (Reporter). (2006, June 28). *Nature Podcast Special: Stem Cells, Interview with David Scadden on stem cell niches.* [Audio podcast]. Retrieved from http://www.nature.com/podcast/stemcells/interviews/scaddon_full.mp3.

11. Schofield, R. (1978). The relationship between the spleen colony-forming cell and the haemopoietic stem cell. *Blood Cells, 4*(1-2), 7-25.

12. Scadden, D. T. (2006). The stem-cell niche as an entity of action. *Nature, 441*(7097), 1075-1079.

13. Chertov, J. L., & Gurevitch, O. A. (1984). *Hematopoietic stem cell and its microenvironment.* Moscow, Russia: Meditzina.

14. Resolution of the presidium of the Russian Academy of Sciences regarding construction of biological institutes in Pushchino. (1962). *Bulletin of the Academy of Sciences of the USSR, 6.*

15. Academics' Case. (n.d.). In *Encyclopaedia of Saint Petersburgh.* Retrieved from http://www.encspb.ru/en/article.php?kod=2804021760.

16. *Intelligence report: The Politburu and Soviet decision-making.* (2007). The Central Intelligence Agency (C.I.A.) Retrieved from http://www.foai.cia.gov/CPE/CAESAR/caesar-53.pdf.

17. Villers, K. (2005, September 18). T.O. stem cell pioneers win "America's Nobel" almost 45 years after a breakthrough stem-cell discovery, a scientific odd couple wins the presitigious Lasker Award. *Gairdner News.* Retrieved from http://www.gairdner.org/Announcements/gairdner/tostemcell.

18. Paste plugs hole in skull. (1966). *Science News, 90*(30), 68.

19. Minutes of Wilsede Meeting, 1988: Alexander J. Friedenstein. On stromal-hematopoietic interrelationships: Maximov's ideas and modern models. (1988). Transcript retrieved from http://www.science-connections.com/books/other/On stromal-hematopoietic interrelationships AJ Friedenstein 1988 Wilsede.pdf.

20. Kellerer, A. M. (2002). The Southern Urals radiation studies. A reappraisal of the current status. *Radiation and Environmental Biophysics, 41*(4), 307-316.

21. McDonald, M. (2004, April 7). Russia finally acknowledging '57 nuclear disaster. *The Seattle Times.* Retrieved from http://seattletimes.nwsource.com/html/nationworld/2001897370_nukeaccident07.html.

22. Svetlana. Elixir of genius for the Soviet leaders. (2009, January 8). [Translation of retrieved website http://omsk.kp.ru/daily/24225.3/424840/].

23. Svetlana, Veligzhanina, A., & Valeev, L. (2005, May 4). Deckman cages – a medicine for an old age? [Translation of retrieved website http://www.kp.ru/daily/23509.3/39545/].

24. Thomas, E. D. (Nobel Lecturer). (1990, December 8). Bone marrow transplantation – Past, present and future. Retrieved from http://nobelprize.org/nobel_prizes/medicine/laureates/1990/thomas -lecture.html.

25. Mathe, O., Jammet, H., Pendic, B., Schwarzenberg, L., Duplan, J. F., Maupin, B., . . . Djukic, Z. (1959). Transfusions et greffes de moelle osseuse homologue chez des humains irradiés à haute dose accidentellement. Extract from *Revue Française d'Etudes Cliniques et Biologiques, 4,* 226-238.

Footnotes

A. Gale, R. (2010, March 17). Personal interview. All quotations in this chapter from Dr. Robert Gale are from this interview unless otherwise indicated.

B. Kharazi, Alex. (2010, February 24). Personal interview. All quotations in this chapter from Dr. Alex Kharazi are from this interview unless otherwise indicated.

C. Tankovich, N. (2010, January). Personal interview. All quotations in this chapter from Dr. Nikolai Tankovich are from this interview unless otherwise indicated.

Chapter 4 Crests and Falls

1. Ebel, R. E., & Center for Strategic and International Studies. (1994). *Chernobyl and its Aftermath: A Chronology of Events.* Washington, DC: Center for Strategic & International Studies.

2. Guskova, A. K., Barabanova, A. V., Baranov, A. Y., Gruszdev, G. P., Pyatkin, Y. K., Nadezhina, N. M., . . . Zykova, I. E.

(1998). *Appendix: Acute Radiation Effects in Victims of the Chernobyl Nuclear Power Plant Accident*. Special Report to the United Nations Scientific Committee on the Effects of Radiation, pp. 617, 622, 630.

3. Gale, R. P. (1987). Immediate Medical Consequences of Nuclear Accidents: Lessons from Chernobyl. *Journal of the American Medical Association, 258*(5), 625-628.

4. Cox, P. (2009). Pathogenetic Stem Cells Poised to Break Through. *Breakthrough Technology Alert*. Retrieved from http://www.internationalstemcell.com/breakingnews/PatrickCox4-09.pdf.

5. Gearheart, J. (2009, May 26). Biography. *Academy of Achievement*. Retrieved from http://www.achievement.org/autodoc/page/gea0bio-1.

6. Green, R. M. (2001). The Stem Cell Debate. *Nova Online*. Retrieved from http://www.pbs.org/wgbh/nova/miracle/stemcells.html.

7. Boyle, A. (2005, June 25). Stem Cell Pioneer Does a Reality Check: James Thomson Reflects on Science and Morality. *MSNBC*. Retrieved from http://www.msnbc.msn.com/id/8393756.

8. Prockop, D. J. (2004). Embryonic Stem Cells Versus Adult Stem Cells: Some Seemingly Simple Questions. In R. Lanza, J. Gearheart, B. Hogan, D. Melton, R. Pedersen, E. D. Thomas, J. Thomson & M. West (Eds.), *Essentials of Stem Cell Biology* (pp. xxiii-xxiv). Burlington, MA: Elsevier Academic Press.

9. Alison, M. R., Poulsom, R., & Wright, N. A. (2002). Editorial: Preface to Stem Cells. *The Journal of Pathology, 197*(4), 417-418.

10. Feng, Q., Lu, S. J., Klimanskaya, I., Gomes, I., Dohoon, K., Chung, Y., . . . Lanza, R. (2010). Hemangioblastic derivatives from human induced pluripotent stem cells exhibit limited expansion and early senescence. *Stem Cells, 28*(4), 704-712.

11. Begley, S. (2010, February 11). Still No Truce in the Stem-Cell Wars: A New Study Finds Serious Problems with Stem Cells Produced from Adult Cells. *Newsweek*. Retrieved from http://www.newsweek.com/2010/02/10/still-no-truce-in-the-stem-cell-wars.html.

12. Tsuji, O., Miura, K., Okada, Y., Fujiyoshi, K., Mukaino, M., Narihito, N., . . . Okano, H. (2007). Therapeutic Potential of Appropriately Evaluated Safe-Induced Pluripotent Stem Cells for Spinal Cord Injury. *Proceedings of the National Academy of Sciences, 107*(28), 12704-12709.

13. Gluckman, E., Broxmeyer, H. E., Auerbach, A. D., Friedman, H. S., Douglas, G. W., Devergie, A., . . . Boyse, E. A. (1989). Hematopoietic Reconstitution in a Patient with Fanconi's Anemia by Means of Umbilical-Cord Blood from an HLA-Identical Sibling. *New England Journal of Medicine, 231*, 1174-1178.

14. University Hospitals of Cleveland. (2001, June 19). Umbilical Cord Blood Transplant: Effective New Leukemia Treatment for Adults. *ScienceDaily*. Retrieved from http://www.sciencedaily.com/releases/2001/06/010614064016.htm.

15. Broxmeyer, H. E. (2010, May 26). Cord Blood Hematopoietic Stem Cell Transplantation StemBook (11: Therapeutic prospects). Retrieved from http://www.ncbi.nlm.nih.gov/bookshelf/br.fcgi?book=stembook&part=cordbloodhematopoieticstmcelltransplantation.

16. Children's Hospital, & Research Center at Oakland. (2009, June 23). Placenta: New Source For Harvesting Stem Cells. *ScienceDaily*. Retrieved from http://www.sciencedaily.com/releases/2009/06/090623091119.htm.

Footnotes

A. Gale, R. (2010, March 17). Personal interview. All quotations in this chapter from Dr. Robert Gale are from this interview unless otherwise indicated.

B. Repin, V. (2009, December). Personal interview in Moscow, RU. All quotations in this chapter from Dr. Vadim Repin are from this interview unless otherwise indicated.

C. Sixty-eight adults, aged 15-58, all having received either intensive chemotherapy or total-body radiation.

D. Daley, G. (2010, April 15). Symposium at Harvard Business School. All quotations in this chapter from Dr. George Daley are from this interview unless otherwise indicated.

Chapter 5 A Quantum Leap

1. Dausset, J. (1981). The Major Histocompatibility Complex in Man – Past, Present, and Future Concepts. *Science, 213*(4515), 1469-1474. (Reprinted from Nobel lecture, University of Paris VII, 1980 December, 8).

2. Gale, R. P. (1987). Immediate Medical Consequences of Nuclear Accidents: Lessons from Chernobyl. *Journal of the American Medical Association, 258*(5), 625-628.

3. Owen, M., & Friedenstein, A. J. (1988). Stromal Stem Cells: Marrow-derived Osteogenic Precursors. In D. Evered & S. Hamlett (Eds.) Ciba Foundation Symposium, *136*, 42-60. *Cell and Molecular Biology of Vertebrate Hard Tissues.* Chichester, UK: Wiley & Sons.

4. Owen, M. E., Cavé, J., & Joyner C. J. (1987). Clonal Analysis In Vitro of Osteogenic Differentiation of Marrow CFU-F. *Journal of Cell Science, 87*(5), 731-738.

5. Parekkadan, B., Palaniappan, S., Van Poll, D., Yarmush, M. L., & Toner, M. (2007). Osmotic Selection of Human Mesenchymal Stem/Progenitor Cells from Umbilical Cord Blood. *Tissue Engineering, 13*(10), 2465-2473. doi:10.1089/ten.2007.0054.

6. Caplan, A. I. (1994). The Mesengenic Process. *Clinics in Plastic Surgery, 21*, 429-435.

7. Lazarus, H. M., Haynesworth, S.E., Gerson, S. L., Rosenthal, N. S., & Caplan A. I. (1995). Ex Vivo Expansion and Subsequent Infusion of Human Bone Marrow-Derived Stromal Progenitor Cells (Mesenchymal Progenitor Cells): Implications for Therapeutic Use. *Bone Marrow Transplantation, 16*(4), 557-564.

8. Koç, O. N., Gerson, S. L., Cooper, B. W., Laughlin, M., Meyerson, H., Kutteh, L., . . . Lazarus, H. M. (2000). Rapid Hematopoietic Recovery After Co-Infusion of Autologous Culture-Expanded Human Mesenchymal Stem Cells (hMSCs) and PBPCs in Breast Cancer Patients Receiving High Dose Chemotherapy. *Journal of Clinical Oncology, 18*(2), 307-316.

9. Koç, O. N., & Lazarus, H. M. (2001). Mesenchymal Stem Cells: Heading Into the Clinic. *Bone Marrow Transplant, 27*(3), 235-239.

10. Götherström, C., West, A., Liden, J., Uzunel, M., Lahesmaa, R., & Le Blanc, K. (2005). Difference in Gene Expression Between Human Fetal Liver and Adult Bone Marrow Mesenchymal Stem Cells. *Haematologica, 90*(8), 1017-1026.

11. Maitra, B., Szekely, E., Gjini, K., Laughlin, M. J., Dennis, J., Haynesworth, S. E., & Koç, O. N. (2004). Human Mesenchymal Stem Cells Support Unrelated Donor Hematopoietic Stem Cells and Suppress T-Cell Activation. *Bone Marrow Transplantation, 33*(6), 597-604.

12. Wagner, W., Rainer, S., & Ho, A. D. (2008). The Stromal Activity of Mesenchymal Stromal Cells. *Transfusion Medicine and Hemotherapy, 35*(3), 185-193.

13. Mbalaviele, G., Jaiswal, N., Meng, A., Cheng, L., Van Den Bos, C., & Thiede, M. (1999). Human Mesenchymal Stem Cells Promote Human Osteoclast Differentiation from CD34+ Bone Marrow Hematopoietic Progenitors. *Endocrinology, 140*(8), 3736-3743.

14. Altman, J. (1962). Are New Neurons Formed in the Brains of Adult Mammals? *Science, 135*(3509), 1127-1128.

15. Altman, J., & Das, G. D. (1967). Postnatal Neurogenesis in the Guinea-Pig. *Nature, 10*(214), 1098 1101.

16. Specter, M. (2001). Rethinking the Brain: How the Songs of Canaries Upset a Fundamental Principle in Science. *The New Yorker, 23*, 42-53.

17. Salk's Fred H. Gage on Neurogensesis in the Adult Brain. (2005). *ScienceWatch, 16*(6). Retrieved from http://www.sciencewatch.com/nov-dec2005/sw_nov-dec2005_page3.htm.

18. Eriksson, P. S., Perfilieva, E., Björk-Eriksson, T., Alborn, A. M., Nordborg, C., Peterson, D. A., & Gage, F. H. (1998). Neurogenesis in the Adult Human Hippocampus. *Nature Medicine, 4*(11), 1313-1317.

19. Ryder, E. F., Snyder, E. Y., & Cepko, C. L. (1990). Establishment and Characterization of Multipotent Neural Cell Lines Using Retrovirus-Mediated Oncogen Transfer. *Journal of Neurobiology, 21*(2), 356-375.

20. Snyder, E. Y., Deitcher, D. L., Walsh, C., Arnold-Aldea, S., Hartwieg, E. A., & Cepko, C. L. (1992). Multipotent Neural Cell Lines Can Engraft and Participate in Development of Mouse Cerebellum. *Cell, 68*(1), 33-51.

21. Kennea, N. L., & Mehmet, H. (2002). Neural Stem Cells. *Journal of Pathology, 197*(4), 536-550.

22. Lois, C., & Alvarez-Buylla A. (1994). Long-Distance Neuronal Migration in the Adult Mammalian Brain. *Science, 264*(5162), 1145-1148.

23. Olanow, C. W., Kordower, J. H., & Freeman, T. B. (1996). Fetal Nigral Transplantation as a Therapy for Parkinson's Disease. *Trends in Neurosciences, 19*(3), 102-109.

24. Rabinovich, S. S., Seledtsov, V. I., Banual, N. V., Poveshchenko, O. V., Senyukov, V. V., Astrakov, S. V.,

. . . Taraban, V. Y. (2005). Cell Therapy of Brain Stroke. *Bulletin of Experimental Biology and Medicine, 129*(1), 126-128.

25. *Science Profile: Dr. Nikolay Mironov, Treating Physician* [Biography/Interview]. Retrieved from http://www.bayerstem cell.com/MedicalTeam.php

26. Mironov, N. (2008). U.S. Utility No. 20090214484, *Stem Cell Therapy for the Treatment of Central Nervous System Disorders*. Washington, DC: U.S. Patent and Trade Mark Office.

27. Ankrum, J., & Karp, J. M. (2010). Mesenchymal stem cell therapy: Two steps forward, one step back. *Trends in Molecular Medicine, 16*(5), 203-209.

Footnotes

A. Repin, V. (2009, December). Personal interview in Moscow, RU. All quotations in this chapter from Dr. Vadim Repin are from this interview unless otherwise indicated.

B. Repin, V. (2009, February 12). Personal interview. All quotations in this chapter, including all those in this paragraph, are from this interview unless otherwise indicated.

C. Kharazi, A. (2010, February 10). Personal interview. All quotations in this chapter from Dr. Alex Kharazi are from this interview unless otherwise indicated.

D. Snyder, E. (2010, March 24). Personal interview. All quotations in this chapter, including all those in this paragraph and occurring hereafter, from Dr. Evan Snyder are from this interview unless otherwise indicated.

E. Howe, M. A. & Mironov, N. (2009, February). Personal communication.

F. Tornambe, P. (2009, December). Personal interview.

Chapter 6 Stroke

1. Stemedica Cell Technologies, Inc. (2009, October). Pre-IND Package. San Diego, CA: David A. Howe.

2. Behle, B. (Writer). (2008). Stem Cell Therapy: The Future of Medicine [Single news story]. In B. Behle (Executive producer), *KMIR6*. Palm Desert, CA: National Broadcasting Company.

3. American Heart Association. (2010). *Heart Disease and Stroke Statistics—2010* Update. Dallas, Texas: American Heart Association.

4. Stroke patients who reach hospitals within "golden hour" twice as likely to get clot-busting drug. (2009). *American Heart Association*. Retrieved from http://www.newsroom.heart.org/index.php?s=43&item=660.

5. Saver, J. L., Smith E. E., Fonarow, G. C., Reeves, M. J., Zhao, X., Olson, D. M., . . . GWTG Stroke Steering Committee and Investigators. (2010). The "golden hour" and acute brain ischemia: Presenting features and lytic therapy in >30,000 patients arriving within 60 minutes of stroke onset. *Stroke, 41*(7), 1431-1439.

6. Gottlieb, A. (2010, January/February). From Victim to Victor: Creating a Stroke Support Group. *Stroke Connection*, pp. 16.

7. Chun, D. (2009). Research Shows Hope for Victims of Stroke. *The Gainesville Guardian*. Retrieved from http://www.gainesville.com/article/20091210/GUARDIAN/912101033?Title=Research showshope-for-victims-of-stroke.

8. Bible, E., Chau, D., Alexander, M., Price, J., Shakesheff, K. M., & Modo, M. (2009). Scaffold particles support neural stem cells transplanted into stroke-induced brain cavities. *Biomaterials, 30*(16), 2985-2994.

9. Paddock, C. (2009, March 9). Stem Cell Scaffolding Makes New Brain Tissue After Stroke Damage. *Medical news Today*. Retrieved from: http://www.medicalnewstoday.com/articles/141510.php.

10. Mick, J. (2009, March 9). Stem Cells Replace Brain Tissue in Stroke-Victim Rats [Web log message]. Retrieved from http://www.dailytech.com/Stem+Cells+Replace+Dead+Brain+Tissue+in+StrokeVictim+Rats/article14520.htm.

11. Salk's Fred H. Gage on Neurogensesis in the Adult Brain. (2005). *ScienceWatch, 16*(6). Retrieved from http://www.sciencewatch.com/nov-dec2005/sw_nov-dec2005_page3.htm.

12. 50, 100, and 150 Years Ago. (1998, November). *Scientific American Magazine*.

13. Snyder, E. Y. (2006). Special issue: The intersection of stem/progenitor cell biology and hypoxic ischemic cerebral injury/stroke. *Experimental Neurology, 199*(1), 1-4.

14. Fagel, D. M., Ganat, Y., Silbereis, J., Ebbitt, T., Stewart, W., Zhang, H., . . . Vaccarino, F. M. (2006). Cortical neurogenesis enhanced by chronic perinatal hypoxia. *Experimental Neuroogy, 199*(1), 77-91.

15. Park, K. I., Hack, M. A., Ourednik, J., Yandava, B., Flax, J. D., Stieg, P. E., . . . Snyder, E. Y. (2006). Acute injury

directs the migration, proliferation, and differentiation of solid organ stem cells: evidence from the effect of hypoxia-ischemia in the CNS on clonal "reporter" neural stem cells. *Experimental Neurology, 199*(1), 156-178

16. Ourednik, J., Ourednik, V., Lynch, W. P., Schachner, M., & Snyder, E. Y. (2002). Neural stem cells display an inherent mechanism for rescuing dysfunctional neurons. *Nature Biotechnology, 20*(11),1103-1110.

17. Rice, J. (2009, January 7). Stem Cells Undo Birth Defects: Transplanted stem cells restore behavior in brain-damaged rodents. *Technology Review*. Retrieved from http://www.technologyreview.com/biomedicine/21930/page1/.

18. Thurston, G., Rudge, J. S., Ioffe, E., Zhou, H., Ross, L., Croll, S. D., . . . Yancopoulos, G. D. (2000). Angiopoietin-1 protects the adult vasculature against plasma leakage. *Nature Medicine, 6*(4), 460 463.

19. Zhang, Z. G., Zhang, L., Jiang, Q., Zhang, R., Davies, K., Powers, C., . . . Chopp, M. (2000). VEGF enchances angiogenesis and promotes blood-brain barrier leakage in the ischemic brain. *Journal of Clinical Investigation, 106*(7), 829-838.

20. Chen, J., Zhang, Z. G., Li, Y., Wang, L., Xu, Y. X., Gautam, S. C., Lu, M., . . . Chopp, M. (2003). Intravenous administration of human bone marrow stromal cells induces angiogenesis in the ischemic boundary zone after stroke in rats. Circulation Research, *92*(6), 692-699.

21. Bai, L., Caplan, A., Lennon, D., & Miller, R. H. (2007). Human mesenchymal stem cells signals regulate neural stem cell fate. *Neurochemical Research, 32*(2), 353-362.

22. Bertani, N., Malatesta, P., Volpi, G., Sonego, P., & Perris, R. (2005). Neurogenic potential of human mesenchymal stem cells revisited: Analysis by immunostaining, time-lapse video and microarry. *Journal of Cell Science, 118*(17), 3925-3936.

23. Wislet-Gendebien, S., Hans, G., Leprince, P., Rigo, J. M., Moonen, G., & Rogister, B. (2005). Plasticity of cultured mesenchymal stem cells: Switch from nestin-positive to excitable neuron-like phenotype. *Stem Cells, 23*(3), 392-402.

24. Lu, P., Blesch, A., & Tuszynksi, M. H. (2004). Induction of bone marrow stromal cells to neurons: Differentiation, transdifferentiation, or artifact? *Journal of Cell Science, 77*(2), 174-191.

25. Keilhoff, G., Goihl, A., Langnäse K., Fansa, H., & Wolf, G. (2006). Transdifferentiation of mesenchymal stem cells into Schwann cell-like myelinating cells. *European Journal of Cell Biology, 85*(1), 11-24.

26. Aleksandrova, M. A., Sukhikh, G. T., Chailakhyan, R. K., Podgornyi, O. V., Marei, M. V., Poltavtseva, R.A., & Gerasimov, Y. U. (2006). Comparative analysis of differentiation and behavior of human neural and mesenchymal stem cells *in vitro* and *in vivo*. *Cell Technologies in Biology and Medicine, 2*(1), 152-160.

27. Hermann, A., Gastl, R., Liebau, S., Popa, O., Fielder, J., Boehm, B., . . . Storch, A. (2004). Efficient generation of neural stem cell-like cells from adult human bone marrow stromal cells. *Journal of Cell Science, 117*(19), 4411-4422.

Footnotes

A. Soto, M. (2010, February). Personal interview. All quotations in this chapter from Dr. Manuel Soto are from this interview unless otherwise indicated.

B. Duncan, P. (2010, March 5). Personal interview. All quotations in this chapter from Dr. Pamela Duncan are from this interview unless otherwise indicated.

Chapter 7 Spinal Cord Injuries

1. Paralysis Resource Center. (2010). *Prevelance of Paralysis*. Christopher & Dana Reeve Foundation. Retrieved from http://www.christopherreeve.org/site/c.mtKZKgMWKwG/b.5184255/k.6D74/Prevalence_of_Paralysis.htm.

2. Bissinger, B. (2010). A lifetime penalty. In Texas, catastrophic spinal injuries aren't enough to change high school football. *Time, 175*(5), 44-45.

3. Stemedica Cell Technologies, Inc. (2009, October). Pre-IND Package. San Diego, CA: David A. Howe.

4. Young, W. (2010). Spinal Cord Injury Levels & Classification. *Spinal Cord Injury Information Pages*. Retrieved from http://www.sci-info-pages.com/levels.html.

5. Huskey, N. (2001, December). Therapeutic uses of stem cells for spinal cord injuries: a new hope. *National Alliance on Mental Illness: Santa Cruz County*. Retrieved from: http://www.namiscc.org/newsletters/December01/SCI-stem-cell-research.htm.

6. Frisén, J., Johansson, C. B., Török, C., Risling, M., & Lendahl, U. (1995). Rapid, widespread, and longlasting

induction of nestin contributes to the generation of glial scar tissue after CNS injury. *Journal of Cell Biology, 131*(2), 453-464.

7. Johansson, C. B., Momma, S., Clarke, D. L., Risling, M., Lendahl, U., & Frisén, J. (1999). Indentification of a neural stem cell in the adult mammalian central nervous system. *Cell, 96*(1), 25-34.

8. Jocelyn, R. (2009, January 7). Stem Cells Undo Birth Defects: Transplanted stem cells restore behavior in brain-damaged rodents. *Technology Review*. Retrieved from http://www.technologyreview.com/biomedicine /21930/page1/.

9. Stichel, C. C., & Müller, H. W. (1998). The CNS lesion scar: new vistas on an old regeneration barrier. Cell and Tissue Research, *294*(1), 1-9.

10. Ramón y Cajal, S. (1991). (R. M. May, Trans.) In J. DeFelipe & E. G. Jones (Eds.), *Degeneration and Regeneration of the Nervous System*. New York, New York: Oxford University Press.

11. Grill, R., Murai, K., Blesch, A., Gage, F. H., & Tuszynski, M. H. (1997). Cellular delivery of neurotrophin-3 promotes corticospinal axonal growth and partial functional recovery after spinal cord injury. *Journal of Neuroscience, 17*(14), 5560-5572.

12. Liu, Y., Kim, D., Himes, B. T., Chow, S. Y., Schallert, T., Murray, M., . . . Fischer, I. (1999). Transplants of fibroblasts genetically modified to express BDNF promote regeneration of adult rat rubrospinal axons and recovery of forelimb function. *Journal of Neuroscience, 19*(11), 4370-4387.

13. McTigue, D. M., Horner, P. J., Stokes B. T., & Gage, F. H. (1998). Neutrophin-3 and brain-derived neutrophic factor induce oligodendrocyte proliferation and myelination of regenerating axons in the contused adult rat spinal cord. *Journal of Neuroscience, 18*(14), 5354-5365.

14. Horner, P. J., & Gage, F. H. (2000). Regenerating the damaged central nervous system. *Nature, 407*(6807), 963-970.

Footnotes

A. Cheng, I. (2010, June 17). Personal interview. All quotations in this chapter from Dr. Ivan Cheng are from this interview unless otherwise indicated.

B. Cheng, I. (2009, December). Personal interview. All quotations in this chapter, occurring hereafter, from Dr. Ivan Cheng are from this interview unless otherwise indicated.

Chapter 8 Traumatic Brain Injury

1. Silver, M. (2009, September 18). Effects of head injury scaring Turley. *Yahoo!Sports*. Retrieved from http://sports.yahoo.com/nfl/news?slug=ms-thegameface091809.

2. Gregory, S. (2010, February 8). The problem with football. Our favorite sport is too dangerous. How to make the game safer. *Time, 175*(5), 46-43.

3. Smith, S. (2009, January 27). Dead athletes' brains show damage from concussions. *CNNhealth*. Retrieved from http://www.cnn.com/2009/HEALTH/01/26/athlete.brains/index.html.

4. Schwarz, A. (2007, January 18). Expert ties ex-player's suicide to brain damage. *The New York Times*. Retrieved from http://www.nytimes.com/2007/01/18/sports/football/18waters.html?_r=2&ref =sports&oref=slogin.

5. Brain Injury Association of Washington. (2009). Lystedt Law – Sports concussion injury. Retrieved from http://www.biawa.org/lystedt.htm.

6. TraumaticBrainInjury.com. (2004). Understanding traumatic brain injury: What are the causes of TBI? (2004). Retrieved from http://www.traumaticbraininjury.com/content/understandingtbi/causesoftbi.html.

7. Hoge, C. W., McGurk, D., Thomas, J. L., Cox, A. L., Engel, C. C., & Castro, C. A. (2008). Mild traumatic brain injury in U.S. Soldiers returning from Iraq. *The New England Journal of Medicine, 358*(5), 453 463.

8. Military Health System & U.S. Department of Defense. (2010). Department of Defense numbers for traumatic brain injury. Retrieved from http://www.health.mil/Research/TBI_Numbers.aspx.

9. American Forces Press Service. (2010, June 22). Kornman, S. (Web Producer). Soldiers struggling with undiagnosed brain injury. *KGUN9-TV, Tuscon*. Retrieved from http://www.kgun9.com/Global/story.asp?S=12690786.

10. Miller, T. C., & Zwerdling, D. (2010, June 9). Top Officer says military takes brain injuries 'extremely seriously'. *ProPublica*. Retrieved from http://www.propublica.org/feature/top-officer-says-military-takes-brain-injuries-extremely-seriously.

11. Miller, T. C., & Zwerdling, D. (2010, June 11). Military mental health probe widens after NPR-ProPublica report. *NPR.* Retrieved from http://www.npr.org/blogs/thetwoway/2010/06/11/127777719/military-mental-health-probe-widens.

12. Miller, T. C., & Zwerdling, D. (2010, June 8). At Fort Bliss, brain injury treatments can be as elusive as diagnosis. *ProPublica.* Retrieved from http://www.propublica.org/feature/at-fort-bliss-brain-injury-treatments-can-be-as-elusive-as-diagnosis.

13. Seledtsov, V. I., Rabinovich, S. S., Parlyuk, O. V., Kafanova, M. Y., Astrakov, S. V., Seledtsova, G. V., . . . Proveschenko, O.V. (2005). Cell transplantation therapy in re-animating severely head-injured patients. *Biomedicine & Pharmacotherapy, 59*(7), 415-420.

14. Seledtsov, V. I., Rabinovich, S. S., Parlyuk, O. V., Poveschenko, O. V., Astrakov, S. V., Samarin, D. M., . . . Kozlov, V. A. (2006). Cell therapy of comatose states. *Bulletin of Experimental Biology and Medicine, 142*(1), 129-132.

15. Mahmood, A., Lu, D., & Chopp, M. (2004). Intravenous administration of marrow stromal cells (MSCs) increases the expression of growth factors in rat brain after traumatic brain injury. *Journal of Neurotrauma, 21*(1), 33-39.

16. Kim, H. J., Lee, J. H., & Kim, S. H. (2010). Therapeutic effects of human mesenchymal stem cells on traumatic brain injury in rats: secretion of neurotrophic factors and inhibition of apoptosis. *Journal of Neurotrauma, 27*(1), 131-138.

17. Xue, S., Zhang, H. T., Zhang, P., Luo, J., Chen, Z. Z., Jang, X. D., & Xu, R. X. (2010). Functional endothelial progenitor cells derived from adipose tissue show beneficial effect on cell therapy of traumatic brain injury. *Neuroscience Letter, 473*(3), 186-191.

Footnotes

A. Interview with patient's personal physician.

Chapter 9 Parkinson's/Alzheimer's & Other Neurological Conditions

1. National Parkinson Foundation. (2010). *Parkinson's Disease (PD) Overview.* Retrieved from http://www.parkinson.org/parkinson-s-disease.aspx.

2. Shihabuddin, L. S., & Aubert, I. (2010). Stem cell transplantation for neurometabolic and neurodegenerative diseases. *Neuropharmacology, 58*(6), 845-854.

3. Lang, A. E., & Lozano, A. M. (1998). Parkinson's disease. First of two parts. *The New England Journal of Medicine, 339*(15), 1044-1053.

4. Alzheimer's Association. (2010). *2010 Alzheimer's Disease Facts and Figures.* Retrieved from http://www.alz.org/alzheimers_disease_facts_figures.asp.

5. Northwest Parkinson's Foundation. (2010). About Parkinson's. Retrieved from http://www.nwpf.org/About Parkinsons.aspx.

6. Lindvall, O., & Kokaia, Z. (2010). Stem cells in human neurodegenerative disorders – time for clinical translation? *The Journal of Clinical Investigation, 120*(1), 29-40.

7. Rothestein, J. D., & Snyder, E. Y. (2004). Reality and immortality – neural stem cells for therapies. *Nature Biotechnology, 22*(3), 283-285.

8. Lindvall, O., & Björkland, A. (2004). Cell replacement therapy: Helping the brain to repair itself. *NeuroRx: The Journal of the American Society for Expermimental NeuroTherapeutics, 1*(4), 379-381.

9. Lindvall, O., & Björkland, A. (2004). Cell therapy in Parkinson's disease. *NeuroRx: The Journal of the American Society for Expermimental NeuroTherapeutics, 1*(4), 382-393.

10. Stemedica Cell Technologies, Inc. (2009, October). Pre-IND Package. San Diego, CA: David A. Howe.

11. Bugaev, V. S. (1999). *Stem Cell Therapy for Treatment of Parkinson's Disease.* (Doctoral dissertation, The Medical Centre of the Russian President's General Management Department, Moscow, Russia).

12. Luo, Y., Kuang, S. Y., & Hoffer, B. (2009). How useful are stem cells in PD therapy? *Parkinsonism & Related Disorders, 15,* S171-175.

13. Alzheimer's Association. (2010). *Inside the Brain: An Interactive Tour.* Retrieved from http://www.alz.org/alzheimers_disease_4719.asp?type=homepageflash.

14. Lee, J. K., Jin, H. K., & Bae, J. S. (2009). Bone marrow-derived mesenchymal stem cells reduce brain amyloid-beta deposition and accelerate the activation of microglia in an acutely induced Alzheimer's disease mouse model.

Neuroscience Letters, 450(2), 136-141.

15. Simard, A. R., & Rivest, S. (2006). Neuroprotective properties of the innate immune system and bone marrow stem cells in Alzheimer's disease. *Molecular Psychiatry, 11*(4), 327-335.

16. Kolata, G. (2011, January 20). F.D.A. sees promise in Alzheimer's imaging drug. *The New York Times*. Retrieved from http://www.nytimes.com/2011/01/21/health/21alzheimers.html.

17. Lee, J. K., Jin, H. K., Endo, S., Schuchman, E. H., Carter, J. E., & Bae, J. S. (2010). Intracerebral transplantation of bone marrow-derived mesenchymal stem cells reduces amyloid-beta deposition and rescues memory deficits in Alzheimer's disease mice by modulation of immune response. *Stem Cells, 28*(2), 329-343.

18. Blurton-Jones, M., Kitazawa, M., Martinez-Coria, H., Castello, N. A., Müller, G. J., Loring, J. F., & LaFerla, F. M. (2009). Neural stem cells improve cognition via BDNF in a transgenic model of Alzheimer disease. *Proceedings of the National Academy of Sciences of the United States of America, 106*(32), 13594-13599.

19. Shihabuddin, L. S., & Aubert, I. (2010). Stem cell transplantation for neurometabolic and neurodegenerative diseases. *Neuropharmacology, 58*(6), 845-854.

20. Nagahara, A. H., Merrill, D. A., Coppola, G., Tsukada, S., Schroeder, B. E., Shaked, G. M., . . . Tuszynski, M. H. (2009). Neuroprotective effects of brain-derived Neurotrophic factor in rodent and primate models of Alzheimer's disease. *Nature Medicine, 15*(3), 331-337.

21. Sanford-Burnham Medical Research Institute. (2010). *Stemedica, Inc. Progress Report*, a commissioned study.

22. Lyketsos, C. G., Steinberg, M., Tschanz, J. T., Norton, M. C., Steffens, D. C., & Breitner, J. C. (2000). Mental and behavioral disturbances in dementia: findings from the Cache County Study on Memory in Aging. *The American Journal of Psychiatry, 157*(5), 708-714.

23. Burns, A., Jacoby, R., & Levy, R. (1990). Psychiatric phenomena in Alzheimer's disease. IV: Disorders of behaviour. *The British Journal of Psychiatry: The Journal of Mental Science, 157*, 86-94.

24. Ryden, M. B. (1988). Aggressive behavior in persons with dementia who live in the community. Alzheimer's Disease and Associated Disorders, *2*(4), 342-355.

25. Alzheimer's Association. (2010). *Mixed Dementia*. Retrieved from http://www.alz.org/alzheimers_disease_mixed_dementia.asp.

26. University of Rochester Medical Center. (2007, September 26). Stem cells show promise for treating Huntington's Disease. *ScienceDaily*. Retrieved from http://www.sciencedaily.com/releases/2007/09/070925090246.htm.

27. Cho, S. R., Benraiss, A., Chmielnicki, E., Samdani, A., Economides, A., & Goldman, S. A. (2007). Induction of neostriatal Neurogenesis slows disease progression in a transgenic murine model of Huntington disease. *Journal of Clinical Investigation, 117*(10), 2889-2902.

28. Bachoud-Lévi, A. C., Gaura, V., Brugières, P., Lefaucheur, J. P., Boissé, M. F., Maison, P., ... Peschanski, M. (2006). Effect of fetal neural transplants in patients with Huntington's disease 6 years after surgery: a long term follow-up study. *Lancet Neurology, 5*(4), 303-309.

29. Freeman, T. B., Cicchetti, F., Hauser, R. A., Deacon, T. W., Li, X. J., Hersch, S. M., . . . Iscacson, O. (2000). Transplanted fetal striatum in Huntington's disease: Phenotypic development and lack of pathology. *Proceedings of the National Academy of Sciences of the United States of America, 97*(25), 13877-13882.

30. Rice, C. M., Mallam, E. A., Whone, A. L., Walsh, P., Brooks, D. J., Kane, N., . . . Scolding, N. J. (2010). Safety and feasibility of autologous bone marrow cellular therapy in relapsing-progressive multiple sclerosis. *Clinical Pharmacology and Therapeutics, 87*(6), 679-685.

31. Whetten-Goldstein, K., Sloan, F. A., Goldstein, L. B., & Kulas, E. D. (1998). A comprehensive assessment of the cost of multiple sclerosis in the United States. *Multiple Sclerosis, 4*(5), 419-425.

32. Chari, D. M. (2007). Remyelination in multiple sclerosis. *International Review of Neurobiology, 79*,589-620.

33. Mazzini, L., Vercelli, A., Ferrero, I., Mareschi, K., Boido, M., Servo, S., . . . Fagioli, F. (2009). Stem cells in amyotrophic lateral sclerosis: state of the art. *Expert Opinion on Biological Therapy, 9*(10), 1245-1258.

34. Deda, H., Inci, M. C., Kürekçi, A. E., Sav, A., Kayihan, K., Ozgün, E., . . . Kocabay, S. (2009). Treatment of amyotrophic lateral sclerosis patients by autologous bone marrow-derived hematopoietic stem cell transplantation: A 1-year follow-up. *Cytotherapy, 11*(1), 18-25.

35. Mazzini, L., Ferrero, I., Luparello, V., Rustichelli, D., Gunetti, M., Mareschi, K., . . . Fagioli, F. (2010). Mesenchymal stem cell transplantation in amyotrophic lateral sclerosis: A Phase I clinical trial. *Experimental Neurology, 223*(1), 229-237.

36. Ende, N., Weinstein, F., Chen, R., & Ende, M. (2000). Human umbilical cord blood effect on sod mice (amyotrophic lateral sclerosis). *Life Sciences, 67*(1), 53-59.

37. Garbuzova-Davis, S., Willing, A. E., Zigova, T., Saporta, S., Justen, E. B., Lane, J. C., . . . Sanberg, P. R. (2003). Intravenous administration of human umbilical cord blood cells in a mouse model of amyotrophic lateral sclerosis: distribution, migration, and differentiation. *Journal of Hematotherapy and Stem Cell Research, 12*(3), 255-270.

38. Garbuzova- Davis, S., Sanberg, C. D., Kuzmin-Nichols, N., Willing, A. E., Gemma, C., Bickford, P. C., . . . Sanberg, P. R. (2008). Human umbilical cord blood treatment in a mouse model of ALS: Optimization of cell dose. *PLoS One, 3*(6), e2494.

39. Corti, S., Locatelli, F., Donadoni, C., Guglieri, M., Papadimitriou, D., Strazzer, S., . . . Comi, G. P. (2004). Wild-type bone marrow cells ameliorate the phenotype of SOD1-G93A ALS mice and contribute to CNS, heart and skeletal muscle tissues. *Brain: A Journal of Neurology, 127*(Pt11), 2518-2532.

40. Vercelli, A., Mereuta, O. M., Garbossa, D., Muraca, G., Mareschi, K., Rustichelli, D., . . . Fagioli, F. (2008). Human mesenchymal stem cell transplantation extends survival, improves motor performance and decrease neuroinflammation in mouse model of amyotrophic lateral sclerosis. *Neurobiology of Disease, 31*(3), 395-405.

41. Xu, L., Yan, J., Chen, D., Welsh, A. M., Hazel, T., Johe, K., . . . Koliatsos, V. E. (2006). Human neural stem cell grafts ameliorate motor neuron disease in SOD-1 transgenic rats. *Transplantation, 82*(7), 865-875.

42. Desphpande, D. M., Kim, Y. S., Martinez, T., Carmen, J., Dike, S., Shats, I., . . . Kerr, D. A. (2006). Recovery from paralysis in adult rats using embryonic stem cells. *Annals of Neurology, 60*(1), 32-44.

43. Corti, S., Locatelli, F., Papdimitriou, D., Del Bo, R., Nizzardo, M., Nardini, M., . . . Comi, G. P. (2007). Neural stem cells LewisX+ CXCR4+ modify disease progression in an amyotrophic lateral sclerosis model. *Brain: A Journal of Neurology, 130*(Pt5), 1289-1305.

44. Corti, S., Locatelli, F., Papadimitriou, D., Donadoni, C., Del Bo, R., Crimi, M., . . . Comi, G. P. (2006). Transplanted ALDHhiS SClo neural stem cells generate motor neurons and delay disease progression of nmd mice, an animal model of SMARD1. *Human Molecular Genetics, 15*(2), 167-187.

Footnotes

A. Patient GR. (2010, June 25). Personal communications, e-mail.

B. Patient GA. (2010, January 22). Personal communications, e-mail.

Chapter 10 Cardiovascular Conditions

1. American Heart Association. (2010). *Heart Disease and Stroke Statistics—2010 Update.* Dallas, Texas: American Heart Association.

2. Cohen, M. (2010, May 11). Sick and desperate fueling 'stem-cell tourism': Patients turn to illegal procedures offshore to help their damaged hearts. *Men's Health.* Retrieved from http://www.msnbc.msn.com/id/36849354/ns/health-heart_health.

3. Ballard, V. L. (2010). Stem cells for heart failure in the aging heart. *Heart Failure Reviews, 15*(5), 447-456.

4. Kajstura, J., Leri, A., Finato, N., Di Loreto, C., Beltrami, C. A., & Anversa, P. (1998). Myocyte proliferation in end-stage cardiac failure in humans. *Proceedings of the National Academy of Science of the United States of America, 95*(15), 8801-8805.

5. Li, Q., Turdi, S., Thomas, D. P., Zhou, T., & Ren, J. (2010). Intra-myocardial delivery of mesenchymal stem cells ameliorates left ventricular and cardiomyocyte contractile dysfunction following myocardial infarction. *Toxicology Letters, 195*(2-3), 119-126.

6. Werner, N., Kosiol, S., Schiegl, T., Ahlers, P., Walenta, K., Link, A., . . . Nickenig, G. (2005). Circulating endothelial progenitor cells and cardiovascular outcomes. *New England Journal of Medicine, 353*(10), 999-1007.

7. Shintani, S., Murohara, T., Ikeda, H., Ueno, T., Honma, T., Katoh, A., . . . Imaizumi, T. (2001). Mobilization of endothelial progenitor cells in patients with acute myocardial infarction. *Circulation, 103*(23), 2776-2779.

8. Werner, L., Deutsch, V., Barshack, I., Miller, H., Keren, G., & George, J. (2005). Transfer of endothelial progenitor cells improves myocardial performance in rats with dilated cardiomyopathy induced following experimental myocarditis. *Journal of Molecular and Cellular Cardiology, 39*(4), 691-697.

9. Kawamoto, A., Gwon, H. C., Iwaguro, H., Yamaguchi, J. I., Uchida, S., Masuda, H., . . . Asahara, T. (2001). Therapeutic potential of ex vivo expanded endothelial progenitor cells for myocardial ischemia. *Circulation, 103*(5), 634-637.

10. Murasawa, S., & Asahara, T. (2008). Cardiogenic potential of endothelial progenitor cells. *Theapeutic Advances in Cardiovascular Disease, 2*(5), 341-348.

11. Abdel-Latif, A., Bolli, R., Tleyjeh, I. M., Montori, V. M., Perin, E. C., Hornung, C. A., . . . Dawn, B. (2007). Adult bone marrow-derived cells for cardiac repair: a systematic review and meta-analysis. *Archives of Internal Medicine, 167*(10), 989-997.

12. Dawn, B., Abdel-Latif, A., Sanganalmath, S. K., Flaherty, M. P., & Zuba-Surma, E. K. (2009). Cardiac repair with adult bone marrow-derived cells: the clinical evidence. *Antioxidant and Redox Signaling, 11*(8), 1865-1882.

13. Chen, S. L., Fang, W. W., Ye, F., Liu, Y. H., Qian, J., Shan, S. J., . . . Sun, J. P. (2004). Effect on left ventricular function of intracoronary transplantation of autologous bone marrow mesenchymal stem cell in patients with acute myocardial infarction. *American Journal of Cardiology, 94*(1), 9295.

14. Cedars-Sinai Medical Center. (2009). First human receives cardiac stem cells in clinical trial to heal damage caused by heart attacks. *MedicalNewsToday.com*. Retrieved from http://www.medicalnewstoday.com/articles/155908.php.

15. Bearzi, C., Rota, M., Hosoda, T., Tillmanns, J., Nascimbene, A., De Angelis, A., . . . Anversa, P. (2007). Human cardiac stem cells. *Proceedings of the National Academy of Sciences of the United States of America, 104*(35), 14068-14073.

16. Magnetic Attraction of Stem Cells to Injured Heart Creates Potent Treatment. (2010, April 12). *DotMedNews.com*

17. Kalka, C., Masuda, H. Takahashi, T., Kalka-Moll, W. M., Silver, M., Kearney, M., . . . Asahara, T. (2000). Transplantation of ex vivo expanded endothelial progenitor cells for therapeutic neovascularization. *Proceedings of the National Academy of Sciences of the United States of America, 97*(7), 3422-3427.

18. Ness, J., & Aronow, W. S. (1999). Prevalence of coexistence of coronary artery disease, ischemic stroke, and peripheral arterial disease in older persons, mean age 80 years, in an academic hospital-based geriatrics practice. *Journal of the American Geriatric Society, 47*(10), 1255-1256.

19. Lawall, H., Bramlage, P., & Amann, B. (2010). Stem cell and progenitor cell therapy in peripheral artery disease. A critical appraisal. *Thrombosis and Haemostasis, 103*(4), 696-709.

20. Tateishi-Yuyama, E., Matsubara, H., Murohara, T., Ikeda, U., Shintani, S., Masaki, H., . . . Therapeutic Angiogenesis using Cell Transplantation (TACT) Study Investigators. (2002). Therapeutic angiogenesis for patients with limb ischemia by autologous transplantation of bone-marrow cells: a pilot study and a randomised controlled trial. *Lancet, 360*(9331), 427-435.

21. Altman, L. K. (2001, November 20). The doctor's world; how to assist failing hearts? New questions emerge. *The New York Times*. Retrieved from http://www.nytimes.com/2001/11/20/science/the-doctor-s-world-how-to-assist-failing-hearts-new-questions-emerge.html.

22. Hughes, S. (2005, September 13). REPAIR-AMI: Stem cells show benefit in MI patients. *Theheart.org*. Retrieved from http://www.theheart.org/article/597863.do.

23. Hare, J. M., Traverse, J. H., Henry, T. D., Dib, N. Strumpf, R. K., Schulman, S. P., . . . Sherman, W. (2009). A randomized, double-blind, placebo-controlled, dose-escalation study of intravenous adult human mesenchymal stem cells (prochymal) after acute myocardial infarction. *Journal of the American College of Cardiology, 54*(24), 2277-2286.

Footnotes

A. Nabil, Dib. (2010, April 22). Personal interview. All quotations in this chapter from Dr. Nabil Dib are from this interview unless otherwise indicated.

B. The only exception being in 1918, when the Spanish Flu epidemic killed over 500,000 Americans.

Chapter 11 Ophthalmic Conditions

1. Fong, D. S, Aiello, L., Gardner, T. W., King, G. L., Blankenship, G., Cavallerano, J. D., . . . American Diabetes Association. (2004). Retinopathy in diabetes. *Diabetes Care, 27*(1), S84-87.

2. Zhang, X., Saaddine, J. B., Chou, C. F., Cotch, M. F., Cheng, Y. J., Geiss, L. S., . . . Klein, R. (2010). Prevalence of diabetic retinopathy in the United States, 2005-2008. *Journal of the American Medical Association, 304*(6), 649-656.

3. American Diabetes Association. Diabetes basics: Diabetes statistics. *Diabetes.org.* Retrieved from http://www.diabetes. org/diabetes-basics/diabetes-statistics/.

4. Rein, D. B., Zhang, P., Wirth, K. E., Lee, P. P., Hoerger, T. J., McCall, N., . . . Saaddine, J. (2006). The economic burden of major adult visual disorders in the United States. *Archives of Ophthalmology, 124*(12), 1754-1760.

5. Ono, M. (2009, October 12). Stem cells used to fight macular degeneration. *R&DMagazine.com* Retrieved from http://www.rdmag.com/Life-Science-Stem-cells-used-to-fight-macular-degeneration/.

6. Marneros, A. G., She, H., Zambarakji, H., Hashizume, H., Connolly, E. J., Kim, I., . . . Olsen, B. R. (2007). Endogenous endostatin inhibits choroidal neovascularization. *The FASEB Journal: Official Publication of the Federation of American Societies for Experimental Biology, 21*(14), 3809-3818.

7. Fulcher, T., Griffin, M., Crowley, S., Firth, R., Acheson, R., & O'Meara, N. (1998). Diabetic retinopathy in Down's syndrome. *British Journal of Ophthamology, 82*(4), 407-409.

8. Zorick, T. S., Mustacchi, Z., Bando, S. Y., Zatz, M., Moreira-Filho, C. A., Olsen, B., & Passos-Bueno, M. R. (2001). High serum endostatin levels in Down syndrome: implications for improved treatment and prevention of solid tumours. *European Journal of Human Genetics, 9*(11), 811-814.

9. Ryeom, S., & Folkman, J. (2009). Role of endogenous angiogenesis inhibitors in Down syndrome. *Journal of Craniofacial Surgery, 20*(1), 595-596.

10. Wang, S., Lu, B., Girman, S., Duan, J., McFarland, T., Zhang, Q. S., . . . Lund, R. (2010). Non-invasive stem cell therapy in a rat model for retinal degeneration and vascular pathology. *PLoS One, 5*(2), e9200.

11. Rice, J. (2009, January 7). Stem cells undo birth defects. *TechnologyReview.com.* Retrieved from http://www.technologyreview.com/biomedicine/21930/?nlid=1627&a=f.

12. Hori, J., Ng, T. F., Shatos, M., Klassen, H., Streilein, J. W., & Young, M. J. (2003). Neural progenitor cells lack immunogenicity and resist destruction as allografts. *Stem Cells, 21*(4), 405-416.

13. ScienceBlog. (2003, July 14). Brain stem cells are not rejected when transplanted. *ScienceBlog.com.* Retrieved from http://scienceblog.com/1828/brain-stem-cells-are-not-rejected-when-transplanted/.

14. Howe, D. (2006). Stemedica treatment sources notebook, "Patient 6" writeup. Stemedica Cell Technologies, Inc.

15. Global Stem Cell Health. (2006). *Diabetic Retinopathy: Alexander Mileshin* [web video]. Available from http://www.bayerstemcell.com/.

16. Tornambe, P. (2009). Synopsis of Review of Stem Cell Study. Stemedica Cell Technologies, Inc.

17. Klein, R., Chou, C. F., Klein, B. E., Zhang, X., Meuer, S. M., & Saaddine, J. B. (2011). Prevalence of age-related macular degeneration in the US population. *Archives of Ophthamology, 129*(1), 75-80.

18. National Eye Institute & National Institutes of Health. (2010). Facts about age-related macular degeneration. *National Eye Institute.* Retrieved from http://www.nei.nih.gov/health/maculardegen/armd_facts.asp.

19. Macrae, F. (2007, June 6). 45-minute operation to restore sight to millions. *DailyMail.co.uk* Retrieved from http://www.dailymail.co.uk/ushome/index.html.

20. The London Project. (2007). Taking the therapy to clinical trials. Retrieved from http://www.thelondonproject.org/OurVision/TheProject/?id=1432.

21. Templeton, S. K. (2009, April 19). Blind to be cured with stem cells. *The Times: The Sunday Times.* Retrieved from http://www.timesonline.co.uk/tol/news/uk/health/article6122757.ece.

22. Saga. (2010). Healthy living: Stem cells to treat AMD. Retrieved from http://www.saga.co.uk/health/healthyliving/bodymatters/stem-cells-to-treat-amd.asp.

23. Sasahara, M., Otani, A., Oishi, A., Kojima, H., Yodoi, Y., Kameda, T., . . . Yoshimura, N. (2008). Activation of bone marrow-derived microglia promotes photoreceptor survival in inherited retinal degeneration. *American Journal of Pathology, 172*(6), 1693-1703.

24. Chan-Ling, T., Baxter, L., Afzal, A., Sengupta, N., Caballero, S., Rosinova, E., & Grant, M. B. (2006). Hematopoietic stem cells provide repair functions after laser-induced Bruch's membrane rupture model of choroidal

neovascularization. *American Journal of Pathology, 168*(3), 1031-1044.

25. Otani, A., Dorrell, M. I., Kinder, K., Moreno, S. K., Nusinowitz, S., Banin, E., . . . Friedlander, M. (2004). Rescue of retinal degeneration by intravitreally injected adult bone marrow-derived linerage-negative hematopoietic stem cells. *Journal of Clinical Investigation, 114*(6), 765-774.

26. MacLaren, R. E., Pearson, R. A., MacNeil, A., Douglas, R. H., Salt, T. E., Akimoto, M., . . . Ali, R. R. (2006). Retinal repair by transplantation of photo receptor precursors. *Nature, 444*(7116), 203-207.

27. Meyer, J. S., Katz, M. L., Maruniak, J. A., & Kirk, M. D. (2006). Embryonic stem cell-derived neural progenitors incorporate into degenerating retina and enhance survival of host photoreceptors. *Stem Cells, 24*(2), 274-283.

28. Columbia University Medical Center. (2010, February 24). Stem cells restore sight in mouse model of retinitis pigmentosa. *ScienceDaily*. Retrieved from http://www.sciencedaily.com/releases/2010/02/100224132737.htm.

Footnotes

A. MA. (2007, September 5). Personal interview. All quotations in this chapter from the patient referred to as MA are from this interview unless otherwise indicated.

B. Tornambe, P. (2009, December). Personal interview. All quotations in this chapter from Dr. Paul Tornambe are from this interview unless otherwise indicated.

Chapter 12 Wound Care

1. Driscoll, P. (2009, December 13). Advanced medical technologies: Incidence and prevalence of wounds by etiology [Web log]. Retrieved from http://mediligence.com/blog/2009/12/13/incidence-and-prevalence-of-wounds-by-etiology/.

2. PRLog. (2008, June 24). Piribo.com: Global wound care market set to hit $12.5bn by 2012 predicts new report. Retrieved from http://www.prlog.org/10082818-piribocom-global-wound-care-market-set-to-hit-125bn-by-2012-predicts-new-report.html.

3. Goldman, R. (2004). Growth factors and chronic wound healing: past, present, and future. *Advances in Skin and Wound Care, 17*(1), 24-35.

4. Alberts, B., Bray, D., Lewis, J., Raff, R., Roberts, K., & Watson, J. D. (1994). *Molecular Biology of the Cell* (3rd ed.) New York, NY: Garland Publishing.

5. Boulton, A. J., Vileikyte, L., Ragnarson-Tennvall, G., & Apelqvist, J. (2005). The global burden of diabetic foot disease. *The Lancet, 366*(9498), 1719-1724.

6. Reiber, G. E., Boyko, E. J., & Smith, D. G. (1995). Lower extremity foot ulcers and amputations in diabetes. *Diabetes in America* (2nd ed.) (pp. 409-428) (NIH Publication No. 95-1468). Bethesda, MD: National Diabetes Information Clearinghouse.

7. National Institute of Diabetes and Digestive and Kidney Diseases. (2008, June). *National Diabetes Statistics, 2007: Complications of Diabetes in the United States* (NIH Publication No. 08-3892). Bethesda, MD: National Diabetes Information Clearinghouse.

8. de la Torre, J. I., & Chambers, J. A. (2008, October 9). Wound healing, chronic wounds. *EMedicine, WebMD*. Retrieved from http://emedicine.medscape.com/article/12984 52-overview.

9. Wu, Y., Chen, L., Scott, P. G., & Tredget, E. E. (2007). Mesenchymal stem cells enhance wound healing through differentiation and angiogenesis. *Stem Cells, 25*(10), 2648-2659.

10. Ramelet, A. A., Hirt-Burri, N., Raffoul, W., Scaletta, C., Pioletti, D. P., Offord, E., . . . Applegate, L.A. (2009). Chronic wound healing by fetal cell therapy may be explained by differential gene profiling observed in fetal versus old skin cells. *Experimental Gerontology, 44*(3), 208-218.

11. Hohlfeld, J., de Buys Roessingh, A., Hirt-Burri, N., Chaubert, P., Gerber, S., Scaletta, C., . . . Applegate, L. A. (2005). Tissue engineered fetal skin constructs for paediatric burns. *The Lancet, 366*(9488) 840-842.

12. Applegate, L. A., Scaletta, C., Hirt-Burri, N., Raffoul, W., & Pioletti, D. (2009). Whole-cell bioprocessing of human fetal cells for tissue engineering of skin. *Skin Pharmacology and Physiology, 22*(2), 63-73.

13. Falanga, V., Margolis, D., Alvarez, O., Auletta, M., Maggiacomo, F., Altman, M., . . . Hardin-Young, J. (1998). Rapid

healing of venous ulcers and lack of clinical rejection with an allogeneic cultured human skin equivalent. Human Skin Equivalent Investigators Group. *Archives of Dermatology, 134*(3), 293-300.

14. Marston, W. A., Hanft, J., Norwood, P., Pollak, R., Dermagraft Diabetic Foot Ulcer Study Group. The efficacy and safety of Dermagraft in improving the healing of chronic diabetic foot ulcers: results of a prospective randomized trial. *Diabetes Care, 26*(6), 1701-1705.

15. Galiano, R. D., Tepper, O. M., Pelo, C. R., Bhatt, K. A., Callaghan, M., Bastidas, N., . . . Gurtner, G. C. (2004). Topical vascular endothelial growth factor accelerated diabetic wound healing through increased angiogenesis and by mobilizing and recruiting bone marrow-derived cells. *American Journal of Pathology, 164*(6), 1935-1947.

16. Asai, J., Takenaka, H., Kusano, K. F., Li, M., Luedemann, C., Curry, C., . . . Losordo, D. W. (2006). Topical sonic hedgehog gene therapy accelerates wound healing in diabetes by enhancing endothelial progenitor cell-mediated microvascular remodeling. *Circulation, 113*(20), 2413-2424.

17. Wu, L., Yu, Y. L., Galiano, R. D., Roth, S. I., & Mustoe, T. A. (1997). Macrophage colony-stimulating factor accelerates wound healing and upregulates TGF-beta1 mRNA levels through tissue macrophages. *Journal of Surgical Research, 72*(2), 162-169.

18. Soler, P. M., Wright, T. E., Smith, P. D., Maggi, S. P., Hill, D. P., Ko, F., . . . Robson, M. C. (1999). In vivo characterization of keratinocyte growth factor-2 as a potential wound healing agent. *Wound Repair and Regeneration, 7*(3), 172-178.

19. Smiell, J. M., Wieman, T. J., Steed, D. L., Perry, B. H., Sampson, A. R., & Schwab, B. H. (1999). Efficacy and safety of becaplermin (recombinant human platelet-derived growth factor-BB) in patients with nonhealing, lower extremity diabetic ulcers: a combined analysis of four randomized studies. *Wound Repair and Regeneration, 7*(5), 335-346.

20. Steed, D. L., Donohoe, D., Webster, M. W., & Lindsley, L. (1996). Effect of extensive debridement and treatment on the healing diabetic foot ulcers. Diabetic Ulcer Study Group. *Journal of the American College of Surgeons, 183*(1), 61-64.

21. Hirt-Burri, N., Scaletta, C., Gerber, S., Pioletti, D. P., & Applegate, L. A. (2008). Wound-healing gene family expression differences between fetal and foreskin cells used for bioengineered skin substitutes. *Artificial Organs, 32*(7), 509-518.

22. Badiavas, E. V., & Falanga, V. (2003). Treatment of chronic wounds with bone marrow-derived cells. *Archives of Dermatology, 139*(4), 510-516.

23. Ichioka, S., Kouraba, S., Sekiya, N., Ohura, N., & Nakatsuka, T. (2005). Bone marrow-impregnated collagen matrix for wound healing: Experimental evaluation in a microcirculatory model of angiogenesis, and clinical experience. *British Journal of Plastic Surgery, 58*(8), 1124-1130.

24. Badiavas, E. V., Ford, D., Liu, P., Kouttab, N., Morgan, J., Richards, A., & Maizel, A. (2007). Long-term bone marrow culture and its clinical potential in chronic wound healing. *Wound Repair and Regeneration, 15*(6), 856-865.

25. Fathke, C., Wilson, L., Hutter, J., Kapoor, V., Smith, A., Hocking A., & Isik, F. (2004). Contribution of bone marrow-derived cells to skin: collagen deposition and wound repair. *Stem Cells, 22*(5), 812-822.

26. Cha, J. & Falanga, V. (2007). Stem cells in cutaneous wound healing. *Clinics in Dermatology, 25*(1), 73-78.

27. Lau, K., Paus, R., Tiede, S., Day, P., & Bayat, A. Exploring the role of stem cells in cutaneous wound healing. *Experimental Dermatology, 18*(11), 921-933.

28. Fang, L. J., Fu, X. B., Sun, T. Z., Li, J. F., Cheng, B., Yang, Y. H., & Wang, Y. X. (2003). An experimental study on the differentiation of bone marrow mesenchymal stem cells into vascular endothelial cells. *Zhonghua Shao Shang Za Zhi, 19*(1), 22-24.

29. Drago, H., Marín, G. H., Sturla, F., Roque, G., Mártire, K., Díaz Aquino, V., . . . Mansilla, E. (2010). The next generation of burns treatment: intelligent films and matrix, controlled enzymatic debridement, and adult stem cells. *Transplantation Proceedings, 42*(1), 345-349.

30. Shumakov, V. I., Onishchenko, N. A., Rasulov, M. F., Krasheninnikov, M. E., & Zaidenov, V. A. (2003). Mesenchymal bone marrow stem cells more effectively stimulate regeneration of deep burn wounds than embryonic fibroblasts. *Bulletin of Experimental Biology and Medicine, 136*(2), 192-195.

31. Mansilla, E., Marin, G. H., Sturla, F., Drago, H. E., Gil, M. A., Salas, E., . . . Soratti, C. (2005). Human mesenchymal stem cells are tolerized by mice and improve skin and spinal cord injuries. *Transplantation Proceedings, 37*(1), 292-294.

32. Sasaki, M., Abe, R., Fujita, Y., Ando, S., Inokuma, D., & Shimizu, H. (2008). Mesenchymal stem cells are recruited into wounded skin and contribute to wound repair by transdifferentiation into multiple skin cell type. *Journal of*

Immunology, 180(4), 2581-2587.

33. Rasulov, M. F., Vasilchenkov, A. V., Onishchenko, N. A., Krasheninnikov, M. E., Kravchenko, V. I., Gorshenin, T. L., . . . Potapov, I. V. (2005). First experience of the use bone marrow mesenchymal stem cells for the treatment of a patient with deep skin burns. *Bulletin of Experimental Biology and Medicine, 139*(1), 141-144.

34. Vojtassák, J., Danisovic, L., Kubes, M., Bakos, D., Jarábek, L., Ulicná, M., & Blasko, M. (2006). Autologous biograft and mesenchymal stem cells in treatment of the diabetic foot. *Neuro Endocrinology Letters, 27*(2), 134-137.

35. Lataillade, J. J., Doucet, C., Bey, E., Carsin, H., Huet, C., Clairand, I., . . . Gourmelon, P. (2007). New approach to radiation burn treatment by dosimetry-guided surgery combined with autologous mesenchymal stem cell therapy. *Regenerative Medicine, 2*(5), 785-794.

36. Falanga, V., Iwamoto, S., Chartier, M., Yufit, T., Butmarc, J., Kouttab, N., . . . Carson, P. (2007). Autologous bone marrow-derived cultured mesenchymal stem cells delivered in a fibrin spray accelerate healing in murine and human cutaneous wounds. *Tissue Engineering, 13*(6), 1299-1312.

37. Yoshikawa, T., Mitsuno, H., Nonaka, I., Sen, Y., Kawanishi, K., Inada, Y., . . . Nonomura, A. (2008). Wound therapy by marrow mesenchymal cell transplantation. *Plastic and Reconstructive Surgery, 121*(3), 860-877.

38. Atala, A. (2006, November 29). Tissue engineering and medicine [Video file]. Retrieved from http://www.zentation. com/viewer/index.php?passcode=9ySbJEKh6w.

39. Hanson, S. E., Bentz, M. L., & Hematti, P. (2010). Mesenchymal stem cell therapy for nonhealing cutaneous wounds. *Plastic and Reconstructive Surgery, 125*(2), 510-516.

40. Jahoda, C. A., & Reynolds, A. J. (2001). Hair follicle dermal sheath cells: Unsung participants in wound healing. *The Lancet, 358*(9291), 1445-1448.

41. Ueda, M., & Nishino, Y. (2010). Cell-based cytokine therapy for skin rejuvenation. *The Journal of Craniofacial Surgery, 21*(6), 1861-1866.

42. Argyris, T. (1976). Kinetics of epidermal production during epidermal regeneration following abrasion in mice. *American Journal of Pathology, 83*(2), 329-340.

43. University of Pennsylvania School of Medicine. (2005, December 1). Hair follicle stem cells contribute to wound healing. *ScienceDaily.* Retrieved from http://www.sciencedaily.com/releases/2005/12/051201224113.htm.

44. Kaur, P. (2006). Interfollicular epidermal stem cells: identification, challenges, potential. *Journal of Investigative Dermatology, 126*(7), 1450-1458.

45. Ohyama, M. (2009, December 3). Hair follicle stem cells – new insights & clinical relevance. *AccessMedicine from McGraw-Hill.* Retrieved from http://www.medscape.com/viewarticle/713341.

46. Yasuyuki, A., Lingna, L., Katsuoka, K., Penman, S., & Hoffman, R. M. (2005). Multipotent nestin-positive, keratin-negative hair-follicle bulge stem cells can form neurons. *The Proceedings of the National Academy of Sciences of the United States of America, 102*(15), 5530-5534.

47. Howard Hughes Medical Institute. (2009, December 8). New skin stem cells surprisingly similar to those found in embryos. *HHMI:Research News.* Retrieved from http://www.hhmi.org/news/miller20091208.html.

48. Move over, Rogaine? (1999, June). *HHMI Bulletin, 12*(2), 6-9. Retrieved from http://www.hhmi.org/fuchs/.

49. Suh, W., Kim, K. L., Kim, J. M., Shin, I. S., Lee, Y. S., Lee, J. Y., . . . Kim, D. K. (2005). Transplantation of endothelial progenitor cells accelerates dermal wound healing with increased recruitment of monocytes/macrophages and neovascularization. *Stem Cells, 23*(10), 1571-1578.

50. Ueda, M. (2007). The use of fibroblasts: Smoothing away wrinkles. *The Biochemist, 29*(6), 11-15.

51. Ueda, M. (2010). Sprayed cultured mucosal epithelial cell for deep dermal burns. *The Journal of Craniofacial Surgery, 21*(6), 1729-1732.

Footnotes

A. Information in the following bullet points is also derived from the reference: Goldman, R. (2004). Growth factors and chronic wound healing: past, present, and future. *Advances in Skin and Wound Care, 17*(1), 24-35.

B. Aficionados will no doubt notice that this protein has been named after a popular videogame character.

Chapter 13 The Future

1. Daley, G., Reeve, B., & Smith, D. (2010, April 15). Bench to bedside: How stem cell R&D will reshape the industry. In R. Higgins (Moderator), *Healthcare Track Event*. Panel conducted at The Harvard Business School Association of Boston in Boston, MA.

2. Kattan, A. (2009, June 16). Adult stem cells are a promising market. *Fortune Magazine*. Retrieved from http://money.cnn.com/2009/06/16/technology/adult_stem_cell_therapy.fortune/index.htm.

3. Furcht, L., & Hoffman, W. (2008). *The Stem Cell Dilemma: Beacons of Hope or Harbingers of Doom?* New York, NY: Arcade Publishing.

4. Kalorama Information. (2009, May 1). *Worldwide wound care: Total market coverage* (Vols. I-III: skin ulcers, burns, surgical and trauma wounds), (4th Ed).

5. Halme, D. G., & Kessler, D. A. (2006). FDA regulation of stem-cell-based therapies. *The New England Journal of Medicine, 355*(16), 1730-1735.

6. Gorman, C. (2005, February 20). Can the FDA heal itself? *Time*. Retrieved from http://www.time.com/time/printout/0,8816,1029866,00.html#.

7. Park, M. (2010, August 12). A mother's plea: Heal my children's skin. *CNNHealth*. Retrieved from http://www.cnn.com/2010/HEALTH/08/12/skin.disease.stem.cell/index.html?iref=NS1.

8. Osiris Therapeutics. (2010, May 5). FDA grants orphan drug status to Osiris Therapeutics' investigational stem cell biologic for type 1 diabetes – update. *CheckOrphan.com*. Retrieved from http://www.checkorphan.org/grid/news/treatment/fda-grants-orphan-drug-status-to-osiris-therapeutics-investigational-stem-cell-biologic-for-type-i-diabetes-update.

9. Vergano, D. (2010, March 3). Stem cells approved to treat 'orphan' disease. *ScienceFair – USAToday*. Retrieved from http://content.usatoday.com/communities/sciencefair/post/2010/03/stem-cells-approved-to-treat-orphan-disease/1.

10. Rare diseases: understanding this public health priority. (2005). EURORDIS. Retrieved from http://www.eurordis.org/IMG/pdf/princeps_document-EN.pdf.

11. Office of Rare Diseases. (2007). Biennial report on rare diseases research activities at the National Institutes of Health – FY2006. *National Institutes of Health – Department of Health and Human Services*. Retrieved from http://rarediseases.info.nih.gov/files/BienniaReportRareDiseasesFY2006Final.pdf.

12. Cyranoski, D. (2005). Far East lays plans to be stem-cell hotspot. *Nature, 438*(7065), 135.

13. Program on Life Sciences, Ethics and Policy, McLaughlin-Rotman Centre for Global Health. (2010, January 8). China leads the way in regenerative stem cell therapy despite skepticism. *Disable-world.com*. Retrieved from http://www.disabled-world.com/news/research/stemcells/china-regenerative-stem-cells.php.

14. Shapiro, A. D. (2010, August 4). China: A new force in stem cell field. *The World – From the BBC, PRI, and WGBH*. Retrieved from http://www.theworld.org/2010/08/04/china-a-new-force-in-stem-cell-field/.

15. Khullar, M. (2009, October 9). Unfettered by regulation, India pulls ahead on stem cell treatments. *GlobalPost*. Retrieved from http://www.globalpost.com/dispatch/india/091009/unfettered-regulation-india-pulls-ahead-stem-cell-treatments.

16. Comarow, A. (2008, May, 1). Saving on surgery by going abroad. *US News*. Retrieved from http://health.usnews.com/health-news/family-health/articles/2008/05/01/saving-on-surgery-by-going-abroad.html.

17. Abramson, H. (2006, February 2). The best money can buy: Medical tourism in the U.S.A. *New America Media*. Retrieved from http://news.newamericamedia.org/news/view_article.html?article_id=5b7c206e74b96be675410f6f369b5113.

18. Ono, D. (2007, May 8). Doctor claims controversial stem cell treatment works. *KABC-TV, Los Angeles*, CA. Retrieved from http://abclocal.go.com/kabc/story?section=news/local&id=5283114.

19. Lindvall, O., & Hyun, I. (2009). Medical innovation versus stem cell tourism. *Science, 324*(5935), 1664-1665.

20. *Guidelines for the clinical translation of stem cells.* (2008, December 3). International Society for Stem Cell Research. Retrieved from http://www.isscr.org/clinical_trans/pdfs/ISSCRGLClinical Trans.pdf.

21. *Patient handbook on stem cell therapies.* (2008, December 3). International Society for Stem Cell Research. Retrieved from http://www.isscr.org/clinical_trans/pdfs/ISSCRPatientHandbook.pdf.

22. Shaw, J. (2010). Tools and tests: The evolution of stem-cell research. *Harvard Magazine, 112*(3), 24-29.

⚭References

23. Gordian, M., Singh, N., Zemmel, R., & Elias, T. (2006). Why products fail in phase III. *In Vivo*. Retrieved from http://www.mckinsey.com/clientservice/pharmaceuticalsmedicalproducts/pdf/why_products_fail_in_phase_III_in_ vivo_0406.pdf.

24. Danielyan, L., Schäfer, R., von Ameln-Mayerhofer, A., Buadze, M., Geisler, J., Klopfer, T., . . . Frey, W. H. 2nd. (2009). Intranasal delivery of cells to the brain. *European Journal of Cell Biology, 88*(6), 315-324.

25. Morrison, D., & National Science Foundation. (2009, September 22). Snorting stem cells: snorting can deliver cells to the brain, research shows. *US News*. Retrieved from http://www.usnews.com/science/articles/2009/09/22/ snorting-stem-cells.html.

26. Ourednik, J., Ourednik, V., Lynch, W. P., Schachner, M., & Snyder, E. Y. (2002). Neural stem cells display an inherent mechanism for rescuing dysfunctional neurons. *Nature Biotechnology, 20*(11), 1103-1110.

27. Atala, A. (2006, November 29). Tissue engineering and medicine [Video file]. Retrieved from http://www.zentation. com/viewer/index.php?passcode=9ySbJEKh6w.

Footnotes

A. All quotations in this chapter, occurring hereafter, from Brock Reeve are from the panel conducted at Harvard Business School on April 15, 2010, unless otherwise indicated.

B. All quotations in this chapter, occurring hereafter, from Robert Higgins are from the panel conducted at Harvard Business School on April 15, 2010, unless otherwise indicated.

C. All quotations in this chapter, occurring hereafter, from Dr. George Daley are from the panel conducted at Harvard Business School on April 15, 2010, unless otherwise indicated.

Index